AF183598

Recent Results in Cancer Research 135

Managing Editors
Ch. Herfarth, Heidelberg · H.-J. Senn, St. Gallen

Associate Editors
M. Baum, London · V. Diehl, Köln
F. Gutzwiller, Zürich · M. F. Rajewsky, Essen
M. Wannenmacher, Heidelberg

Founding Editor
R. Rentchnik, Geneva

O. D. Wiestler U. Schlegel
J. Schramm (Eds.)

Molecular Neuro-oncology and Its Impact on the Clinical Management of Brain Tumors

With 39 Figures and 9 Tables

Springer-Verlag
Berlin Heidelberg New York
London Paris Tokyo
Hong Kong Barcelona
Budapest

Prof. Dr. O. D. Wiestler
Institut für Neuropathologie
Universitätskliniken Bonn
Sigmund-Freud-Straße 25
53105 Bonn

Dr. U. Schlegel
Neurologische Universitätsklinik
Sigmund-Freud-Straße 25
53105 Bonn

Prof. Dr. J. Schramm
Neurochirurgische Universitätsklinik
Sigmund-Freud-Straße 25
53105 Bonn

ISBN-13:978-3-642-85041-7 e-ISBN-13:978-3-642-85039-4
DOI: 10.1007/978-3-642-85039-4

This work is subject to copyright. All rights are reserved, whether the whole or part of the material is concerned, specifically the rights of translation, reprinting, reuse of illustrations, recitation, broadcasting, reproduction on microfilm or in any other way, and storage in data banks. Duplication of this publication or parts thereof is permitted only under the provisions of the German Copyright Law of September 9, 1965, in its current version, and permission for use must always be obtained from Springer-Verlag. Violations are liable for prosecution under the German Copyright Law.

© Springer-Verlag Berlin Heidelberg 1994
Softcover reprint of the hardcover 1st edition 1994

The use of general descriptive names, registered names, trademarks, etc. in this publication does not imply, even in the absence of a specific statement, that such names are exempt from the relevant protective laws and regulations and therefore free for general use.

Product Liability: The publishers cannot guarantee the accuracy of any information about dosage and application contained in this book. In every individual case the user must check such information by consulting the relevant literature.

Data conversion by RTS, Wiesenbach
19/3130-5 4 3 2 1 0 – Printed on acid-free paper

Contents

*List of Contributors**

* The address of the principal author is given on the first page of each contribution.
[1] Page on which contribution begins.

Introduction

O. D. Wiestler[1], U. Schlegel[2], and J. Schramm[3]

[1]Institut für Neuropathologie, Universitätskliniken Bonn, Sigmund-Freud-Str. 25, 53127 Bonn, Germany
[2]Neurologische Universitätsklinik, Sigmund-Freud-Str. 25, 53127 Bonn, Germany
[3]Neurochirurgische Universitätsklinik, Sigmund-Freud-Str. 25, 53127 Bonn, Germany

In contrast to various other neoplastic disorders, there has still been no dramatic progress in the treatment of gliomas. Modern microsurgical and imaging techniques have made more tumors surgically accessible and have allowed a more extensive surgical resection. However, these new developments have not improved the clinical outcome. Recently, molecular biological studies on genes and genetic loci affected in tumors of the nervous system have yielded significant new insights into pathogenetic machanisms. Many neuro-oncologists are therefore looking forward to translating molecular genetic findings into novel diagnostic and therapeutic strategies for the management of these devastating neoplasms. We have produced this volume with the intention of highlighting major developments in both molecular and clinical neuro-oncology and of stimulating the communication and cooperation between these two fields.

Two major families of growth-controlling genes have emerged from the past decade of intense research on the molecular genetics of tumors: oncogenes and tumor suppressor genes. Oncogenes are characterized by their potential to stimulate the growth of susceptible cells whereas tumor suppressor genes share a growth-inhibiting property. A stringently controlled interplay between these two regulatory mechanisms is required to maintain a stable composition of tissues. Mutational activation or inactivation of genes implicated in these pathways appear to play a major role in the process of tumor formation.

One of the first neural tumors for which specific molecular defects have been identified was the peripheral neuroblastoma. Manfred Schwab (Heidelberg) who was among the pioneers in this field summarizes the current status of the neuroblastoma work. This tumor frequently exhibits amplification of the N-*myc* oncogene which results in significant over-production of the N-*myc* gene product. The amplified N-*myc* gene has received much attention from pediatric oncologists since it was clearly demonstrated that N-*myc* amplification is among the most significant prognostic factors for children affected by this neoplasm. The association between an amplified N-*myc* locus, and aggressive behavior of neuroblastomas is so significant that adjuvant chemotherapy is now recommended for all patients exhibiting this molecular genetic alteration irrespective of the clinical stage of the tumor. There is also recent evidence for a tumor suppressor gene in neuroblastoma on the short arm of chromsome 1. Several laboratories are in the process of identifying and cloning this tumor suppressor gene.

Among the most common and most devastating tumors of the brain is the glioblastoma multiforme. Even with intensive multimodal treatment, average survival rarely exceeds 9 months. A significant fraction of glioblastomas show amplification of the epidermal growth factor (EGF) receptor oncogene. These data are summarized by Peter Collins (Stockholm) who also provides evidence for specific mutational changes of the EGF receptor gene in malignant gliomas. Since this gene encodes a receptor protein with a prominent extracellular domain at the cell surface, attempts are currently being made to devise immunotherapy regimens with a monoclonal antibody directed to the EGF-receptor protein.

In contrast to oncogenes, which so far have been associated only with peripheral neuroblastoma and glioblastoma multiforme and not with other tumors of the nervous system, there is ample evidence for an involvement of putative or already identified tumor suppressor genes in these neoplasms. The p53 suppressor gene which appears to be altered in a substantial number of diverse human tumors, has been extensively analyzed in tumors of the brain. Paul Kleihues et al. (Zurich) present a comprehensive study on point mutations in the p53 gene in a large series of human brain tumors which includes all major tumor entities. This study clearly indicates that p53 is frequently involved in astrocytomas and glioblastoma multiforme of adult patients, not, however, in pilocytic astrocytomas and most other neoplasms of the central and peripheral nervous system. One of the conclusions is that p53 exerts a tropism for astroglia in the brain. Clinical neuro-oncologists are particularly interested in a potential prognostic relevance of p53 mutations and other molecular genetic changes for individual patients. This issue was addressed by Uwe Schlegel et al. (Bonn) in a large retrospective study on human astrocytomas and glioblastomas. Their findings strongly suggest that there is no prognostic significance of p53 mutations in patients with astrocytic gliomas. A similar study on overexpression of the EGF receptor also failed to demonstrate a significant prognostic impact of this oncogene in malignant gliomas.

With the identification of increasing numbers of genes and genetic loci associated with human gliomas, it is now possible to examine individual tumors for specific patterns and combinations of genetic lesions. This analysis may ultimately evolve into a powerful tool for the characterization and prognostic evaluation of tumor samples. Andreas von Deimling and coworkers (Boston, Bonn, Zurich) report elegant examples to underline the potential of this strategy. By comparing specific lesions on chromosme 17p, chromosome 10, and the EGF receptor gene, they obtained strong evidence for at least two genetically distinct variants of glioblastoma multiforme. These differ not only in their molecular genetic imprint but also in clinical features such as age of the patient and, potentially, postoperative survival. This work has also nicely demonstrated that pilocytic astrocytomas, which have long been viewed by neuro-oncologists and neuropathologists as a separate astrocytic tumor entity, show distinct patterns of molecular genetic defects, in particular the involvement of a locus on chromosome 17q, presumably the NF1 tumor suppressor gene.

Significant progress has been made in experimental strategies to study specifically modified tumor-related genes in animal models. The generation of transgenic mice yields important insights into the molecular biology of tumors. An alternative in vivo strategy for studying tumor-associated genes in the brain is introduced by Otmar Wiestler et al. (Bonn, Zurich). This procedure employs retrovirus-mediated gene transfer into fetal brain transplants. Introduction of a variety of activated oncogenes with potential neurotropism into neural grafts has produced intriguing neoplastic changes and models for human brain tumors, in particular medulloblastomas/primitive neuroectodermal tumors and glioblastoma multiforme.

Cell biologists have been able to identify the origin and differentiation pathways of major cell types of the central nervous system. Mark Noble (London) gives an overview of many years of work on glial cell lineages in the brain. Elegant studies in the rat optic nerve have identified two functionally and histogenetically distinct propulations of astrocytes, one of which shares a common progenitor cell with oligodendroglia. Several laboratories are currently studying the impact of this concept on our understanding of the histogenesis of gliomas.

Immunological and molecular biological studies have recently succeeded in uncovering the pathogenesis of paraneoplastic disorders of the nervous system. Jerome Posner (New York), a pioneer in this field, gives an overview on paraneoplastic encephalomyelopathy and sensory neuropathy in patients with small cell lung cancer. It was found that the serum and the cerebrospinal fluid of affected patients contain an antibody immunoreactive with both cells of the patient's tumor and neurons of the central and peripheral nervous systems. A similar mechanism has been identified in other paraneoplastic disorders, and the antigens have been characterized molecularly using antibodies derived from cerebrospinal fluid and serum for expression cloning.

It is generally agreed that malignant gliomas require adjuvant postoperative treatment. In the field of radiotherapy there has been excitement recently about stereotactic external beam irradiation, a technique which theoretically should allow a more precise targeting of small focal lesions in the brain while sparing the adjacent normal tissue. The development and potential of this technique is critically reviewed in this issue by Michael Brada (London). His paper emphasizes the potential of this technique but also points to limitations which may ultimately hamper a broader use of stereotactic external beam radiotherapy. Stereotactic neurosurgeons and radiotherapists are reporting progress with an alternative approach of focal high dose irradiation, i.e. interstitial implant radiotherapy of brain tumors. Christoph Ostertag (Freiburg) outlines the development of this field during the past decade. Animal experiments have been conducted to study dosage effects and the reaction to the implanted radioisotope of neoplastic and normal brain tissue, a variety of different radioisotopes have been comparatively evaluated and numerous tumors of diverse histogenetic origin and different histopathological grades have been treated by sterotaxic implantation of radioactive seeds. Many authors now agree that interstitial implant radiotherapy should be restricted to low grade gliomas at certain sites within the brain. If stringent selection criteria are met, there may be dramatic effects in individual patients. Yet another radiotherapeutic approach is presented by Mark Malkin (New York) who summarizes the Memorial Sloan-Kettering Cancer Center experience with interstitial brachytherapy through a stereotactically placed cathether which harbors a radioisotope. This cathether is left in situ for a period of approx. seven days. Preliminary data indicate that selected patients with high grade gliomas may benefit from this mode of focal irradiation.

Several authors deal with the issue of chemotherapy of gliomas. For a long time this field has been rather discouraging. However, recent observations appear to indicate that certain neural tumors may exhibit a significant chemosensitivity. The reports by Gregory Cairncross (London, Ontario) on the striking response of oligodendrogliomas to chemotherapy have received considerable attention. These findings are summarized in his contribution to this volume. Additional patients are currently enrolled in a trial to further substantiate this unexpected response. The situation is much less promising with glioblastomas. Peter Krauseneck (Bamberg) summarizes the results of a large German-Austrian multicenter trial on the effect of chemotherapeutic treatment on anaplastic astrocytomas and glioblastoma multiforme. This trial focused particularly on the agents BCNU (carmustine) and VM26 (teniposide), neither of which appeared to be significantly effective. A new regimen is introduced by Allesandro Olivi (Baltimore) in his report on local BCNU wafer therapy. Continuous local application of a drug into the surgical cavity should circumvent pharmacokinetic problems and reduce some of the chemotherapy side effects. A final evaluation of this approach will be possible only after completion of controlled clinical trials. In contrast to malignant gliomas, primary CNS lymphomas usually show a dramatic initial response to combined radio- and chemotherapy. The current debate centers on the proper sequence for administration of the two modalities, the optimal combination of chemotherapeutic agents to be used, and the risks and benefits of intrathecal chemotherapy. These issues are comprehensively dealt with in the contribution by Lisa deAngelis (New York).

What is the current status of experimental therapeutic startegies based on molecular biological and recent immunological findings? The amplification and overexpression of the EGF receptor oncogene in a significant fraction of glioblastomas has prompted pilot studies with monoclonal antibodies targeted to the receptor protein. The observation that normal brain tissue does not express significant amounts of the EGF receptor appears to favor this approach. However, there still remains considerable uncertainty about the most effective route of administration of moncolonal antibodies and the most efficient mechanisms of antibody-mediated cytotoxicity. Another potential problem concerns the considerable heterogeneity of receptor expression within individual tumors. A phase I trial employing systemic injection of a monoclonal antibody to the EGF receptor, which appears to confer antibody-dependent cellular cytotoxicity, has recently been initiated in Germany. The coordinator of this study, Manfred Westphal (Hamburg) presents an overview of the current experience.

More than a decade of intense search for tumor-specific antigens or antibodies has produced disappointing results. On the other hand, critical mechanisms of the specific and unspecific activation of cellular and humoral immune responses have now been identified. Some of these developments may allow the specific modulation of immune reactions and the targeting of immune responses to specific cell types such as tumor cells. An elegant novel strategy is presented by Gundram Jung and coworkers (Munich), who clearly show that an effective and specific immune attack can be directed to the surface of tumor cells if bispecific monoclonal antibodies are used as mediating reagents. It remains to be demonstrated that successful targeting of activated T cells can also be achieved in tumors of the brain.

There is now a broad consensus that the multistage process of tumor development is fundamentally associated with mutations and abnormal regulation of growth-controlling genes. A specific postoperative treatment will therefore be possible only if the affected genes and gene products can be effectively controlled or restored. A few examples for such pathogenetically based therapeutic approaches are already emerging. Some of these are presented in this volume. Many more should follow in the near future. This development will require a close collaboration between both basic and clinical oncologists. We hope that the present volume will contribute to initiating and maintaining the spirit for collaborative studies in this field.

Human Neuroblastoma: Amplification of the N-myc Oncogene and Loss of a Putative Cancer-Preventing Gene on Chromosome 1p

M. Schwab

German Cancer Research Center, Division of Cytogenetics, Im Neuenheimer Feld 280, 69120 Heidelberg, Germany

Introduction

The nervous system is the most common site for the development of solid neoplasms in childhood. Neuroblastoma represents a tumor developing at peripheral sites from primitive neuroectodermal cells derived from the neural crests. It very often has a rapidly progressive clinical course. Many advances have been made in understanding the genesis and biology of this tumor which have been translated into better clinical management; however, little improvement in survival rates has been achieved, at least for the large group of patients who have metastatic tumor.

Neuroblastoma is the most frequent solid tumor of childhood, with an annual incidence of 9 cases per million white children under 15 years of age (Michaelis and Kaatsch 1986; Kramer et al. 1983). Various studies have revealed a median age of presentation of under 2 years. The incidence of neurblastoma *in situ*, defined as nodules of primitive neuroblastic cells in the adrenal, appears to be much higher (1 out of 179 and 1 out of 259; Beckwith and Perrin 1971; Hasegawa et al. 1982), as suggested by random autopsy studies of infants under 3 months of age. It is possible that these cells have retained their potential to undergo differentiation, a process that results in regression of *in situ* neuroblastoma. In fact, spontaneous regression is one of the most unusual aspects of neuroblastoma and occurs particularly in infants with a small primary tumor, in spite of extensive liver involvement and the presence of subcutaneous nodules. This group of patients, defined according to Evans et al. (1971) as having stage IV disease, have a survival rate of 70% (an excellent comprehensive picture of the biology of neuroblastoma has been recently presented by Berthold et al. 1990).

The mechanisms contributing to the development of neuroblastomas are largely unclear, but nonrandom chromosomal changes identified in recent years suggest the involvement of genetic alterations. This review discusses both the approaches that have led to the identification of genetic alterations in neuroblastoma and their possible role in tumorgenesis, and it outlines as a paradigm the potential use of a genetic alteration for determining the prognosis of neuroblastoma patients.

Oncogene Amplification

Amplification of cellular oncogenes is one of the major genetic alterations that appear to contribute to the development of animal and human tumors (for reviews see Alitalo and Schwab 1986; Schwab and Amler 1990). Originally the presence of amplified DNA was indicated by conspicuous karyotypic abnormalities, the extrachromosomal double minutes (DMs) and the intrachromosomal homogeneously staining regions (HSRs). Either abnormality has been found in animal and human tumor cells to represent the cytogenetic manifestation of multiple copies of cellular oncogenes. The first instances in which this association could be established include the c-*myc* gene in a human colonic carcinoma cell line COLO 320 (Alitalo et al. 1983) and the K-*ras* gene in the murine adrenocortical tumor cell line Y1 (Schwab et al. 1983).

Amplification of N-*myc* in Neuroblastomas

While most cell lines and tumors that have been analyzed show sporadic amplification of cellular oncogenes, the frequency of amplification of N-*myc* in neuroblastomas is striking. Suspicion for the presence of an amplified oncogene was originally raised by the earlier observation that human neuroblastomas, both cell lines and tumors, carry DMs or HSRs at significant frequency (Cox et al. 1965; Brodeur et al. 1981). As yet, N-*myc* has been identified as the only amplified oncogene in all neuroblastomas carrying DMs or HSRs. It is fair to assume, therefore, that N-*myc* represents the gene providing the selective force for maintaining the amplified DNA within the genome of the neuroblastoma cell.

N-*myc* has been found amplified between five and séveral hundred-fold in neuroblastoma cell lines and tumors (Schwab et al. 1983; Kohl et al. 1983; Brodeur et al. 1984). The amplified DNA has a much greater complexity than the size of the N-*myc* transcription unit. Mapping studies using pulsed-field gel electrophoresis have established that the amplified DNA encompassing the N-*myc* transcription unit can be from approximately 100 kbp to more than 1500 kbp in size (Amler and Schwab 1989; Amler and Schwab 1992). The individual amplicons are often arranged in a regular pattern, where variable numbers of N-*myc* amplicons are repeated at unit length in 5'ó 3' direction. Although some models and speculations have been offered to rationalize the pathway leading to this regular arrangement, the initial events as well as the processing of amplified DNA in the neuroblastoma cell have escaped elucidation, mainly due to the lack of experimental models that would allow analysis of the amplification mechanisms under reproducible conditions. It is not clear, however, whether models of gene amplification related to drug resistance can provide a fair picture of what might be happening during amplification of cellular oncogenes. As far as N-*myc* amplification in neuroblastomas are concerned there are three elements that appear to be important: (a) amplification involves transposition of N-*myc* from its normal position at chromosome 2p24 to apparently random sites on other chromosomes where the HSR appears (Schwab et al. 1984); (b) the architecture of the amplified DNA is stable over long periods of time (Amler and Schwab 1989); and (c) a regular pattern of amplified N-*myc* is the predominant structure seen (Schwab and Amler 1989).

Amplification of N-*myc* in other types of tumors is less frequent than in neuroblastomas. Few cases have been reported for medulloblastomas (Fuller and Bigner 1992), retinoblastomas (Lee et al. 1984), astrocytomea (Garson et al. 1985), and small cell lung cancers (Nau et al. 1986). Particularly interesting is the setting of small cell lung cancers where two other members of the *myc* gene family have been found amplified, c-*myc* and L-*myc* (Nau et al. 1986). It is not clear whether differential amplification of various *myc* family genes might define biologically or clinically different subset of small cell lung cancers. As a general rule, N-*myc* has been found amplified only in tumors with neuronal qualities, and it appears fair to assume that the function of the N-*myc* gene is normally in growth control or differentiation of certain neuronal cells.

N-*myc* Amplification as a Prognostic Marker

An important prognostic parameter for patients with neuroblastoma is the clinical stage. Patients with stage I or II tumors generally have a good prognosis, with 75%–90% achieving 2-year disease-free survival. In contrast, patients with stage III or IV tumors have poor prognosis, with 10%–30% 2-year survival. Surveys of several hundered patients with neuroblastoma have revealed a strong correlation between N-*myc* amplification and stage III and IV tumors (Brodeur et al. 1984; Bartram and Berthold 1987; Berthold 1990; Nakagawara et al. 1988; Seeger et al. 1985). The prognostic significance of N-*myc* amplification becomes most obvious from the follow-up of patients with stage I and II tumors positive for amplification. In most instances these tumors, which on the basis of clinical stage were of good prognosis, progressed later and became fatal. A peculiar type of stage IV tumors which is characterized by frequent spontaneous regression without clinical intervention rarely shows amplification. Three patients with stage IV tumors have been reported as positive for amplification (Carlsen et al. 1986; Cohn et al. 1987; Tonini et al. 1987). All tumors progressed later and were fatal. Collectively, these observations demonstrate that N-*myc* amplification is a reliable prognostic parameter for poor prognosis of patients with stage I, II, or IV tumors.

The possibility of identifying a subset of patients with poor prognosis, among a group that should have good prognosis by clinical parameters, could represent a valuable setting for improved therapeutic approaches. Current strategies for the treatment of neuroblastoma depend on the prognosis for survival which is evaluated on the basis of tumor stage and the degree to which the tumor can be surgically removed. An additional parameter introduced recently is genomic analysis to identify the status of N-*myc*. The pilot study of the German Neuroblastoma Study Group advises treatment of patients according to protocols that are specific for each of four risk groups (Table 1). Risk group A includes patients with localized tumor that can be surgically removed to at least 90% (the prognosis for these patients for survival is between 80% and 100%). Risk group B includes patients with a localized tumor that extends beyond the area of the organ of origin, and which therefore cannot be removed completely (prognosis 65%–80%). Risk group C includes patients carrying either a metastatic tumor or a localized tumor that cannot be found to regress after four cycles of chemotherapy (prognosis 20%–30%). Finally, risk group D includes only patients with stage IV tumor, which usually regresses spontaneously without therapeutic intervention. Patients originally assigned on clinical and histopathological grounds to risk groups A or B are transferred to group C if they are positive for amplification).

Functions of the N-Myc Protein

N-*myc* encodes two polypeptides that result from alternative use of two translational start codons (Mäkelä et al. 1989) The relative masses of the two proteins are 62 and 64 kDa, respectively. The two proteins are localized in the nucleus of the cell and are phosphorylated. Under in vitro conditions casein kinase efficiently carries out phosphorylation in the central region and at serine 367 (Hamann et al. 1991).

Two evolutionarily conserved regions of the protein appear particularly suitable to address the question of protein function. One is the carboxy-terminal region containing a helix-loop-helix (HLH) and a leucine zipper motif (Zip), and the other is the N-terminus carrying what has been referred to as "*myc*-boxes" (Schwab 1988).

The Helix-Loop-Helix/Leucine Zipper Motif

Proteins encoded by the proto-oncogenes c-*myc*, L-*myc*, and N-*myc* contain at their carboxy-terminus a tripartite segment comprising a basic DNA binding region, an HLH, and a Zip, which are believed to be involved in DNA binding and protein-protein interaction. Using a monoclonal antibody directed against an N-terminal epitope of the N-Myc protein in immunoprecipitations performed with extracts of neuroblastoma cells, our laboratory was the first to demonstrate data that support the in vivo association of two nuclear phosphoproteins p20/22 with N-Myc (Wenzel et al. 1991). These p20/22 proteins turned out to be identical to another protein, Max, that was identified independently through an in vitro reconstruction assay (Blackwood and Eisenman 1991). Time course experiments showed the presence of the complex in cellular extracts immunoprecipitated within a 5-min interval after the preparation of the cell extract. While the expression of N-*myc* is restricted, expression of Max(p20/22) has been observed in cells of diverse human and murine embryonal lineages, as detected by heterologous complex formation. By introduction of expression vectors containing the wild-type N-*myc* gene or N-*myc* genes with in-frame deletions or point mutations into recipient cells and subsequent immunoprecipitation of the resulting N-Myc proteins it could be shown that the HLH-Zip region is essential to the formation of the N-Myc-p20/22 complex in vivo (Wenzel et al. 1991). Recently an alternatively spliced messenger RNA has been identified that encodes a form of Max truncated at the C-terminus (Mäkelä et al. 1992). This DMax protein retains the ability to bind to the CACGTG motif in a complex with c-*myc* but lacks the nuclear localization signal. In a *myc-ras* cotransformation assay using rat embryo cells *max* suppressed, but D*max* enhanced, the transformation efficiency. Thus the *max* gene appears to encode both a negative and a positive regulator of Myc function. It is not clear at this point whether D*max* is expressed also in human neuroblastoma cells. An important question therefore that cannot be answered at this point is how the elevated level of N-Myc, consequent to N-*myc* gene amplification, is involved in the development of neuroblastoma. Due to overexpression N-Myc could act as a scavanger and eliminate p20/22, thus its tumor-suppressing potential. Alternatively, if D*max* is expressed, the elevated level of N-Myc protein could result in a larger number of positive growth-activating complexes. These questions are currently under investigation.

The *myc*-Boxes

The two *myc*-boxes were originally defined as short, roughly 60 and 40 nucleotides long, and in the first coding exon of the *myc* genes (Schwab et al. 1983; Schwab 1988). These boxes are highly conserved over a broad evolutionary range ranging from chicken to man. Kato and collaborators (1990) were the first to identify the amino terminal portion of a Myc protein, c-Myc, as a transcription-activating domain. In an extension of these studies we asked whether the transcription activation might be directed by the *myc*-boxes. As the experimental approach we have substituted the transcription-activating domain in the transcription factor Gal4 from yeast by the complete or incomplete N-Myc protein. The various mutant N-Myc constructs were generated through site-directed mutagenesis, followed by construction of deletions. Recombinant genes consisting of the DNA binding domain of Gal4 and of N-Myc were expressed in various human cells, and it was tested whether portions of N-Myc are capable of stimulating transcription of a reporter gene attached to Gal4 binding sites that are the target of the DNA-binding domain of Gal4. Two observations were of particular interest (Cziepluch et al., manuscript submitted). First, expression of the complete N-Myc protein did not result in stimulation of transcription, but deletion of the C-terminal half did. These results indicate that N-Myc may act as a transcription factor, and that the C-terminus can act as a repressor of this activity. This observation is in line with similar effects seen for other proteins, such as Myb, c-Myc, and p53 (Kato et al. 1990; Weston and Bishop 1989; O'Rourke et al. 1990). Second, the amino-terminal regions conferring transcription activation map to the *myc*-boxes. Also interesting is the ability of the protein RB1 encoded by the retinoblastoma gene to bind to the amino-terminal portion of N-Myc where the transactivation regions are localized (Rustgi et al. 1991). Most likely RB1 is not required to the transcription-activation because this effort could also be observed in retinoblastoma line WERI, which lacks RB1 (Cziepluch et al. manuscript submitted). It remains to be established, however, whether N-Myc is a transcription factor on its own in the sense that it can bind to the promoter region of a specific gene and modulate its transcription.

Significance of N-*myc* Amplification Versus Other Genetic Alterations

Amplification of N-*myc* is seen in a relatively small proportion of neuroblastomas, predominantly of stage III and IV. Two additional genetic alterations have been reported: deletion at chromosome 14q and deletion at chromosome 1p.

Chromosome 14q

Deletion of chromosome 14q was originally detected by loss-of-heterozygosity (LOH) studies using a probe that detects the locus D14S1 (Suzuki et al. 1989). The incidence of deletion was around 50%. In a somewhat more detailed study LOH was observed in 40% of 25 informative cases, with the commonly deleted region distal to the D14S13 locus (14q32-ter) (Takayama et al. 1992). The deleted region must be fairly small, the cytogenetic analyses of neuroblastoma cells as yet have not revealed 14q deletions at significant frequency.

Chromosome 1p

Alterations of chromosome 1p constitute the most frequent genetic change in neuroblastoma, reaching a frequency of more than 70% on the basis of cytogenetic analyses (Brodeur et al. 1981). Alterations of 1p are also seen at significant frequency in other types of cancers, including colon cancer (Fearon et al. 1987; Leister et al. 1990), alveolar rhabdomyosarcoma (Douglass et al. 1991), Merkel cell tumor (Harnett et al. 1991), malignant glioma (Lindström et al. 1991), hepatoblastoma (Lindström et al. 1991; Simon et al. 1991), malignant mesothelioma (Flejter et al. 1989), and ductal carcinoma of the breast (Genuardi et al. 1989). Altogether the state of present information indicates that the distal portion of chromosome 1p contains genetic information whose alteration may contribute to the development of cancer.

Because the alterations at chromosome band 1p36 involve mostly deletions and translocations, the search for a putative tumor suppressor gene can be pursued under two perspectives. First, the smallest overlapping region of deletion can be mapped through LOH studies, and, second, DNA sequences at translocation breakpoints can be defined through molecular cloning. Either approach requires the availability of a large panel of molecular probes from the altered genomic region.

We generated a panel of DNA probes closely positioned to each other by establishing a microclone library specific for the distal part of the p arm of chromosome 1 (Martinsson et al. 1989). The dense distribution of probes should be advantageous in several respects. Firstly, small deletions should be detectable with a higher probability because of the ability to detect allelic loss in cases where adjacent loci were not informative due to homozygosity. Secondly, it should be possible to define the borders of deleted regions within narrow limits and to determine a small region commonly deleted in different tumors.

Applying this strategy it was possible to discover allelic deletions in a high proportion of stage III and IV tumors (at least 90%) analyzed (Weith et al. 1989). These studies revealed that distal 1p material was indeed lost from the genome of the tumor cells. In another study of chromosomal deletions in neuroblastomas, loss of heterozygosity was also detected in band 1p36, although the frequency described was lower (28%) than indicated by cytogenetic analyses (Fong et al. 1989). The higher overall frequency of loss of genetic material from the 1p arm among stage III and IV tumors in our studies is probably due to the fact that probes generated by microcloning are from within the consensus deletion and are located closer to the putative suppressor gene related to neuroblastoma. The number of tumors displaying allelic loss with these probes exceeded that showing cytogenetically detectable rearrangements. One may suspect that small deletions are likely to remain undetectable upon microscopic investigation.

In our series several tumors obviously had interstitial 1p deletion that allowed delineation of a smallest region of overlap at subbands 1p36.1–2. A rough estimate can be made of the size of this deleted DNA segment. The entire 1p36 band comprises about 0.7% of the total haploid chromosome length. Predicting an even distribution of the DNA along the chromosomes, 1p36 would contain about 20 Mbp of DNA (0.7% of totally 3×10^9 bp as the haploid DNA content). Roughly half of the 1p36 band is represented by 1p36.1–1p36.2. Hence the genomic region included in the common deletion would span about 10 Mbp óf DNA. Future studies should result in establishing a long-range restriction map of this region with pulsed-field gel electrophoresis. This long-range map will provide information on the presence and location of CpG-rich islands, which often signify the 5' regions of genes and will therefore be a tool for the identification of transcription units in this region.

The significance of genetic alteration in chromosome band 1p36 for neuroblastoma is dramatized by the finding of translocation breakpoints which could be mapped through both Giemsa banding (Savelyeva et al., manuscript submitted) and fluorescence in situ hybridization with flanking probes to a site within the smallest overlapping deletion (Barker et al., manuscript in preparation). In this region a constitutional translocation (2;17)(p36;q12–21) has also been found in a patient with neuroblastoma (Laureys et al. 1990). Approaches are now in progress to isolate the corresponding DNA sequences by employing a combination of yeast artificial chromosomes (YAC). If mapping combined with pulsed-field gel electrophoretic analyses. The results should soon be at hand and tell us whether specific genetic information is commonly altered in neuroblastomas, and, if so, what its significance is for tumorigenesis and for its practical clinical use in the differential diagnosis of small round cell tumors of children that often are difficult to diagnose.

Conclusion

Pediatric cancers have been particularly valuable settings to define basic principles concerning the significance of genetic alterations for human cancers. Two instances characterize this particularly well. First, the concept of tumor suppressor genes was developed for one pediatric cancer, retinoblastoma, and the first tumor suppressor gene has been isolated from there. Second, the significance of oncogene amplification was recognized for the first time for another pediatric tumor, neuroblastoma. Amplification of N-*myc* has turned out to be a paradigm for a genetic alteration that can be of clinical use as a prognostic marker.

Acknowledgements. Work in the author's laboratory is supported by the Deutsche Forschungsgemeinschaft, the Dr. Mildred Scheel Stiftung, the Heidelberg-Mannheim Comprehensive Cancer Center and the DKFZ-Israel Cooperation.

References

Alitalo K, Schwab M (1986) Oncogene amplification in tumor cells. Adv Cancer Res 47:235

Alitalo K, Schwab M, Lin CC, Varmus H, Bishop JM (1983) Homogeneously staining chromosomal regions contain amplified copies of an abundantly expressed cellular oncogene (c-*myc*) in malignant neuroendocrine cells from a human colon carcinoma. Proc Natl Acad Sci USA 80:1707

Amler LC, Schwab M (1989) Amplified N-myc in human neuroblastoma cells is often arranged as clustered tandem repeats of differently recombined DNA. Molec Cell Biol 9:4903

Amler LC, Schwab M (1992) Multiple amplicons of discrete sizes encompassing N-*myc* in neuroblastoma cells evolve through differential recombination from a large precursor DNA. Oncogene 7:807

Bartram CR, Berthold F (1987) Amplification and expression of the N-*myc* gene in neuroblastoma. Eur J Pediatr 146:162

Beckwith JB and Perrin EV (1963) *In situ* neuroblastomas: a contribution to the natural history of neural crest tumors. Am J Pathol 43:1089

Berthold F (1990) Overview Biology of neuroblastoma. In: Neuroblastoma: Tumor Biology and Therapy. Pochadly, Tebbi, (eds) CRC Press Inc, Boca Raton, p 1

Blackwood EM, Eisenman RN (1991) Max: A helix-loop-helix zipper protein that forms a sequence-specific DNA-binding complex with Myc. Science 251:1211

Brodeur G, Seeger RC, Schwab M, Varmus HE, Bishop JM (1984) Amplification of N-*myc* in untreated human neuroblastomas correlates with advanced disease stage. Sience 224:1121

Brodeur GM, Green AA, Hayes FA, Williams KG, Williams DL, Tsiatis AA (1981) Cytogenetic features of human neuroblastomas and cell lines. Cancer Res 41:4678

Carlsen NLT, Christiansen IJ, Schroeder H, Bro PV, Hesselberg K, Jensen KB, Nielsen KH (1986) Prognostic value of different staging systems in neuroblastomas and completeness of tumour exision. Arch Die Child 61:832

Cohn SL, Herst CV, Maurer HS, Rosen ST (1987) N-*myc* amplification in an infant with stage IV-s neuroblastoma. J Clin Oncol 5:1441

Cox D, Yuncken C, Spriggs A (1965) Minute chromatin bodies in malignant tumours of childhood. Lancet 2:55

Douglass EC, Rowe ST, Valentine M, Parham DM, Berkow R, Bowman WP, Maurer HM (1991) Variant translocations of chromosome 13 in alveolar rhabdomyosarcoma. Genes, Chromosomes & Cancer 3:480

Evans AE, D'Angio GB, Randolph J (1971) A proposed staging for children with neuroblastoma. Cancer 27:374

Fearon ER, Hamilton SH, Vogelstein B (1987) Clonal analysis of human colorectal tumours. Science 238:193

Flejter WL, Li FP, Antman KH, Testa JR (1989) Recurring loss involving chromosomes 1, 3 and 22 in malignant mesothelioma: Possible sites of tumor suppressor genes. Genes, Chromosomes and Cancer 1:148

Fong CT, Dracopoli NC, White PS, Merril PT, Griffith RC, Housman DE, Brodeur GM (1989) Loss of heterozygosity for the short arm of chromosome 1 in human neuroblastomas: Correlation with N-myc amplification. Proc Natl Acad Sci USA 86:3753

Fuller G, Bigner S (1992) Amplified cellular oncogenes in neoplasms of the central nervous system. Mut Res 276:299
Garson JA, McIntyre PG, Kemshead JT (1985) N-myc amplification in malignant astrocytoma. The Lancet 8457:718
Genuardi M, Tshihira H, Anderson DE, Saunders GF (1989) Distal deletion of chromosome 1p in ductal carcinoma of the breast. Amer J Hum Genet 45:73
Hamann U, Wenzel A, Frank R, Schwab M (1991) The MYCN protein of human neuroblastoma cells is phosphorylated by casein kinase II in the central region and at serine 367. Oncogene 6:1745
Harnett PR, Kearsley JH, Hayward NK, Dracopoli NC, Kefford RF (1991) Loss of allelic heterozygosity on distal chromosome 1p in Merkel Cell Carcinom. Cancer Genet Cytogenet 54:109
Hasegawa R, Tatematsu M, Imaida K et al. (1982) Neuroblastoma *in situ*. Acta Pathol Jpn 32:537
Kato GJ, Barrett J, Villa-Garcia M, Dang CV (1990) An amino-terminal c-*myc* domain required for neoplastic transformation activities transcription. Mol Cell Biol 10:5914
Kohl NE, Kanda N, Schreck RR, Bruns G, Latt SA, Gilbert F, Alt FW (1983) Transposition and amplification of oncogene-related sequences in human neuroblastomas. Cell 35:359
Koufos A, Hansen MF, Copeland NG, Jenkins NA, Lampkin BC, Cavanee WK (1985) Loss of heterozygosity in three embryonal tumors suggest a common pathogenetic mechanism. Nature 316:330
Kramer S, Meadows AT, Jarrett P, Evans AE (1983) Incidence of childhood cancer: experience of a decade in a population-based registry. J Natl Cancers Inst 70:49
Laureys G, Speleman F, Opdenakker G, Benoit Y, Leroy J (1990) Constitutional translocation t(1;17)(p36;q12–21) in a patient with neuroblastoma. Genes, Chromosomes and Cancer 2:252
Lee WH, Murphree AL, Benedict WF (1984) Expression and amplification of the N-*myc* gene in primary retinoblastoma. Nature 309:458
Leister I, Weith A, Brüderlein S, Cziepluch C, Schlag P, Schwab M (1990) Human colorectal cancer: high frequency of deletions at chromosome 1p35. Cancer Res 50:7232
Lindström E, Salford LG, Heim S, Mandahl N, Strömblad S, Brun A, Mitelman F (1991) Trisomy 7 and sex chromosome loss need not be representative of tumor parenchyma cells in malignant glioma. Genes, Chromosomes & Cancer 3:474
Mäkelä, TP, Saksela K, Alitalo K (1989) Two N-myc polypeptides with distinct amino termini encoded by the second and third exons of the gene. Mol Cell Biol 9:1545
Mäkelä TP, Koskinen PJ, Västrik I, Alitalo K (1992) Alternative forms of Max as enhancers of suppressors of *myc-ras* cotransformation. Science 256:373
Martinsson T, Weith A, Cziepluch C, Schwab M (1989) Chromosome 1 deletions in human neuroblastomas: Generation and fine mapping of microclones from the distal 1p region. Genes, Chromosomes and Cancer 1:67
Michaelis J, Kaatsch P (1986) Cooperative documentation of childhood malignancies in the FRG. System design and five-year results. Monogr Paediatr 18:56
Nakagawara A, Ikeda K, Tsuda T, Higashi K (1988) Biological characteristics of NMYC amplified neuroblastomas in patients over one year of age. In: Advances in neuroblastoma research; Evans, D'Angio, Seeger (eds). Alan R Liss, Inc. New York, p 31
Nau M, Brooks B, Carney D, Gazdar A, Batey J, Sausville E, Minna J (1986) Human small-cell lung cancers show amplification and expression of the N-myc gene. Proc Natl Acad Sci USA 83:1092
O'Rourke RW, Miller CW, Kato GJ, Simon KJ, Chen D-L, Dang CV, Koeffler HP (1990) A potential transcriptional activation element in the p53 protein. Oncogene 5:1829
Rustgi AK, Dyson N, Bernards R (1991) Amino-terminal domains of c-myc and N-myc proteins mediate binding to the retinoblastoma gene product. Nature 352:541
Schwab M (1988) The MYC-box oncogenes. In: The Oncogene Handbook; Reddy, Skalka, Curran (eds) Elsevier Science Publishers BV, p 381
Schwab M, Amler LC (1990) Amplification of cellular oncogenes: A predictor of clinical outcome in human cancer. Genes, Chromosomes and Cancer 1:180
Schwab M, Alitalo K, Klempnauer KH, Varmus HE, Bishop JM, Gilbert F, Brodeur G, Goldstein M, Trent J (1983) Amplified DNA with limited homology to myc cellular oncogene is shared by human neuroblasoma cell lines and a neuroblastoma tumor. Nature 305:245
Schwab M, Alitalo K, Varmus KH, Bishop JM, George D (1983) A cellular oncogene (c-Ki-ras) is amplified, overexpressed, and located within karyotypic abnormalities in mouse adrenocortical tumor cells. Nature 303:497

Schwab M, Varmus HE, Bishop JM, Grzeschik KH, Naylor S, Sakaguchi A, Brodeur G, Trent J (1984) Chromosome localization in normal human cells and neuroblastomas of a gene related to c-myc. Nature 308:288

Seeger RC, Brodeur GM, Sather H, Dalton A, Siegel SE, Wong KY, Hammond D (1985) Association of multiple copies of the N-myc oncogene with rapid progression of neuroblastomas. N Engl J Med 313:1111

Simon D, Knowles B, Weith A (1991) Abnormalities of chromosome 1 and loss of heterozygosity on 1p in primary hepatomas. Oncogene 6:765

Suzuki T, Mugishima H, Fujisawa T, Okumi M, Okabe I, Yokota J, Terada M (1991) Loss of heterozygosity on chromosome 14 in neuroblastoma. In: Advances in Neuroblastoma Reserach; Evans AE, D'Angio GJ, Knudson Jr AG, Seeger RC (eds) Wiley-Liss, Inc, p135

Takayama H, Suzuki T, Mugishima H, Fujisawa T, Ookuni M, Schwab M, Gehring M, Nakamura Y, Sugimura T, Terada M, Yokota J (1992) Deletion mapping of chromosomes 14q and 1p in human neuroblastoma. Oncogene 7:1185

Tonini GP, Verdona G, de Bernardi B, Sansone R, Massimo L, Cornaglia-Ferraris P (1987) N-*myc* oncogene amplification in a patient with IV-s neuroblastoma. Am J Pediatr Hematol Oncol 9:8

Weith A, Martinsson T, Cziepluch C, Brüderlein S, Amler LC, Berthold F, Schwab M (1989) Neuroblastoma consensus deletion maps to chromosome 1p36.1–2. Genes, Chromosomes and Cancer 1:159

Wenzel A, Cziepluch C, Hamann U, Schürmann J, Schwab M (1991) The N-Myc oncoprotein is associated *in vivo* with the phosphoprotein Max(p20/22) in human neuroblastoma cells. EMBO J 10:3703

Weston K, Bishop JM (1989) Transcriptional activation by the v-myb oncogene and its cellular progenitor, c-myb. Cell 58:85

Epidermal Growth Factor Receptor Gene and Its Transcripts in Glioblastomas

V. P. Collins

Division of Neuropathology, Department of Pathology, Sahlgrenska Hospital, 41345 Gothenburg, Sweden and Ludwig Institute for Cancer Research, Stockholm Branch, Karolinska Hospital, S-17176 Stockholm, Sweden

Introduction

The astrocytic variants of the gliomas, comprising astrocytoma, anaplastic astrocytoma, and glioblastoma, form the most common group of these tumours in adults (Walker et al. 1985) and together account for approximately 50% of primary intracranial tumours. Glioblastomas make up almost half of these and are unfortunately the most malignant tumours of the series (Mahaley et al. 1989). Thus, due to their frequency the astrocytic group of gliomas has received most attention, with the glioblastomas being particularly well studied, due to their abundance and biological aggressiveness.

The cytogenetic observation that many glioblastomas had multiple double-minute chromosomes(DMs) was the first evidence that amplification of genes might be occurring in glioblastomas (Bigner et al. 1984). The presence of DMs had been shown to be associated with gene amplification (Kaufman and Schimke 1981). More recent cytogenetic studies of gliomas have shown DMs to be present in up to 50% of glioblastoas (Bigner et al. 1988; Bigner et al. 1990).

Almost simultaneously the epidermal growth factor receptor gene (EGFR) was shown to be amplified in malignant gliomas (Libermann et al. 1984, 1985). At that time the amplified gene was also suggested to be rearranged due to the presence of variable restriction fragments in the tumour DNAs. The fragments observed in the initial reports have proved to be common sequence polymorphisms within the normal gene (Lee et al. 1988). When normal leucocyte DNA from individual patients was used as a control for constitutional polymorphisms, rearrangement of the EGFR gene was shown to occur in association with amplification (Malden et al. 1988; Sugawa et al. 1990; Wong et al. 1992). EGFR amplification has been studied in so many astrocytic gliomas that reliable estimates for its incidence in this group of brain tumours can be made. Astrocytomas (malignancy grade II) have been studied in least numbers, and only single cases have been reported to show amplification (Libermann et al. 1985; Helseth et al. 1988; Diedrich et al. 1991; Ekstrand et al. 1991). Greater numbers of anaplastic astrocytomas (malignancy grade III) have been examined, and the cumulative results suggest that the incidence lies well under 10%

(Wong et al. 1987; Diedrich et al. 1991; Ekstrand et al. 1991). More than 200 cases of glioblastomas (malignancy grade IV) have been examined, and the cumulative incidence of amplification of the EGFR gene lies around 40% (Libermann et al. 1985; Wong et al. 1987; Helseth et al. 1988; James et al. 1988; Malden et al. 1988; Diedrich et al. 1991; Ekstrand et al. 1991; Tuzi et al. 1991). This would leave 10% of glioblastomas with no gene amplification to account for their DMs. There have, however, been reports of the amplification of other genes including the MYCN gene (Wong et al. 1987; Diedrich et al. 1991; Ekstrand et al. 1991), the GLI gene (Kinzler et al. 198), and the platelet-derived growth factor receptor A (PDGFRA) gene (Ekstrand et al., in preparation; Collins et al. 1991; Flemming et al. 1992; Kumabe et al. 1992) . In addition, there have been single reports of amplification of MYC (Trent et al. 1986; Bigner et al. 1988), MYB (Welter et al. 1990) and K-*ras* (Bigner et al. 1988)genes in glioblastoma cell lines or xenografts.

The EGFR Gene and Transcript

The human EGFR gene covers a region of at least 110 kDa, has 26 exons (average size 170 bases) and is located on the p arm of chromosome 7p13–p11 (Merlino et al. 1985; Haley et al. 1987). The first intron is large, probably exceeding 20 kb. Two transcripts approximately 5.6 and 10 kb in size have been identified (Ullrich et al. 1984). In human brain and in gliomas almost exclusively the 10-kb transcript is seen (Ekstrand et al. 1991). The transcripts have a short 5' non-coding sequence, followed by a signal peptide sequence and a coding sequence of 3816 bases (Ullrich et al. 1984). This is followed in both transcripts by non-coding 3' sequences with no known function. A 5532-nucleotide cDNA has been cloned (Ullrich et al. 1984). In the coding region the exon-exon borders have been estimated (Haley et al. 1987).

The Functional Regions of the Receptor Protein

The EGFR protein has received much attention, and the protein has been divided into a number of functional domains (Fig. 1). There is the extracellular domain, which is divided into four regions, an N-terminal domain, believed to be a minor contributor to the ligand binding region, the first of two cystine-rich domains, followed by a cystine-poor sequence that is a major contributor to the ligand binding domain and a further cystine rich region (Ullrich and Schlessinger 1990). The transmembrane domain is made up of 23 amino acids. The cytoplasmic region has a short stretch of 49 amino acids containing a threonine at position 654, the phosphorylation of which inhibits the action of the receptor. This is followed by the tyrosine kinase domain (Ullrich and Schlessinger 1990), and the short segment responsible for internalization and calcium control following ligand binding (Wells et al. 1990; Chang et al. 1991) and finally by the control region with its many phosphorylation sites (Ullrich and Schlessinger 1990).

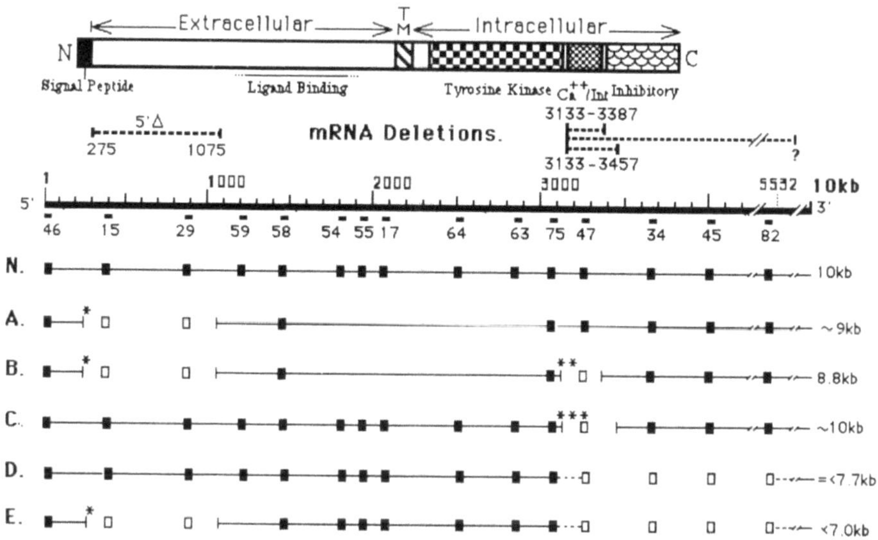

Fig. 1. The EGFR protein and transcripts. *Above*, the protein is depicted with its N-terminal signal peptide, extracellular domain, major ligand binding domain, transmembrane domain (*TM*) and intracellular C-terminal region. The intracellular region is divided into the tyrosine kinase domain, the internalization (*Int*) and calcium control region (Ca^{2+}) and, nearest the C-terminal, the inhibitory region with its phosphorylation sites. Below the protein are shown the transcript deletions described by Sugawa et al. (1990) and Ekstrand et al. (1992). The 10-kb transcript (almost exclusively observed in brain) is depicted with the 50-mer oligonucleotides used for the differential hybridization studies directly below. *Below*, the different transcripts found in the tumours (*N, A-E*). The untranslated sequences, translated sequences and sequences deleted from the various transcripts detected in glioblastomas are depicted. *N*, normal 10-kb transcript; *A*, the commonest aberrant transcript with the loss of 801 bases near the 5' end, which appears to occur in about 20% of all glioblastomas (Yamazaki et al. 1988, 1990; Humphrey et al. 1990; Sugawa et al. 1990; Ekstrand et al. 1992), B-E the transcripts with abnormalities of the 3' end (Ekstrand et al. 1992). Further aberrant transcripts have been described (Wong et al. 1992). These aberrant transcripts could be found in different combinations in the same tumour (see Ekstrand et al. 1992) but only when there was evidence of EGFR gene amplification. In one tumour, which was studied at primary presentation and at recurrence 1 year later, the D transcript had been further mutated to the E variant (Ekstrand et al. 1992)

Amplification of the EGFR Gene in Gliomas

Amplification of the EGFR occurs mainly in glioblastomas and there in approximately 40%. In the few cases studied that have shown both amplification and restriction fragment length polymorphisms of the gene, only one allele of the gene is amplified (Sugawa et al. 1990). Overexpression of the transcript or the EGFR protein has been documented in all cases where amplification was determined molecular biologically (Ekstrand et al. 1991). Expression levels of the receptor transcript or its protein vary markedly in cases with no evidence of amplification (Ekstrand et al. 1991). Immunohistochemistry with the currently available excellent monoclonal antibodies and antisera can adequately survey biopsy material for the occurrence of high levels of EGFR (see for example Reifenberger et al. 1989; Reifenberger et al., in preparation).

However, this technology, which can easily be introduced into routine pathology, cannot determine whether this is due to amplification or other phenomena effecting expression levels.

Rearrangements of the Amplified EGFR Gene

Rearrangements of the amplified EGFR genes were first noted at the 5' end (coding for the extracellular domain) in primary tumours and xenografts (Malden et al. 1988; Yamazaki et al. 1988). Further studies, using series of oligonucleotides to identify short cDNA sequences, showed that amplified aberrant restriction fragments occur, and that these can be identified using oligonucleotides to exon 8 (Sugawa et al. 1990). In these cases both Southern and northern blot analysis, using oligonucleotides complementary to exons 2–7, generally gave a signal much below that expected and observed when oligonucleotides complementary to the coding sequences outside this region were used (Sugawa et al. 1990). Restriction fragments of variable aberrant size, amplified to variable degrees, were noted in the individual cases. The normal restriction fragments were always present and amplified to a degree particular to the case. It is concluded that the normal gene is always amplified to some degree, and that the aberrant variant has occurred during the amplification processes with the aberrant gene then being further amplified (Sugawa et al. 1990; Ekstrand et al. 1992). Further study has shown that a series of other rearrangements may also occur involving the extracellular or the cytoplasmic domains (Ekstrand et al. 1992; Wong et al. 1992). The rearrangements at the 5' end of the EGFR gene have, however, been shown to be the most common.

EGFR Transcripts in Glioblastomas with Abnormalities of the 5' End of the Transcript

Gliomas express transcripts for the pre-pro-proteins of the ligands transforming growth factor-a and epidermal growth factor, as well as the EGFR, opening the possibility of autocrine, paracrine, or juxtacrine stimulation of growth in these tumours (Ekstrand et al. 1991). Detailed study of the transcripts for EGFR in glioblastomas has shown that cases with amplification of the gene have higher transcript levels (Ekstrand et al. 1991). Differential hybridisation of a series of oligonucleotides complementary to the coding region of the transcripts gave different levels of signal, under standardized conditions, suggesting that there was loss of coding sequence complementary to some regions in a proportion of the mRNA molecules (Sugawa et al. 1990; Ekstrand et al. 1992; see Fig. 1) The region most commonly found to be lacking was at the 5' end (Sugawa et al. 1990). A fragment of the aberrant transcript was amplified using reverse-transcriptase polymerase chain reaction (PCR) technology, with the primers in the flanking regions to the sequences noted to be missing. From a normal transcript the PCR product would be approximately 1185 bp while the product from the cases with aberrant differential hybridization patterns showed a fragment of normal size *and*, in addition, a shorter 384 bp (loss of 801 bp) PCR product. Careful northern blotting demonstrated the shorter transcript, although at 10 kb it is difficult to demonstrate such small changes in sequence length. Sequencing of the PCR-amplified cDNA showed that the coding sequence was identical in the different tumours despite the fact that the gene rearrangement had been shown to be different. The coding sequence of the transcript was normal until the end of the first exon (base 274), after which there was the loss of the 801 bases. This loss does not result in a reading frame shift but codes for 267 amino acids. The sequence then continued at base 1076 in all cases. The sequence lost divides the two flanking codons, resulting in a unique amino acid at this position, after which the sequence continues in frame. The amino acid sequence coded by the rearranged transcript is unique and is not present on any normal cell. Similar studies of the gene and transcripts have been carried out independently by other groups who have reported similar findings (Amazaki et al. 1988; Humphrey et al. 1990; Yamazaki et al. 1990; Wong et al. 1992).

The consistent transcript sequence aberration in different tumors which had variable genomic rearrangements was difficult to explain. Studies using the PCR-based exon-exon connection strategy showed that base 1076 was the first base of an exon after a 1.7kb intron (Sugawa et al. 1990). The consistent transcript abnormality in tumours with variable genetic rearrangements could thus be explained on the basis of the aberrant splicing of exon 1 to exon 8 (Sugawa et al. 1990).

Further studies of a large series of glioblastomas have shown that this aberration of the extracellular domain of the receptor is detectable, at variable levels, in at least half of the glioblastomas with amplification of the EGFR (Sugawa et al., in preparation).

Other EGFR Transcript Abnormalities in Glioblastomas

While the most common abnormality of the EGFR transcripts in glioblastomas is the loss of 801 bases coding for the external domain of the receptor described above, further abnormalities have been observed. These may effect the extracellular region as has been described by Wong et al. (1992) or the cytoplasmic domains as described by Ekstrand et al.(1992). The cytoplasmic domain abnormalities are more complex than those effecting the sequences coding for the extracellular domain. The genomic rearrangements are in these cases also variable, yet give rise to similar transcripts due to aberrant splicing. In some cases cryptic splice sites in coding sequence are used. They can occur alone or together with the 5' rearrangement described above. The consequences of these 3' rearrangements is in most cases aberrant splicing with a frame shift. This results in the truncation of the receptor just after the tyrosine kinase domain. In one of our cases (see Fig. 1. transcript B), a cryptic splice site was used to produce a transcript with no frame shift but the loss of codons for the 87 amino acids which form the region involved in internalization of the receptor following ligand binding (Wells et al. 1990; Chang et al. 1991). Such a receptor would not down-regulate once it had bound ligand – a scenario shown in experimental studies to result in transformation when ligand is available, which is the case in gliomas (Chen et al. 1989; Wells et al. 1990; Ekstrand et al. 1991). The majority of the rearrangements resulted in aberrant splicing with a frame shift, or the 3' sequence of the transcript was indeterminable as it continued 3' with unknown sequences and as a result could not be amplified by the PCR technique. ,The frequency of these rearrangements is lower than that of the 5' rearrangement. The different transcript variants documented in glioblastomas are shown in Fig. 1 B–E.

Is There Any Correlation Between Amplification, Rearrangement, Histopathology, and Patient Survival?

In a series of 64 gliomas, 28 of which had EGFR amplification, Bigner et al. (1988) evaluated the tumours for a variety of morphological characteristics. There were no morphological correlates to EGFR amplification. In situ hybridization showed that all of the many morphologically different cell types found in the glioblastomas had evidence of amplification (Bigner et al. 1988). In addition, attempts to correlate patient survival to EGFR amplification have so far proved fruitless (Bigner et al. 1988; Diedrich et al. 1991). No attempts to correlate the amplified and rearranged EGFR gene to survival have been reported.

Implications of the Findings for the Treatment of Gliomas

Amplification and rearrangement of the EGFR receptor in glioblastomas is only one of the multitude of molecular abnormalities which combine to make this malignant cell. Only by understanding these events can we hope to design treatment modalities which specifically kill malignant cells and leave normal cells unharmed. Optimistically one might hope that the overexpression of the EGFR protein could be used to effectively target treatment. Clinical trials are underway using antibodies to the normal EGFR protein. The aberrant form of the EGFR protein should also prove interesting in this regard as it is present on the surface of the tumour cells of approximately 20% of glioblastomas and represents a tumour-specific epitope which does not exist on any normal cell.

*Acknowledgements.*Supported by the Swedish Cancer Fund and the Inga Britt and Arne Lundbergs Research Foundation.

References

Bigner SH, Mark J, Mahaley JM S, Bigner DD (1984) Patterns of the early gross chromosomal changes in malignant human gliomas. Hereditas 101:103–113

Bigner SH, Burger PC, Wong AJ, Werner MH, Hamilton SR, Muhlbaier LH, Vogelstein B, Bigner DD (1988) Gene amplification in malignant human gliomas: clinical and histopathologic aspects. J Neuropathol Exp Neurol 47 (3):191–205

Bigner SH, Vogelstein B, Bigner DD (1988) Chromosomal abnormalities and gene amplification in malignant gliomas. ISI Atlas of Sci Biochem1:333–336

Bigner SH, Humphrey PA, Wong AJ, Vogelstein B, Mark J, Friedman HS, Bigner DD (1990) Characterization of the epidermal growth factor receptor in human glioma cell lines and xenografts. Cancer Res 50 (24):8017–22

Chang C, Kao JPY, Lazar CS, Walsh BJ, Wells A, Wiley HS, Gill GN, Rosenfeld MG (1991) Ligand-induced internalization and increased cell calcium are mediated via distinct structural elements in the carboxyl terminus of the epidermal growth factor receptor. J Biol Chem 266 (34):23467–23470

Chen WS, Lazar CS, Lund KA, Welsh JB, Chang C.-P, Walton GM, Der CJ, Wiley HS, Gill GN, Rosenfeld MG (1989) Functional independence of the epidermal growth factor receptor from a domain required for ligand induced internalization and calcium regulation. Cell 59:33–43

Collins VP, Ekstrand J, James CD (1991) A Glioblastoma with high-level amplification of the PDGF-alfa receptor. Proceedings of Ninth International Conference on Brain Tumor Research and Therapy Asilomar California October 15–18 1991:

Diedrich U, Soja S, Behnke J, Zoll B (1991) Amplification of the c-erb-B oncogene is associated with malignancy in primary tumors of neuroepithelial tissue. JNeurol, 238:221–224

Ekstrand AJ, James CD, Cavenee WK, Seliger B, Pettersson RF, Collins VP (1991) Genes for epidermal growth factor receptor, transforming growth factor alpha and epidermal growth factor and their expression in human gliomas in vivo. Cancer Res 51 (8):2164–72

Ekstrand AJ, Sugawa N, James CD, Collins VP (1992) Amplified and rearranged epidermal growth factor receptor genes in human glioblastomas reveal deletions of sequences encoding portions of the N- and/or C-terminal tails. Proc Natl Acad Sci 89:4309–4313

Flemming TP, Saxena A, Clark WC, Robertson JT, Oldfield EH, Aaronson SA, Unnisa Ali I (1992) Amplification and or overexpression of platlet-derived growth factor receptors and epidermal growth factor receptor in human glial tumors. Cancer Res 52:4550–4553

Haley JD, Whittle N, Bennett P, Kinchington D, Ullrich A, Waterfield MD (1987) The human EGF receptor gene: Structure of the 110 kb locus and identification of sequences regulating its transcription. Onc Res1:375–396

Helseth PA, Unsgaard G, Dalen A, Fure H, Skandsen A, Öedegaard A, Vik R (1988) Amplification of the epidermal growth factor gene in biopsy specimens from human intracranial tumours. Br J Neurosurg 2:217–225

Humphrey PA, Wong AJ, Vogelstein B, Zalutsky MR, Fuller GN, Archer GE, Friedman HS, Kwatra MM, Bigner SH, Bigner DD (1990) Anti-synthetic peptide antibody reacting at the fusion junction of deletion-mutant epidermal growth factor receptors in human glioblastoma. Proc Natl Acad Sci USA 87 (11):4207–11

James CD, Carlbom E, Dumanski JP, Hansen MF, Nordenskjöld M, Collins VP, Cavanee W (1988) Clonal genomic alterations in glioma malignancy stages. Cancer Res 48:5546–5555

Kaufman RJ, Schimke RT (1981) Amplification and loss of dihydrofolate reductase genes in a chinese hamster ovary cell line. Mol Cell Biol 1:1069–1076

Kinzler KW, Bigner SH, Bigner DD, Trent JM, Law ML, O'Brien SJ, Wong AJ, Vogelstein B (1987) Identification of an amplified highly expressed gene in a human glioma. Science 236 (4797):70–3

Kumabe T, Sohma Y, Kayama T, Yoshimoto T, Yamamoto T (1992) Amplification of alpha-platelet-derived growth factor receptor gene lacking an exon coding for a portion of the extracellular region in a primary brain tumor of glial origin. Oncogene 7 (4):627–33

Lee JS, Ro JS, Eisbruch A, Shtalrid M, Ferrell RE, Gutterman JU, Blick M (1988) Multiple restriction fragment length polymorphisms of the human epidermal growth factor receptor gene. Cancer Res 48 (14):4045–8

Libermann TA, Nusbaum HR, Razon N, Kris R, Lax I, Soreq H, Whittle N, Waterfield MD, Ullrich A, Schlessinger J (1985) Amplification enhanced expression and possible rearrangement of EGF receptor genein primary human brain tumors of glial origin. Nature 313:144–147

Libermann TA, Razon N, Bartal AD, Yarden Y, Schlessinger J, Soreq H (1984) Expression of epidermal growth factor receptors in human brain tumors. Cancer Res 44:753–760

Mahaley MS, Mettlin C, Natarajan N, Lawes ER, Peace BB (1989) National survey of patterns of care for brain-tumor patients. JNeurosurgery 71:826–836

Malden LT, Novak U, Kaye AH, Burgess AW (1988) Selective amplification of the cytoplasmic domain of the epidermal growth factor receptor gene in glioblastoma multiforme. Cancer Res 48:2711–2714

Merlino GT, Ishii S, Whang-Peng J, Knutsen T, Xu YH, Clark AJ, Stratton RH, Wilson RK, Ma DP, Roe BA et al (1985) Structure and localization of genes encoding aberrant and normal epidermal growth factor receptor RNAs from A431 human carcinoma cells. Mol Cell Biol 5:1722–1734
Reifenberger G, Prior R, Deckert M, Wechsler W (1989) Epidermal growth factor receptor expression and growth fraction in human tumours of the nervous system. Virchows Arch A Pathol Anat Histopathol 414 (2):147–55
Sugawa N, Ekstrand AJ, James CD, Collins VP (1990) Identical splicing of aberrant epidermal growth factor receptor transcripts from amplified rearranged genes in human glioblastomas. Proc Natl Acad Sci USA 87 (21):8602–6
Trent J, Meltzer P, Rosenblum M, Harsh G, Kinzler K, Mashal R, Feinberg A, Vogelstein B (1986) Evidence for rearrangement amplification and expression of c-myc in a human glioblastoma. Proc Natl Acad Sci USA 83 (2):470–3
Tuzi NL, Venter DJ, Kumar S, Staddon SL, Lemoine NR, Gullick WJ (1991) Expression of growth factors in human brain tumors. Br J Cancer 63:227–233
Ullrich A, Schlessinger J (1990) Signal transduction by receptors with tyrosine kinase activity. Cell 61 (April):203–212
Ullrich A, Coussens L, Hayflick JS, Dull TJ, Gray A, Tam AW, Lee J, Yarden Y, Libermann TA, Schlessinger J, Downward J, Mayes EL, Whittle N, Waterfield MD, Seeburg PH (1984) Human epidermal growth factor receptor cDNA, sequence and aberrant expression of the amplified gene in A431 epidermoid carcinoma cells. Nature 309: 418–425
Walker AE, Robins M, Weinfeld FD (1985) Epidemology of brain tumors: The national survey of intracranial neoplasms. Neurology 35:219–226
Wells A, Welsh JB, Lazar CS, Wiley HS, Gill GN, Rosenfeld MG (1990) Ligand-induced transformation by a noninternalizing epidermal growth factor receptor. Science 247:962–964
Welter C, Henn W, Theisinger B, Fischer H, Zang KD, Blin N (1990) The cellular myb oncogene is amplified rearranged and activated in human glioblastoma cell lines. Cancer Letters 52: 57–62
Wong AJ, Bigner SH, Bigner D, Kinzler KW, Hamilton SR, Vogelstein B (1987) Increased expression of the epidermal growth factor receptor gene in malignant gliomas is invariably associated with gene amplification. Proc Natl Acad Sci USA 84:6899–6903
Wong AJ, Ruppert JM, Bigner SH, Grzeschik CH, Humphrey PA, Bigner DS, Vogelstein B (1992) Structural alterations of the epidermal growth factor receptor gene in human gliomas. Proc Natl Acad Sci USA 89 (7):2965–9
Yamazaki H, Fukui Y, Ueyama Y, Tamaoki N, Kawamoto T, Taniguchi S, Shibuya M (1988) Amplification of the structurally and functionally altered epidermal growth factor receptor gene (c-erbB) in human brain tumors. Mol Cell Biol 8:1816–1820
Yamazaki H, Ohba Y, Tamaoki N, Shibuya M (1990) A deletion mutation within the ligand binding domain is responsible for activation of epidermal growth factor receptor gene in human brain tumors. Jpn J Cancer Res 81:773–779

Type and Frequency of p53 Mutations in Tumors of the Nervous System and Its Coverings

P. Kleihues[1], H. Ohgaki[1], R. H. Eibl[1], M. B. Reichel[1], L. Mariani[1], M. Gehring[2], I. Petersen[1], T. Höll[1], A. von Deimling[3], O. D. Wiestler[3], and M. Schwab[2]

[1]Institute of Neuropathology, Department of Pathology, University Hospital, Schmelzbergstr. 12, 8091 Zurich, Switzerland
[2]Institute of Experimental Pathology, German Cancer Research Center, Im Neuenheimer Feld 280, 69120 Heidelberg, Germany
[3]Institute of Neuropathology, University of Bonn, Sigmund-Freud-Str. 25, 53127 Bonn, Germany

Introduction

The p53 tumor suppressor gene encodes a nuclear phosphoprotein which is involved in the regulation of cell proliferation (Boyd and Barrett 1990). The wild-type p53 gene acts as a tumor suppressor gene, whereas some p53 mutations occurring within highly conserved regions not only cause loss of tumor suppressor function but may activate p53 to an oncogene in a dominant negative fashion (Finlay et al. 1989; Eiyahu et al. 1989). A variety of human tumors have been shown to contain either a loss of both alleles of the p53 gene, a loss of one allele of the p53 gene, and one p53 allele with an associated point mutation, insertion, or deletion of the remaining allele or an inactivation of the p53 gene in one allele but a normal (wild-type) sequence in the other. The rapidly accumulating data on p53 genetic alterations indicate that it may constitute the gene most frequently involved in human oncogenesis (Hollstein et al. 1991; Levine et al. 1991). In this review, we summarize all the available data on p53 mutations in human nervous system tumors.

p53 Mutations in Astrocytomas

Frequency of p53 Mutations

Two studies have shown that 3 out of 8 (38%) and 3 out of 11 (27%) of low-grade astrocytoma contain p53 mutations (von Deimling et al. 1992; Ohgaki et al. 1993), whereas Fults et al. (1992) found no mutation in a total of 6 cases. Together, these three independent studies revealed the presence of p53 mutations in 6 out of 25 cases, i.e., an overall incidence of 24%. Anaplastic astrocytomas (WHO grade III) often develop over a course of several years from low-grade astrocytomas but may also arise de novo, i.e., without clinical or histopathological evidence of a preceding benign glioma. Two studies have demonstrated that anaplastic astrocytomas contain p53 mutations in 9 out of 28 cases, i.e., at an overall incidence of 32% (von Deimling et al. 1992; Louis et al. 1993). Glioblastomas frequently develop from low-grade or anaplastic astrocytomas (secondary glioblastoma) but may also arise primarily after a short history of only weeks or a few months, with no evidence of a less malignant precursor lesion (primary glioblastoma). In three independent studies, altogether 24 p53 mutations were identified in a total of 72 glioblastomas, i.e., in 33% of cases (Fults et al. 1992; Louis et al. 1993; Frankel et al. 1992). The observation that p53 mutations are present in low grade astrocytomas, anaplastic astrocytomas, and glioblastoma multiforme may indicate that this gene is involved during a rather early stage of neoplastic transformation. Sidransky et al. (1992) reported that the progression to glioblastoma is characterized by a clonal expansion of cells carrying a p53 mutation, presumably due to a selective growth advantage. This view is supported by a report by Hayashi et al. (1991) who found p53 mutations only in progressive recurrent gliomas. However, both studies are based on a few cases and require confirmation in a larger series of tumors.

Pilocytic astrocytomas (WHO grade I) are circumscribed, grow slowly, and very rarely progress to malignancy. They typically manifest in children, with a peak incidence around the age of 10–12 years, and in young adults and are preferentially located in midline structures, for example, basal ganglia, temporal lobe, optic nerve, brain stem, and cerebellum. It has been clearly shown that pilocytic astrocytomas do not contain mutations in the highly conserved regions of the p53 gene (Ohgaki et al. 1993), suggesting a different genetic basis from astrocytomas grade II, III, or glioblastoma multiforme for this benign childhood neoplasm.

Distribution and Nature of p53 Mutations

Mutations were located in the highly conserved region of the gene (Ohgaki et al. 1993), with clusters at codons 175 (7.5%), 248 (17.5%), and 273 (7.5%). These three codons have also been reported to be hot spots for mutations in colon cancer (Levine et al. 1991).

Among the types of p53 mutations in these astrocytic brain tumors, G→A transitions (38%) prevail, followed by C→T transitions (18%) and frameshift mutations (18%) as shown in Table 1. G→A transitions are also the most frequent type of p53 mutation in small cell lung cancer, colon cancer, and lymphoid malignancies (Hollstein et al. 1991). The p53 mutations in astrocytic human brain tumors are located predominantly at CpG sites (55%), similar to a variety of other human neoplasms (Levine et al. 1991), including colon carcinoma (61%), sarcomas (53%), lymphomas/leukemias (47%), bladder carcinoma (33%) , and small cell lung carcinoma (31%).

Model for Malignant Progression of Astrocytomas

There is increasing evidence that in human astrocytomas multiple genetic events may occur in a typical sequence which parallels histopathologically defined stages of malignant progression (Bigner and Vogelstein 1990). It appears that in low-grade

Table 1. Nature of *p53* gene base substitutuion mutations in astrocytic human brain tumors.

Mutations at G:C		Mutations at A:T		Mutations at C:G		Mutations at T:A	
→A:T	→T:A	→G:C	→A:T	→T:A	→G:C	→G:C	→C:G
38%	5%	5%	3%	18%	5%	5 %	5%

Summary of p53 mutations in the 40 published cases of astrocytomas grade II and III, and glioblastoma multiforme. G→A transition (38%), C→T transition (18%) are most frequent. In addition, there were 7 cases (18%) with frameshift mutations.

astrocytomas (WHO grade II), p53 mutations with or without loss of heterozygosity on chromosome 17p are the principle detectable change although isolated cases with loss of heterozygosity on chromosomes 13 and 22 have been reported (James et al. 1988). In addition to p53 mutations and the loss of heterozygosity of 17p, the involvement of a second, yet unidentified tumor suppressor gene on chromosome 17p distinct from the p53 gene has been suggested for malignant astrocytomas (Frankel et al. 1992; Saxena et al. 1992). More than 40% of anaplastic astrocytomas show loss of heterozygosity on chromosome 19q (von Deimling et al. 1992b) while loss of heterozygosity on chromosomes 9p, 13, and 22 appears to be a rare event (James et al. 1988). In addition to p53 mutations, more than 70% of glioblastoma multiforme show the loss of chromosome 10 (von Deimling et al. 1992c). In contrast to low-grade and anaplastic astrocytomas, glioblastomas contain, in approximately one-third of cases, amplification of the epidermal growth factor receptor gene (EGFR), sometimes in a truncated form (Bigner and Vogelstein 1990; von Deimling et al. 1992c; Ekstrand et al. 1991; Bigner et al. 1988). All glioblastomas with EGFR amplification also show loss of chromosome 10 (von Deimling et al. 1992c).

p53 Mutations in Nonastrocytic Tumors of the Human Nervous System

A variety of nervous system tumors have recently been screened for p53 mutations. As summarized in Table 2, the results obtained clearly indicate that loss of function of the p53 gene is infrequently, if at all, involved in the evolution of nonastrocytic tumors of the nervous system and its coverings.

Oligodendrogliomas are glial tumors, typically located in the cerebral hemispheres. Two of 17 (12%) oligodendrogliomas have been reported to contain p53 mutations (Ohgaki et al. 1991). Medulloblastomas are malignant embryonal cerebellar tumors with a peak incidence between 7 and 12 years of age. Two out of 19 (11%) medulloblastomas have been reported to contain p53 mutations (Ohgaki et al. 1991) The meningeal hemangiopericytoma is a rare tumor which, in contrast to meningiomas, has a tendency for recurrence and metastasis to distant sites. Its histogenesis has remained enigmatic. One of the 7 hemangiopericytomas (14%) contained a p53 mutation (Ohgaki et al. 1993). Schwannomas (synonymously termed neurinomas) are benign neoplasms originating from Schwann's cells of cranial or peripheral nerves. The ten cases examined were all located in the acoustic nerve and did not

Table 2. p53 Mutations in tumors of the nervous system and its coverings

	Mutations in exon 5	6	7	8	Total (%)	Reference
Pilocytic astrocytoma	0	0	0	0	0/12 (0%)	Ohgaki et al. 1993
Low grade astrocytoma	1	0	1	1	3/11 (27%)	Ohgaki et al. 1993
	2	0	1	1	3/8 (38%)[a]	von Deimling et al. 1992
	0	0	0	0	0/6 (0%)	Fults et al. 1992
Anaplastic astrocytoma	1	1	1	1	4/14 (29%)	von Deimling et al. 1992
	2	1	1	1	5/14 (36%)	Fults et al. 1992
Glioblastoma multiforme	0	0	4	0	4/14 (29%)	Louis et al. 1992
	6	1	4	1	13/33 (39%)[b]	Frankel et al. 1992
	2	2	1	2	7/25 (28%)	Fults et al. 1992
Hemangiopericytoma	0	0	1	0	1/7 (14%)	Ohgaki et al. 1993
Meningioma	1	0	0	0	1/8 (13%)	Mashiyama et al. 1991
	0	0	0	0	0/22 (0%)	Ohgaki et al. 1993
Oligodendroglioma	1	0	1	0	2/17 (12%)	Ohgaki et al. 1991
Medulloblastoma	0	2	0	0	2/19 (11%)	Ohgaki et al. 1991
	0	0	0	0	0/12 (0%)	Saylors et al. 1991
Central neurocytoma	0	0	0	0	0/12 (0%)	Ohgaki et al. 1993
Choroid plexus tumor	0	0	0	0	0/10 (0%)	Ohgaki et al. 1993
Ependymoma	0	0	0	0	0/17 (0%)	Ohgaki et al. 1991
Schwannoma	0	0	0	0	0/13 (0%)	Ohgaki et al. 1993
Neuroblastoma	0	0	0	0	0/30 (0%)	Ohgaki et al. 1993

[a]One astrocytoma grade II had two mutations in exon 5.
[b]One glioblastoma contained a mutation in exon 4.

contain p53 mutations (Ohgaki et al. 1993). Loss of heterozygosity of chromosome 22 (Fiedler et al. 1991) and coexpression of c-*sis* and c-*fos* have been observed in this lesion (Riva and Larizza 1992). The central neurocytoma, a recently identified rare supratentorial brain tumor of young adults, is characterized by its intraventricular location, a usually benign clinical course and a consistent tendency for neuronal differentiation (Hassoun et al. 1982; von Deimling et al. 1990). No evidence for the involvement of p53 mutations has been found in the development of this neoplasm. Meningiomas are usually benign neoplasms originating from meningothelial cells. They are genetically characterized by loss of chromosome 22 (Collins et al. 1990) and an enhanced expression of c-*myc*, *sis*, and *fos* (Riva and Larizza 1992; Kazumoto et al. 1990; Amidt et al. 1991). One study showed a p53 mutation in one of 8 (13%) meningiomas (Mashiyama et al. 1991) whereas another showed no mutation in 22 (15 benign and 7 atypical) cases (Ohgaki et al. 1993). Choroid plexus tumors are epithelial tumors derived from the choroid plexus of the cerebral ventricles. No p53 mutation was detected in 6 papillomas and 4 carcinomas (Ohgaki et al. 1993). Neuroblastomas of the adrenal gland and the sympathetic nervous system are rare malignant embryonal tumors composed of neuroblasts or cells with incipient neuronal differentiation. Amplification of the N-*myc* gene is a frequent event in neuroblastomas (Schwab 1990) and appears to be correlated with clinical outcome (Schwab 1990; Brodeur 1990). In addition, tumor suppressor genes associated with neuroblastomas have been mapped on chromosomes 1p and 14q (Schwab 1990; Takayama et al. 1992; Fong et al. 1992; Ellmeier et al. 1992). Although high levels of p53 protein were reported for some neuroblastoma cell lines (Sidell and Koeffer 1988; Davidoff et al. 1992), no evidence of a mutational inactivation of the p53gene was found in 30 neuroblastomas (Ohgaki et al. 1993). Ependymomas develop from the neuroepithelial lining of the ventricles and the central canal of the spinal cord and are composed predominantly of neoplastic ependymal cells. No p53 mutations were observed in 15 ependymomas (Ohgaki et al. 1991).

Conclusion

Among tumors of the human nervous system, mutations of the p53 tumor suppressor gene have been shown to be largely restricted to neoplasms of astrocytic origin. Several studies demonstrate that p53 mutations are common (24%–33% incidence) in low-grade astrocytoma (WHO grade II), anaplastic astrocytoma (WHO grade III), and in the glioblastoma multiforme (WHO grade IV) but do not occur in juvenile pilocytic astrocytomas (WHO grade I), suggesting a basic difference in the molecular pathogenesis of these neoplasms. The low incidence of p53 mutations in medulloblastomas, oligodendrogliomas, meningeal hemangiopericytomas, and meningiomas and the complete absence in the remainder of the nervous system tumors investigated in this study suggest that the p53 gene may not play a crucial role in their development. It should be added that the present work was restricted to the search for mutational inactivation of the p53 suppressor gene. Different mechanisms of inactivation, i.e., complex formation of the p53 protein with viral (Boyd and Barrett 1990; Levine et al. 1991) or mammalian (mdm2; Momand et al. 1992) oncoproteins, may also occur but have, to date, not been identified in neoplasms of the human nervous system.

References

Amidt M, Dumanski JP, Collins VP, Ratner L (1991) Structure and expression of the c-*sis* gene and its relationship to sporadic meningiomas. Cancer Res 15:4295–4298

Bigner SH, Burger PC, Wong AJ, Werner MH, Hamilton SR, Muhlabier LH, Vogelstein B, Bigner DD (1988) Gene amplification in malignant human gliomas: Clinical and histopathologic aspects. J Neuropathol Exp Neurol 47:191–205

Bigner BH, Vogelstein B (1990) Cytogenetic and molecular genetics of malignant gliomas and medulloblastoma. Brain Pathol 1:12–18

Boyd JA, Barrett JC (1990) Tumor suppressor genes: possible functions in the negative regulation of cell proliferation. Mol Carcinogenesis 3:325–329

Brodeur GM (1990) Neuroblastoma-clinical applications of molecular parameters. Brain Pathol 1: 47–54

Collins VP, Nordenskjoeld M, Dumanski JP (1990) The molecular genetics of meningiomas. Brain Pathol 1:19–24

Davidoff AM, Pence JC, Shorter NA, Iglehart JD, Marks JR (1992) Expression of p53 human neuroblastoma-and neuroepithelioma-derived cell lines. Oncogene 7:127–133

Eiyahu D, Michalovitz D, Eiyahu S, Pinhash-Kimhi O, Oren M (1989) Plasmids encoding wild type p53 can inhibit oncogenic-mediated transformation. Proc Natl Acad Sci USA 86:8763–8767

Ekstrand AJ, James CD, Cavenee WK, Seliger B, Pettersson RF, Collins VP (1991) Genes for epidermal growth factor receptor, transforming growth factor alpha, and epidermal growth factor and their expression in human gliomas in vivo.Cancer Res 15:2164–2172
Ellmeier W, Aguzzi A, Kleiner E, Kurzbauer R, Weith A (1992) Mutually exclusive expression of a helix-loop-helix gene and N-*myc* in human neuroblastomas and in normal development. EMBO J 11:2563–2571
Fiedler W, Claussen U, Ludecke HJ, Senger G, Horsthemke B, Geurts Van Kessel A, Goertzen W, Fahsold, R (1991) New markers for the neurofibromatosis-2 region generated by microdissection of chromosome 22. Genomics 10:786–791
Finlay C, Hinds P, Levine AJ (1989) The p53 protooncogene can act as a suppressor of transformation. Cell 57:1083–1093
Fong C, White PS, Peterson K, Sapienza C, Cavenee WK, Kern SE, Vogelstein B, Cantor AB, Look AT, Brodeur GM (1992) Loss of heterozygosity for chromosome 1 or 14 defines subsets of advanced neuroblastomas. Cancer Res 52:1780–1785
Frankel RH, Bayona W, Koslow M, Newcomb EW (1992) p53 Mutations in human malignant gliomas: Comparison of loss of heterozygosity with mutation frequency. Cancer Res 52:1427–1433
Fults D, Brockmeyer D, Tullous MW, Pedone CA, Cawthon RM (1992) p53 Mutation and loss of heterozygosity on chromosome 17 and 10 during human astrocytoma progression. Cancer Res 52: 674–679
Hassoun J, Gambarelli D, Grisoli F, Pellet W, Salamon G, Pellisier JF, Toga M (1982) Central neurocytoma. Acta Neuropathol 56:151–156
Hayashi Y, Yamashita J, Yamaguchi K (1991) Timing and role of p53 gene mutation in the recurrence of glioma. Biochem Biophis Res Commun 180:1145–1150
Hollstein MC, Sidransky D, Vogelstein B, Harris CC (1991) p53 mutations in human cancers. Science 253:49–53
James CD, Carlbom E, Dumanski JP, Hausen M, Nordenskjöld MD, Collins VP, Cavenee WK (1988) Clonal genomic alterations in glioma malignancy stages. Cancer Res 48:5546–5551
Kazumoto K, Tamura M, Hoshino H, Yuasa Y (1990) Enhanced expression of the *sis* and c-*myc* oncogenes in huma meningiomas. J Neurosurg 72:786–791
Levine AJ, Momand J, Finlay CA (1991) The p53 tumor suppressor gene. Nature 351:453–456
Louis DN, von Deimling A, Chung RY, Rubio MP, Whaley JH, Eibl RH, Ohgaki H, Wiestler OD, Thor AD, Seizinger BR (1993) Comparative study of p53 gene and protein alterations in human astrocytomas. Journal of Neuropathology & Experimental Neurology 52:31–38
Mashiyama S, Murakami Y, Yoshimoto T, Sekiya T, Hayashi K (1991) Detection of p53 gene mutations in human brain tumors by single-strand conformation polymorphism analysis of polymerase chain reaction products. Oncogene 6:1313–1318
Momand J, Zambetti GP, Olson DC, George D, Levine AJ (1992) The mdm-2 oncogene product forms a complex with the p53 protein and inhibits p53-mediated transactivation. Cell 69: 1237–1245
Ohgaki H, Eibl RH, Wiestler OD, Yasargil MG, Newcomb EW, Kleihues P (1991) p53 mutations in nonastrocytic human brain tumors. Cancer Res 51:6202–6205
Ohgaki H, Eibl RH, Schwab M, Reichel M, Mariani L, Gehring M, Petersen I, Holl T, Wiestler O D and Kleihues P (1993) Mutations in tumor suppressor gene p53 in neoplasms in human nervous system. Mol. Carcinogenesis 8:74–80
Orita M, Suzuki Y, Sekiya T, Hayashi K (1989) A rapid and sensitive detection of point mutations and genetic polymorphisms using polymerase chain reaction. Genomics 5:874–879
Riva P, Larizza L (1992) Expression of c-*sis* and c-*fos* genes in human meningiomas and neurinomas. Int J Cancer 30:873–877
Saxena A, Clark WC, Robertson JT, Ikejiri B, Oldfield EH, Ali IU (1992) Evidence for the involvement of a potential second tumor suppressor gene on chromosome 17 distinct from p53 in malignant astrocytomas. Cancer Res 52:6716–1721
Saylors III RL, Sidransky D, Friedman HS, Bigner SH, Bigner DD, Vogelstein B, Brodeur GM (1991) Infrequent p53 gene mutations in medulloblastomas. Cancer Res 51:4721–4723
Schwab M (1990) Amplification of the MYCN oncogene and deletion of putative tumor suppressor gene in human neuroblastomas. Brain Pathol 1:41–46
Sidell N, Koeffer HP (1988) Modulation of Mr 53,000 protein with induction of differentiation of human neuroblastoma cells.Cancer Res 48:2226–2230

Sidransky D, Mikkelsen T, Schwechheimer K, Rosenblum ML, Cavanee W, Vogelstein B (1992) Clonal expansion of p53 mutant cells is associated with brain tumor progression. Nature 355: 846–847

Takayama H, Suzuki T, Mugishima H, Fujisawa T, Ookuni M, Schwab M, Gehring M, Nakamura Y, Sugimura T, Terada M, Yokota J (1992) Deletion mapping of chromosomes 14q and 1p in human neuroblastoma. Oncogene 7:1185–1189

von Deimling A, Kleihues P, Saremaslani P, Yasargil MG, Spörri O, Suedhof TC, Wiestler OD (1991) Histogenesis and differentiation potential of central neurocytomas. Lab Invest 64:585–591

von Deimling A, Eibl RH, Ohgaki H, Louis DN, von Ammon K, Peterson I, Kleihues P, Chung RY, Wiestler OD, Seizinger BR (1992a) p53 mutations correlate with 17p allelic loss in grade II and grade III astrocytoma. Cancer Res 52:2897–2990

von Deimling A, Louis DN, von Ammon K, Petersen I, Wiestler OD, Seizinger BR (1992b) Evidence for a tumor suppressor gene on chromosome 19q associated with human astrocytomas, oligodendrogliomas, and mixed gliomas. Cancer Res 52:4277–4299

von Deimling A, Louis DN, von Ammon K, Petersen I, Höll T, Chung RY, Martuza RL, Schoenfeld DA, Yasargel Gazi M, Wiestler OD, Seizinger BR (1992c) Association of epidermal growth factor receptor gene amplification with loss of chromosome 10 in human glioblastoma multiforme. J Neurosurg 77:295–301

Astrocytic Gliomas: Characterization on a Molecular Genetic Basis

A. von Deimling[1], D. N. Louis[2], J. Schramm[3], and O. D. Wiestler[1]

[1]Institut für Neuropathologie, Universitätskliniken Bonn, Sigmund-Freud-Str. 25, 53127 Bonn, Germany
[2]Molecular Neuro-oncology Laboratory, Massachusetts General Hospital, 149 13th St., Charlestown, MA 02129-9142 U.S.A.
[3]Neurochirugische Universitätsklinik,Universitätskliniken Bonn, Sigmund-Freud-Str. 25, 53127 Bonn, Germany

Introduction

Astrocytic tumors are the most common primary human central nervous system tumors. Histopathological parameters have been employed to distinguish four grades of malignancy: pilocytic astrocytoma (WHO grade I), astrocytoma (WHO grade II), anaplastic astrocytoma (WHO grade III), and glioblastoma multiforme (GBM; WHO grade IV; Kleihues et al. 1993). While classical histopathological methods have not been able to characterize pathogenic factors contributing to tumor formation in the brain, molecular analyses have revealed frequent chromosomal alterations that may indicate specific molecular genetic mechanisms. The involvement of oncogenes and tumor suppressor genes in neoplastic disorders has now been firmly established (Bishop 1991; Marshall 1991). Several characteristic genomic alterations have been identified in astrocytic gliomas. Loss of portions of the short arm of chromosome 17 is observed in grade II and III astrocytoma and GBM (El-Azouzi et al. 1989; Fults et al. 1989; James et al. 1989; von Deimling et al. 1992), while loss of chromosome 10 and amplification of the epidermal growth factor receptor (EGFR) gene are essentially restricted to GBM (Libermann et al. 1984; Bigner et al. 1988; James et al. 1988; Fujimoto et al. 1989; Fults et al. 1990; Watanabe et al. 1990; von Deimling et al. 1992).

Recent reports have drawn attention to the possibility of subdividing human tumors on the basis of genetic differences. Initially the presence of oncogene amplification was demonstrated to be of prognostic relevance and allowed the separation of certain tumors into subgroups with or without oncogene amplification. For instance, in neuroblastomas, N-*myc* amplification corresponds with higher grade and with differential chemotherapeutic susceptibilities (Brodeur 1990), and in breast carcinomas those tumors with *neu*/*erbB2* amplification have a poorer prognosis than those without amplification (Slamon et al. 1987; Thor et al. 1989). Attempts to correlate the frequently occurring amplification of the EGFR gene with histopathological parameters and patient survival have produced conflicting results (Bigner et al. 1988; Hurtt et al. 1992). Neither study succeeded in correlating EGFR gene amplification with histopathological features. Analysis of tumor suppressor gene inactivation, rather than oncogene activation, may also be useful in subdividing tumors. For instance, mutations in the p53 tumor suppressor gene have been shown to correlate with the behavior of breast carcinomas (Thor et al. 1992), and may allow the separation of breast carcinomas into those with and those without p53 mutations. In addition, in soft-tissue sarcomas expression of the retinoblastoma tumor suppressor gene product may be an important prognostic variable (Cance et al. 1990). Loss of heterozygosity (LOH) studies are a convenient means to analyze the involvement of potential tumor suppressor genes in human neoplasms. The loss of chromosomal alleles, as demonstrated by LOH studies, is thought to unmask the presence of mutant tumor suppressor genes. LOH studies have therefore been used to subclassify tumors. In renal carcinoma the loss of potential tumor suppressor genes on either chromosome 3 in the clear cell type or chromosome 17 in the granular cell type can be used to subdivide these tumors on a molecular genetic basis (Ogawa et al. 1992). Furthermore, recents studies in neuroblastoma have suggested that differential loss of loci on chromosome 1 or chromosome 14 may characterize different groups of neuroblastoma (Fong et al. 1992). Finally, it may be possible to divide tumors by combined analysis of oncogenes and tumor suppressor genes. To this end, it has recently been suggested that some malignant melanoma cell lines can be separated into those with *ras* mutations and those with neurofibromatosis type 1 gene mutations (Andersen et al. 1992).

The involvement of already identified cloned genes (EGFR, p53) and putative tumor suppressor genes raises the question of whether astrocytic gliomas can also be classified on the basis of their molecular genetic alterations. We here present the compiled data of our recent studies based on the analysis of 108 astrocytic gliomas (20 pilocytic astrocytomas WHO grade I, 8 astrocytomas WHO grade II, 14 astrocytomas WHO grade III, and 66 glioblastomas). All tumors were examined for structural genetic alterations in the most frequently affected regions on chromosomes 10, 17, 19q and in the EGF-receptor gene (von Deimling et al. 1992a–c,1993a,b).

Pilocytic Astrocytoma WHO Grade I

Pilocytic astrocytomas are astrocytic brain tumors of low malignancy that occur predominantly in childhood and adolescence. Typical sites for this tumor entity are the cerebellar hemispheres and midline structures of the central nervous system such as the hypothalamus, brain stem, and optic nerves (Russell and Rubinstein 1989). Pilocytic astrocytomas usually follow a benign course and may be cured by surgical resection. These tumors occur both sporadically and in association with neurofibromatosis type 1 (NF1, von Recklinghausen's neurofibromatosis). One-third of all patients with pilocytic astrocytomas of the optic nerve (optic glioma) have NF1 (Garner and Klinworth 1982), and 15% of all patients with NF1 develop optic glioma (Lewis et al. 1984). The histopathological features of pilocytic astrocytomas are identical in the sporadic and NF1-associated forms and include elongated "piloid" cells, coarse glial fibrillary matrix, microcysts, Rosenthal fibers, and granular bodies. The clinical and pathological features readily distinguish pilocytic astrocytomas from adult supratentorial astrocytomas, which are often clinically and histologically malignant tumors.

In our series of 20 pilocytic astrocytomas, four (20%) showed LOH on chromosome 17 (von Deimling et al. 1993). Three of these tumors had allelic losses confined to the long arm, and one had lost the entire chromosome. Analysis with multiple probes mapped on chromosome 17q defined a commonly affected region, extending from the centromere to 17q21. These allelic losses suggest the involvement of a tumor suppressor gene on the long arm of chromosome 17, located between the centromere and 17q21, in the pathogenesis of pilocytic astrocytoma. Allelic loss on chromosome 17q was not associated with any of the special histopathological features of pilocytic astrocytoma such as Rosenthal fibers, protein droplets, or microcystic change and was observed in both supratentorial and infratentorial pilocytic astrocytomas. Only one of the four tumors with LOH 17q was from a documented NF1 patient.

The long arm of chromosome 17 harbors several genes that are involved in tumorigenesis. Among these genes, the NF1 tumor suppressor gene is a particularly interesting candidate since patients afflicted with NF1 are prone to developing pilocytic astrocytomas (Lewis et al. 1984). The NF1 gene exhibits GTPase-activating protein (GAP) activity, interacts with the *ras* proto-oncogenes and may be involved in the control of cell growth (Xu et al. 1990; Han et al. 1991; DeClue et al. 1992). Alterations in the NF1 gene in patients with NF1 and in tumors from patients with NF1 have been detected in only a few cases (Cawthon et al. 1990; Viskochil et al. 1990; Wallace et al. 1990; Stark et al. 1991; Li et al. 1992). However, large regions of the gene have not been studied in detail. Our one patient with NF1 demonstrated LOH on 17q that included the NF1 locus, but the remaining copy of the NF1 gene has not yet been examined. Studies to analyze the NF1 gene in sporadic and NF1-related pilocytic astrocytomas are currently in progress.

LOH on the short arm of chromosome 17 has been noted frequently in adult astrocytomas (Fults et al. 1989; James et al. 1989; von Deimling et al. 1992). However, only one of the 20 pilocytic astrocytomas in this study, displayed LOH on 17p. Allelic losses on the long arm of chromosome 17, while found in 20% of the pilocytic astrocytomas, have not been detected in our series of adult grade II and III astrocytoma. Furthermore, allelic losses on chromosomes 10 and 19q, and amplification of the EGFR gene, which are frequent events in adult astrocytomas, have not been observed in pilocytic astrocytomas (von Deimling et al. 1992; von Deimling et al. 1992). These molecular genetic findings support the clinicopathological separation of pilocytic astrocytomas from adult astrocytomas.

Astrocytoma WHO Grade II and Anaplastic Astrocytoma WHO Grade III

Astrocytoma WHO grade II and grade III typically arise in middle-aged patients. Grade II astrocytomas frequently progress to grade III astrocytoma within a period of several years. The most commonly encountered genetic alteration in these tumors is LOH 17p, which occurs in approximately half of all grade II and grade III astrocytomas. This genomic region includes the p53 tumor suppressor gene. Mutations in the conserved regions of the p53 gene, which span exons 5–8, have been identified in numerous human malignancies, such as carcinomas of the breast, lung, and colon (Nigro et al. 1989; Takahashi et al. 1990; Hollstein et al. 1991). These mutations are often associated with a corresponding loss of the second copy of chromosome 17 (Nigro et al. 1989; Baker et al. 1990), thus meeting the classical paradigm of recessive tumor suppressor gene inactivation (Knudsen 1976). In several human tumors it has been suggested that p53 mutations are relatively late steps in tumorigenesis (Baker et al. 1990; Menon et al. 1990). However, the recent identification of germline p53 mutations in the hereditary cancer syndrome of Li-Fraumeni suggests that p53 mutations may be important in tumor initiation as well (Malkin et al. 1990; Srivastava et al. 1990).

Because LOH on chromosome 17p is frequently observed in lower-grade astrocytomas, we explored the possibility that p53 mutations may occur in grade II and III astrocytomas. We analyzed 22 astrocytic tumors (8 grade II astrocytomas and 14 grade III anaplastic astrocytomas) for mutations in the conserved regions of the p53 gene by single-strand conformation polymorphism (SSCP) analysis and direct DNA sequencing. In addition, we evaluated all tumors for LOH of chromosome 17p by Southern blot restriction fragment length polymorphism analysis to assess the relationship of p53 mutations to allelic loss on chromosome 17p.

SSCP analysis revealed eight tumors with an abnormal migration pattern in one of the examined p53 exons. Four of these cases were astrocytomas WHO grade II (4/8) and four were anaplastic astrocytomas WHO grade III (4/14). p53 mutations in exons 5–8 were observed in 7 of 11 tumors with LOH on 17p. p53 mutations were not detected in any tumor which had maintained both 17p alleles. The association of p53 mutations with LOH on 17p was statistically significant (Fisher's exact test, p 0.01).

By direct DNA sequencing we have demonstrated p53 mutations in 3 of 8 grade II astrocytomas and 4 of 14 grade III anaplastic astrocytomas. Southern blot restriction fragment length polymorphism (RFLP) analysis showed that 50% of astrocytomas and anaplastic astrocytomas had LOH of 17p (4/8 grade II and 7/14 grade III). These results show that loss of chromosome 17p is more common in lower grade astrocytomas than had been previously suggested (El-Azouzi et al. 1989; Fults et al. 1989; Venter and Thomas 1991). In addition, the percentage of LOH 17p does not appear to differ between grade II and grade III astrocytoma, implying that loss of chromosome 17p may be involved in an early stage of astrocytoma formation. All cases with p53 mutations had LOH of 17p, while four cases had LOH of 17p without detectable p53 mutations. These data reveal that p53 mutations are not restricted to the grade IV GBM but are found in lower grade astrocytic tumors as well. In addition, they demonstrate an association between p53 mutations and LOH of 17p, which suggests that the genetic locus on chromosome 17p affected in the tumors is the p53 gene. An interesting problem not yet resolved concerns the nature of alternative tumor-associated genes which substitute for p53 mutations in those astrocytomas without detectable lesions on chromosome 17p.

Progression from grade II to grade III astrocytoma may involve several additional genes. Evidence for such putative "progression genes" on chromosomes 9p and 19q has been presented (James et al. 1991; Olopade et al. 1992; von Deimling et al. 1992).

Glioblastoma Multiforme WHO Grade IV

GBM are the most frequent and most malignant astrocytic gliomas. They occur predominantly in older patients. GBM can arise in patients with a previously diagnosed lower-grade astrocytoma or apparently de novo, as primary high-grade tumors. Although the histopathological appearance of GBM is extremely heterogeneous, it has not been possible to differentiate by light microscopy those GBMs that arise from previous astrocytomas from those that arise de novo (Burger and Green 1987). Neither immunohistochemical nor ultrastructural analyses have provided evidence for subdividing GBM into clinically or biologically distinct entities.

Young age of the patient at the time of diagnosis and high Karnofsky performance status score are favorable prognostic parameters in GBM (Gehan and Walker 1977; Burger and Green 1987). In addition, GBM patients with a history of a previous lower grade tumor (so-called "secondary GBM") appear to have better prognoses than those whose tumors arose in a clinically de novo manner (so-called "primary GBM;" Winger et al. 1989). These observations thus hint at the possibility of subdividing GBMs and suggest that younger patients with a clinical history or histological evidence of a previous lower grade tumor (i.e., patients with "secondary GBM") may represent a more favorable subgroup of GBM.

Several LOH studies in astrocytomas have demonstrated specific defects, most frequently involving chromosomes 9p, 10, 17p, 19q, and 22 (James et al. 1988; El-Azouzi et al. 1989; Fujimoto et al. 1989; Fults et al. 1989; James et al. 1989; Fults et al. 1990; Watanabe et al. 1990; von Deimling et al. 1992). Most investigators have observed a tendency for chromosome 10 deletions to be associated with high-grade astrocytoma, predominantly GBM, and chromosome 17 deletions to be associated with both lower grade diffuse astrocytomas and GBMs. While studies of LOH have not been able to subdivide GBMs, they have suggested that molecular genetic data may contribute to the debate on the origin of GBM, i.e., whether GBM arises through dedifferentiation from lower grade tumors or arises de novo (James et al. 1988). Using Southern blot analysis, we have investigated the incidence of LOH of chromosomes 10, 17, 19q, and amplification of the EGFR gene in 66 GBMs to determine whether these tumors can be subtyped on a genetic basis. Our findings show that LOH on chromosome 17p and EGFR gene amplification rarely occur together in GBM ($p = 0.01$). This allows the separation of GBMs into at least two distinct genetic subsets (see Figs. 1, 2). Loss of chromosome 10, however, was present in all patients with EGFR gene amplification and in many patients with loss of chromosome 17 and was therefore not useful for subdividing GBMs. From these data we propose a model of at least two molecular pathways resulting in distinct variants of GBM.

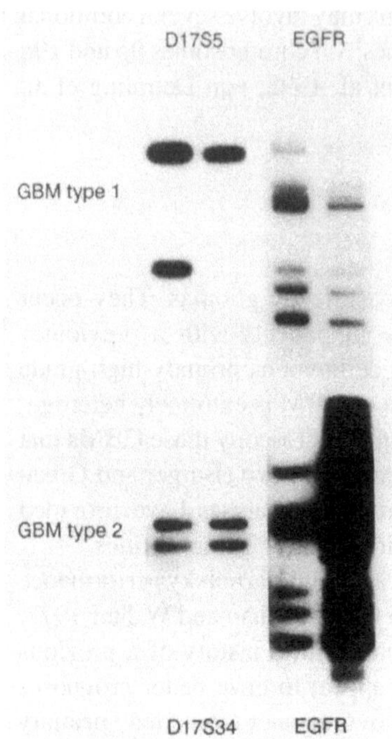

Fig. 1. Representative Southern blots demonstrating the characteristic molecular genetic features of GBM type 1 and type 2. *Above*, loss of heterozygosity at D17S5 without EGFR gene amplification in GBM type 1; *below*, maintenance of heterozygosity at D17S34 with amplification of the EGFR gene in GBM type 2. In each panel: *left lane*, constitutional DNA; *right lane*, tumor DNA. (From von Deimling 1993)

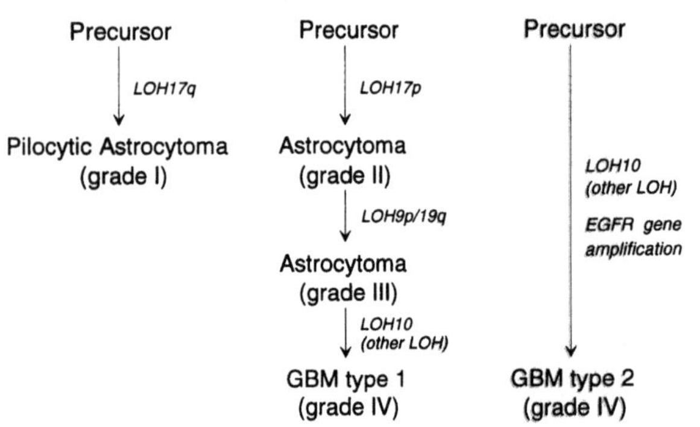

Fig. 2. Schematic illustration of hypothetical genetic pathways leading to pilocytic astrocytoma WHO grade I, astrocytoma WHO grade II and WHO grade III, and GBM type 1 and type 2

The genetic pathway to GBM type 1 is associated with loss of genetic material on the short arm of chromosome 17. Since loss of chromosome 17p and mutations of the corresponding p53 gene both occur as commonly in grade II and III astrocytomas as in GBM, 17p loss and p53 mutations most likely represent early steps in astrocytoma formation (James et al. 1989; von Deimling et al. 1992). Those GBM that have allelic loss of chromosome 17p may, therefore, arise through progression from lower grade astrocytic lesions. In some cases, the precursor lesion may be a microscopic focus that is not clinically symptomatic. Progression to GBM may involve further genetic alterations, such as loss of chromosome 10.

The genetic pathway to GBM type 2 involves EGFR gene amplification subsequent to loss of chromosome 10. We have shown that amplification of the EGFR gene is closely associated with loss of chromosome 10, and have suggested that loss of a tumor suppressor gene on chromosome 10 precedes EGFR gene amplification (von Deimling et al. 1992). These tumors can also exhibit LOH on other chromosomes, such as 19q (von Deimling et al. 1992). It is tempting to speculate that such tumors arise de novo, without a preceding lower grade astrocytoma. None of the patients in our study with EGFR gene amplification had a history of an earlier lower grade astrocytoma.

In our series patients with GBM type 1 had a mean age of 40.5 years, whereas patients with GBM type 2 had a mean age of 56.3 years. The observation that GBM type 1 occurs in significantly younger patients than GBM type 2 ($p = 0.001$) lends further support to the genetic subclassification of GBMs. These data may indicate that the age-based difference in prognosis reflects the predominance of GBM type 1 in the younger population of astrocytoma patients. In addition, it is possible that those anaplastic glioma patients with a previous history of lower grade glioma that do better clinically (Winger et al. 1989) are also our GBM type 1.

Despite the identification of putatively distinct genetic subsets of GBM, histological evaluation failed to reveal any association of specific histological features with the two genetic subsets. This implies that the histological heterogeneity of GBM is a common phenotype and may not reflect the different genetic pathways. It further suggests that histological means of separating GBMs may not provide the same differential information as genetic analyses.

Conclusions

Molecular genetic analysis has already provided evidence for specific genetic mechanisms in the pathogenesis of gliomas. The data available show that genetic analysis may contribute significantly to classifying and subgrouping astrocytic gliomas (Table 1). The model in Fig. 2 emphasizes the different genetic pathways of tumor formation in pilocytic astrocytoma, grade II, and grade III astrocytoma and GBM. Pilocytic astrocytoma may be characterized by LOH on 17q, a genetic feature not seen in grade II and grade III astrocytoma and only rarely observed in GBM. This emphasizes an independent pathway in the formation of these tumors which may involve the NF1 tumor suppressor gene. Grade II and grade III astrocytomas are characterized by a high incidence of LOH on 17p and p53 mutations. Progression from grade II to grade III astrocytoma may involve loci on chromosomes 9p and 19q. GBM may be divided into at least two subsets. One subset is characterized by loss of the short arm of chromosome 17 and absence of EGFR gene amplification. This type of GBM occurs primarily in younger patients (GBM type 1) and may arise through progression from low-grade astrocytomas. The other subset is characterized by EGFR gene amplification without loss of chromosome 17 and occurs primarily in older patients (GBM type 2).

Table 1. Summary of genetic data on patients with astrocytic brain tumors

Diagnosis	*n*	LOH 10	LOH 17p	LOH 17q	LOH 19q	*EGFR* amp	*p53* mut
Pilocytic astrocytoma WHO grade I	20	0/18	1/20	4/20 (20%)	0/10	0/14	–
Astrocytoma WHO grade II	8	0/8	4/8	0/5	0/6	0/8	3/8
Anaplastic satrocytoma WHO grade III	14	0/14	7/14 (50%)	0/12	4/9 (44%)	0/14	(38%)
Glioblastoma multiforme WHO grade IV	66	46/64 (72%)	18/66 (27%)	7/47 (15%)	11/46 (24%)	24/66 (36%)	5/27 (19%)

amp, Amplification; mut, mutation; –, not examined.

Future studies will need to demonstrate the prognostic relevance of genomic alterations in astrocytic gliomas and identify novel genes associated with tumorigenesis in the brain.

Acknowledgements. We would like to gratefully acknowledge the colleagues who have contributed to these studies, in particular K. v. Ammon, P. Kleihues, H. Ohgaki, I. Petersen, B. R. Seizinger and M. G. Yasargil. Our projects were supported by grants from the NIH, ACS, DFG and by a center grant from the University of Bonn Medical Center and the State of Nordrhein-Westfalen.

References

Andersen L, Fountain J, Gutmann D, Tarle S, Glover T, Dracopoli N, Housman D, Collins F (1992) Neurofibromatosis 1 DNA, RNA and protein abnormalities in malignant melanoma. Am J Hem Genet 51:A56

Baker SJ, Preisinger AC, Jessup JM, Paraskeva C, Markowitz S, Wilson JKV, Hamilton SR, Vogelstein B (1990) p53 mutation occur in combination with 17p allele deletions as late events in colorectal tumorigenesis. Cancer Res 50:7717–7722

Bigner SH, Burger PC, Wong AJ, Werner MH, Hamilton SR, Muhlbaier LH, Vogelstein B, Bigner DD (1988) Gene amplification in malignant human gliomas: clinical and histopathologic aspects. J Neuropath Exp Neurol 47:191–205

Bigner SH, Mark J, Burger PC, Mahaley SM, Bullard DEJ, Muhlbaier LH, Bigner DD (1988) Specific chromosomal abnormalities in malignant human gliomas. Cancer Res 48:405–411

Bishop JM (1991) Molecular themes in oncogenesis. Cell 64:235–248

Brodeur GM (1990) Neuroblastoma – clinical applications of molecular parameters. Brain Pathol 1:47–54

Burger PC, Green SB (1987) Patient age, histologic features, and length of survival in patients with glioblastoma multiforme. Cancer 59:1617–1625

Cance WG, Brennan MF, Dudas ME, Huang CM, Cordon-Cardo C (1990) Altered expression of the retinoblastoma gene product in human sarcomas. New Engl J Med 323:1457–1462

Cawthon RM, Weiss R, Xu G, Viskochil D, Culver M, Stevens J, Robertson M, Dunn D, Gesteland R, O'Connell P, White R (1990) A mayor segment of the neurofibromatosis type 1 gene: cDNA sequence, genomic structure, and point mutations. Cell 62:193–201

DeClue JE, Papageorge AG, Fletcher JA, Diehl SR, Ratner N, Vass WC, Lowy DR (1992) Abnormal regulation of mammalian p21ras contributes to malignant tumor growth in von Recklinghausen (type 1) neurofibromatosis. Cell 69:265–273

El-Azouzi M, Chung RY, Farmer GE, Martuza RL, Black PM, Rouleau GA, Hettlich C, Hedley-Whyte ET, Zervas NT, Panagopoulos K, Nakamura Y, Gusella J, Seizinger BR (1989) Loss of distinct regions on the short arm of chromosome 17 associated with tumorigenesis of human astrocytomas. Proc Natl Acad Sci USA 86:7186–7190

Fong C-T, White PS, Peterson K, Sapienza C, Cavenee WK, Kern SE, Vogelstein B, Cantor AB, Look AT, Brodeur GM (1992) Loss of heterozygosity for chromosome 1 or 14 defines subsets of advanced neuroblastomas. Cancer Res 52:1780–1785

Fujimoto M, Fults DW, Thomas GA, Nakamura Y, Heilbrun MP, White R, Story JL, Naylor SL, Kagan-Hallet KS, Sheridan PJ (1989) Loss of heterozygosity on chromosome 10 in human glioblastoma. Genomics 4:210–214

Fults D, Tippets RH, Thomas GA, Nakamura Y, White R (1989) Loss of heterozygosity for loci on chromosome 17p in human malignant astrocytoma. Cancer Res 49:6572–6577

Fults D, Pedone CA, Thomas GA, White R (1990) Allelotype of human malignant astrocytoma. Cancer Res 50:5784–5789

Garner A, Klinworth GK (1982) Tumors of the orbit, optic nerve and lacrimal sace. Marcel Dekker New York

Gehan EA, Walker MD (1977) Prognostic factors for patients with brain tumors. In: Modern concepts in brain tumor therapy. National Cancer Institute Monograph No 46 pp 189–195

Han J-W, McCormick F, Macara IG (1991) Regulation of ras-GAP and the neurofibromatosis 1 gene product by eicosanoids. Science 252:576–579

Hollstein M, Sidransky D, Vogelstein B, Harris CC (1991) p53 mutations in human cancers. Science 253:49–53

Hurtt MR, Moossy J, Donovan-Peluso M, Locker J (1992) Amplification of epidermal growth factor receptor gene in gliomas: histopathology and prognosis. J Neuropath Exp Neurol 51:84–90

James CD, Carlblom E, Dumanski JP, Hansen M, Nordenskjold M, Collins VP, Cavenee WK (1988) Clonal genomic alterations in glioma malignancy stages. Cancer Res 48:5546–5551

James CD, Carlbom E, Nordenskjold M, Collins VP, Cavenee WK (1989) Mitotic recombination of chromosome 17 in astrocytomas. Proc Natl Acad Sci USA 86:2858–2862

James CD, He J, Carlbom E, Nordenskjold M, Cavenee WK, Collins VP (1991) Chromosome 9 deletion mapping reveals interferon a and interferon b-1 gene deletions in human glial tumors. Cancer Res 51:1684–1688

Kleihues P, Burger PC, Scheithauer BW (1993) Histological Typing of Tumours of the Central Nervous System. In: (ed) 2 Springer-Verlag Berlin Heidelberg, New York, London, Paris, Tokyo, Barcelona

Knudsen AG (1976) Genetics and the etiology of childhood cancer. Pediatr Res 10:513–517

Lewis RA, Gerson LP, Axelson KA, Riccardi VM, Whitford RP (1984) Von Recklinghausen neurofibromatosis. II. Incidence of optic gliomata. Ophthalmology 91:929

Li Y, Bollag G, Clark R, Stevens J, Conroy L, Fults D, Ward K, Friedman E, Samowitz W, Robertson M, Bradley P, Cawthon R (1992) Somatic mutations in the neurofibromatosis 1 gene in human Tumors. Cell 69:275–281

Libermann TA, Nusbaum HR, Razon N, Kris R, Lax I, Soreq H, Whittle N, Waterfield MD, Ullrich A, Schlessinger J (1984) Amplification, enhanced expression and possible rearrangement of EGF receptor in primary human brain tumors of glial origin. Nature 313:144–147

Malkin D, Li FP, Strong LC, Fraumeni JF, Nelson C, Kim DH, Kassel J, Gryka MA, Bishoff FZ, Taisky MA, Friend SH (1990) Germ line p53 mutations in a familial syndrome of breast cancer, sarcomas, and other neoplasms. Science 250:1222–1228

Marshall CJ (1991) Tumor supressor genes. Cell 64:313–326

Menon AG, Anderson KM, Riccardi VM, Chung RY, Whaley JM, Yandell DW, Farmer GE, Freiman RN, Lee JK, Li FP, Barker DF, Ledbetter DH, Kleider A, Martuza RL, Gusella JF, Seizinger BR (1990) Chromosome 17p deletions and p53 gene mutations associated with the formation of malignant neurofibrosarcomas in Recklinghausen neurofibromatosis. Proc Natl Acad Sci USA 87:5435–5439

Nigro JM, Baker SJ, Preisinger AC, Jessup JM, Hostetter R, Cleary K, Bigner SH, Davidson N, Baylin S, Devilee P, Glover T, Collins FC, Weston A, Modali R, Harris CC, Vogelstein B (1989) Mutations in the p53 gene occur in diverse tumor types. Nature 342:705–708

Ogawa O, Habuchi T, Kakehi Y, Koshiba M, Sugiyama T Yoshida, O (1992) Allelic losses at chromosome 17p in human renal carcinoma are inversely related to allelic losses at chromosome 3p. Cancer Res 52:1881–1885

Olopade OI, Jenkins RB, Ransom DT, Malik K, Pomykala H, Nobori T, Cowan JM, Rowley JD, Diaz MO (1992) Molecular analysis of deletions of the short arm of chromosome 9 in human gliomas. Cancer Res 52:2523–2529

Slamon DJ, Clark GM, Wong SG, Levin WJ, Ullrich A, McGuire WL (1987) Human breast cancer: correlation of relapse and survival with amplification of the HER-2/neu oncogene. Science 235:177–182

Srivastava S, Zou Z, Pirollo K, Blattner W, Chang EH (1990) Germ-line transmission of a mutated p53 gene in a cancer-prone family with Li-Fraumeni syndrome. Nature 348:747–749
Stark M, Assunm G, Krone W (1991) A small deletion and an adjacent base exchange in a potential stem-loop region of the neurofibromatosis 1 gene. Hum Gen 87:685–687
Takahashi T, D'Amico D, Chiba I, Buchhagen DL, Minna JD (1990) Identification of intronic point mutations as an alternative mechanism for p53 inactivation in lung cancer. J Clin Invest 86:363–369
Thor AD, Schwartz LH, Koerner FC, Edgerton SM, Skates SJ, Yin S, McKenzie SJ, Panicali DL, Marks PJ, Fingert HJ, Wood WC (1989) Analysis of c-erbB-2 expression in breast carcinomas with clinical follow-up. Cancer Res 49:7147–7152
Thor AD, Moore DH, Edgerton SM, Chen L-C, Ngo J, Kawasaki ES, Reihsaus E, Schwartz L, Smith HS (1992) Increased accumulation of the p53 suppressor gene product is an independent prognostic variable for breast cancer. J Natl Canc Inst 84:845–855
Venter DJ, Thomas DGT (1991) Multiple sequential molecular abnormalities in the evolution of human gliomas. Br J Cancer 63: 753–757
Viskochil D, Buchberg AM, Xu G, Cawthon RM, Stevens J, Wolff RK, Culver M, Carey JC, Copeland NG, Jenkins NA, White R, O'Connell P (1990) Deletions and a translocation interupt a cloned gene at the neurofibromatosis type 1 locus. Cell 62:187–192
von Deimling A, Eibl RH, Ohgaki H, Louis DN, von Ammon K, Petersen I, Kleihues P, Chung RY, Wiestler OD, Seizinger BR (1992) p53 mutations are associated with 17p allelic loss in grade II and grade III astrocytoma. Cancer Res 52:2987–2990
von Deimling A, Louis DN, von Ammon K, Petersen I, Hoell T, Chung RY, Martuza R, Schoenfeld D, Yasargil MG, Wiestler OD, Seizinger BR (1992) Association of epidermal growth factor receptor gene amplification with loss of chromosome 10 in human glioblastoma multiforme. J Neurosurg 77:295–301
von Deimling A, Louis DN, von Ammon K, Petersen I, Wiestler OD, Seizinger BR (1992) Evidence for a tumor suppressor gene on chromosome 19q associated with human astrocytomas, oligodendrogliomas and mixed gliomas. Cancer Res 52:4277–4279
von Deimling A, von Ammon K, Schoenfeld D, Wiestler OD, Seizinger BR, Louis DN (1993) Subsets of glioblastoma multiforme defined by molecular genetic analysis. Brain Pathol 3:19–26
von Deimling A, Louis DN, Menon AG, von Ammon K, Petersen I, Ellison D, Wiestler OD, Seizinger BR (1993) Deletions on the long arm of chromosome 17 in pilocytic astrocytoma. Acta Neuropathol (in press)
Wallace MR, Marchuk DA, Andersen LB, Letcher R, Odeh HM, Saulino AM, Fountain JW, Brereton A, Nicholson J, Mitchell AL, Brownstein BH, Collins FS (1990) Type 1 neurofibromatosis gene: identification of a large transcript disrupted in three NF1 patients. Science 249:181–186
Watanabe K, Nagai M, Arai T, Kawashima K (1990) Loss of constitutional heterozygosity in chromosome 10 in human glioblastoma. Acta Neuropathol 80:251–254
Winger MJ, Macdonald DR, Cairncross JG (1989) Supratentorial anaplastic gliomas in adults. J Neurosurg 71:487–493
Xu G, O'Connell P, Viskochil D, Cawthon R, Robertson M, Culver M, Dunn D, Stevens J, Gesteland R, White R, Weiss R (1990) The neurofibromatosis type 1 gene encodes a protein related to GAP. Cell 62:599–608

Prognostic Relevance of Transforming Genes

U. Schlegel[1], J. Neumann[2], D. Kindermann[3], H. K. Wolf, A. Baumann[4], F. Forster[1], and R. Fimmers[1]

[1]Neurologische Universitätsklinik, Sigmund-Freud-Str. 25, 53127 Bonn, Germany
[2]Neurochirugische Universitätsklinik, Sigmund-Freud-Str. 25, 53127 Bonn, Germany
[3]Pathologisches Institut, Universitätskliniken Bonn, Sigmund-Freud-Str. 25, 53127 Bonn, Germany
[4]Institut für Neuropathologie, Universitätskliniken Bonn, Sigmund-Freud-Str. 25, 53127 Bonn, Germany

Introduction

Malignant transformation is considered the result of a multipstep process in which cells aquire mutations of genes that are critical for the regulation of cell proliferation and differentiation (Bishop 1987; Weinberg 1989). In astrocytic gliomas several different mutations have been identified, some of which are confined to certain grades of malignancy (Collins 1990). Amplification and overexpression of the gene encoding the epidermal growth factor receptor (EGFR) is nearly exclusively present in glioblastomas (Libermann 1985; Ekstrand 1991; Agosti 1992). Amplification of EGFR gene fragments with large deletions encoding a truncated receptor has been described as well as amplification of the intact gene encoding a functional receptor (Yamazaki 1988; Humphrey 1990,1991; Ekstrand 1992). An amplified and overexpressed EGFR may or may not be capable of being activated by its main ligand transforming growth factor-α (TGF-α, Yamazaki 1988; Humphrey 1991). In many astrocytic gliomas TGF-α itself has been found to be overexpressed in a large number of these tumors without evidence of genetic alteration (Schlegel 1990; Ekstrand 1991), and an autocrine mechanism of growth stimulation by the EGFR/TGF-α system has been postulated in glioma cells (Ekstrand 1991). Mutations and allelic loss of the tumor suppressor gene p53 have been reported in astrocytic gliomas (Nigro 1989; v. Deimling 1992; Frankel 1992; Fults 1992). It has been reported that in low-grade astrocytomas cells with mutations of the p53 gene represent a minority. The fact that these cells may undergo clonal expansion in recurrent malignant gliomas suggests that p53 mutations play a significant role in malignant progression (Sidransky 1992).

Oncogene mutations and oncoprotein expression have been reported to be of prognostic relevance in some somatic cancers: N-myc amplifications in neuroblastomas are confined to grade III and IV tumors (Schwab, this volume); the presence of K-*ras* point mutations in adenocarcinomas of the lung correlates with a poor outcome (Slebos 1990); c-erbB2 oncoprotein expression in breast cancer has been reported to be be associated with short survival time (Slamon 1987). However, investigations on possible correlations between oncogene mutation/expression and clinical course in brain tumors are sparse and are confined to rather small numbers of tumors (Bigner 1991;

Hurtt 1992; Jaros 1992; Reiffenberger 1993). The present work was carried out to investigate a possible prognostic relevance of EGFR, TGF-α, and p53 expression in gliomas of different tumor grades. Additionally, mutations and aberrant expression of the p53 tumor suppressor gene were studied in low-grade astrocytomas and in the corresponding high-grade recurrences in the same patients to elucidate a possible influence of these mutations on malignant transformation and on clinical outcome.

Material and Methods

Tissue Specimens and Histopathology. Specimens of 72 primary tumors (24 WHO grade II astrocytomas, 19 WHO grade III astrocytomas, and 29 glioblastomas) and nine recurrent malignant tumors of the initially low-grade astrocytomas (five anaplastic astrocytomas, four glioblastomas) were taken from the neuropathological archives. Each tumor specimen had been obtained by partial or gross total tumor resection and was rereviewed and classified for the purpose of this study by two neuropathologists according to the revised WHO classification for brain tumors (Kleihues 1993). The only selection criteria were availability of tumor material and sufficient clinical follow-up. All primary tumors were untreated prior to operation, none of the low-grade tumors was irradiated or treated with chemotherapy after operation. Control nontumorous brain for immunohistochemistry was obtained from autopsy cases. Normal control DNA was extracted from white blood cells of healthy individuals. The majority of patients included in this study were followed in the local outpatient brain tumor service. In the other cases information on clinical course, time, and cause of death were obtained by correspondence with physicians at other institutions. All primary tumors had been operated on between 1975 and 1989. Thus complete clinical follow-up information was available for periods of 2–15 years.

Oncoprotein Expression. The expression of EGFR, TGF-α, and p53 was detected immunohistochemically using the indirect Streptavidin-biotin-peroxidase method. Primary antibodies used were monoclonal antibody E30 against the extracellular domain of human EGFR (Merck), monoclonal antibody 213.-4.4 against TGF-α (Oncogene Science), monoclonal antibody 1801 against human p53 (Oncogene Science; Banks 1986) and polyclonal rabbit antisera CM1 against p53 (Medac: Midgley 1992). In order to semiquantitatively express the extent of positive immunoreaction for each tumor, two reviewers who were not involved in the experimental procedures independently evaluated the percentage of immunopositive tumor cells using the following grading system: 0, no immunoreaction; 1, up to 10% of tumor cells stained; 2; 10%–50% of tumor cells stained; 3; 50%–90% of tumor cells stained; 4; more than 90% of tumor cells stained.

Genetic Mutations. Exons 5–8 of the p53 gene, which harbor more than 95% of mutations published (de Fromentel 1992), were screened for the presence of mutations by single-strand conformation polymorphism (SSCP) analysis as described elsewhere (Schlegel 1992).

Results

Immunohistochemistry. Immunohistochemical staining was carried out with anti EGFR and anti-TGF-α antibodies for the primary tumors and with the two anti-p53 antibodies for all primary and recurrent tumors. The scores of the two reviewers were in agreement in 60% of cases, there was a difference in staining score of 1 in 30%, and one of greater than 1 in 10% of the cases. No bias of either reviewer for a higher or lower staining score was found. Figure 1 depicts the staining score for p53 (AB CM1), EGFR, and TGF-α as given by reviewer 1.

p53. Due to its extremely short half-life, the normal p53 protein is not detectable with standard immunohistochemical techniques (Bartek 1990). Some mutant forms, however, are much more stable, and a large variety of human tumors reveal aberrant p53 expression, as shown by immunohistochemistry (Bartek 1992). Therefore, a positive immunoreaction strongly suggests the presence of abnormal p53 protein. Mouse monoclonal antibody 1801 recognizes a denaturation resistant epitope between amino acid residues 32 and 79 of human wild-type and mutant p53 (Banks 1986). CM1 is a polyclonal rabbit antiserum, raised against human p53 expressed in *Escherichia coli* (Midgley 1992). Differences in staining between the two antibodies were found in six of the 72 primary tumors and in none of the nine recurrent tumors. In three cases antibody 1801 revealed a positive immunoreaction and CM1 did not; in three other tumors the results were vice versa. Aberrant p53 expression was detected in: 9/24 (AB 1801) 10/24(AB CM1) = 40% of WHO II astrocytomas; 5/19 (AB 1801) 6/19 (AB CM1) = 35% of WHO III astrocytomas; 7/29 (AB 1801) 5/29 (AB CM1) = 21% of glioblastomas; and 6/9 (AB 1801) 6/9 (AB CM1) = 67% of recurrent gliomas. In two cases the primary tumor did not show a positive immunoreaction, whereas the corresponding malignant recurrent tumor did. In one case the primary tumor showed aberrant p53 expression and the recurrent malignant tumor did not. As depicted in Fig. 1a, the presence and extent of a positive immunoreaction were not dependent of tumor grade. Immunoreactivity was found exclusively in nuclei and most frequently showed a granular staining pattern (Fig. 2a). Immunoreactive cells were distributed uniformly throughout the tumors. With neither antibody was there immunoreactivity in the nontumorous control cortex. No immunoreactivity was seen when either tumor or control tissues were incubated with normal mouse IgG or normal rabbit serum.

Epidermal Growth Factor Receptor. Four of 24 WHO grade II astrocytomas were weakly immunoreactive for EGFR. In these cases the clinical course was not worse than in cases without EGFR immunoreactivity. Seven of 19 (37%) of the WHO grade III and 14 of 29 (48%) of the glioblastomas showed a positive immunoreaction. The staining was slightly more pronounced in grade IV gliomas (Fig. 1b). The immunostaining was cytoplasmic or membranous and was distributed heterogeneously across the sections (Fig. 2c).

Transforming Growth Factor-α. With the exception of two low-grade astrocytomas all gliomas revealed TGF-α expression to some extent (Fig. 1c). The nontumorous control

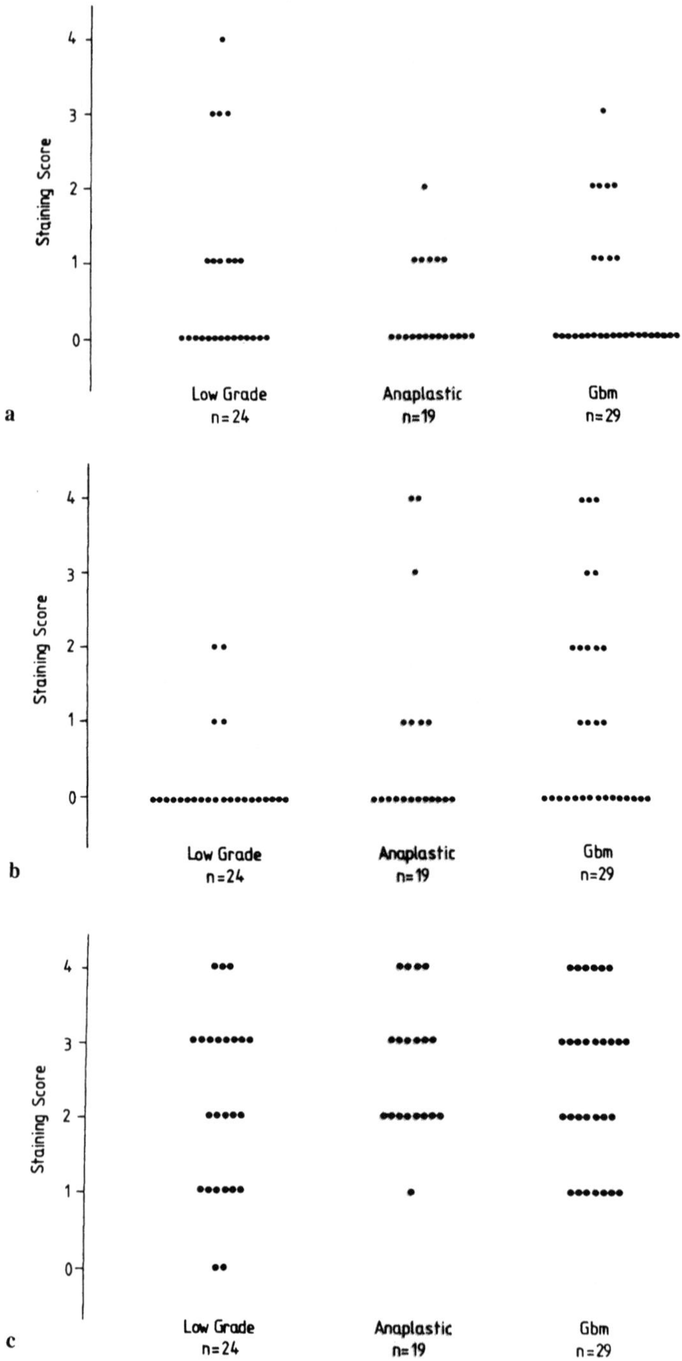

Fig. 1. The arbitrary staining score as given by reviewer 1 for p53 (**a**), EGFR (**b**), and TGF-α (**c**) is depicted for astrocytic gliomas of different tumor grade

a

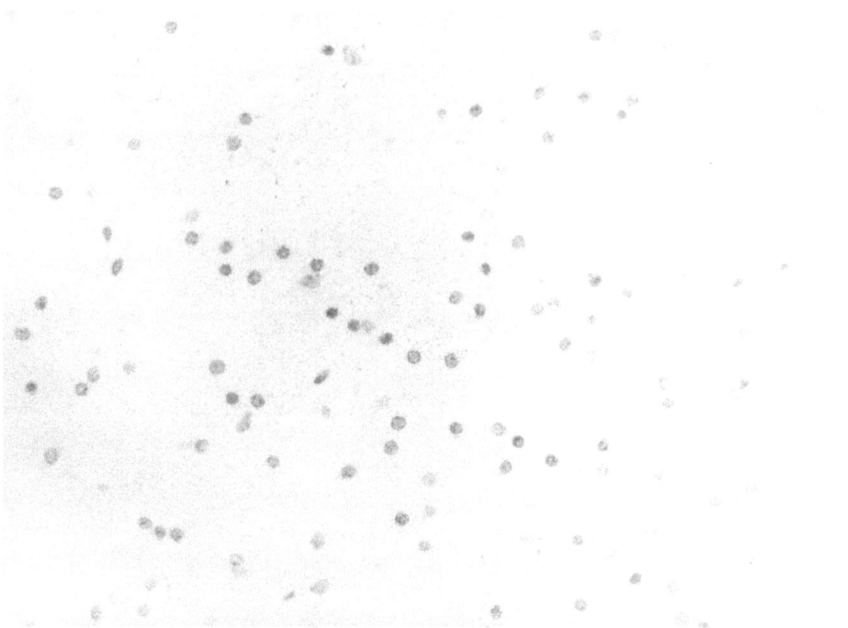

b

Fig. 2. a Positive immunoreaction of nuclei in a WHO grade II astrocytoma using antibody 1801 against human p53. **b** No immunoreaction was detected in normal cortex or in the same tumor with nonimmune mouse IgG (data not shown)

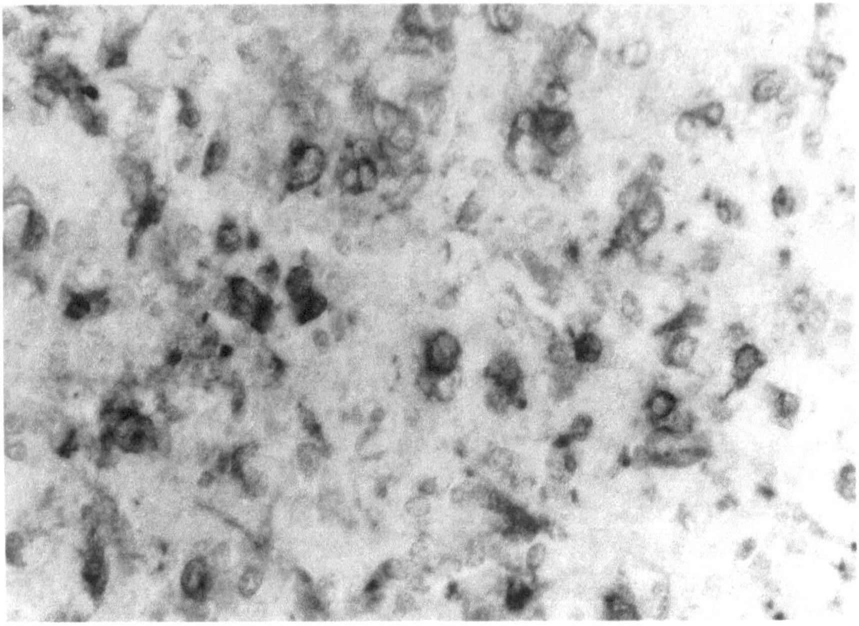

c

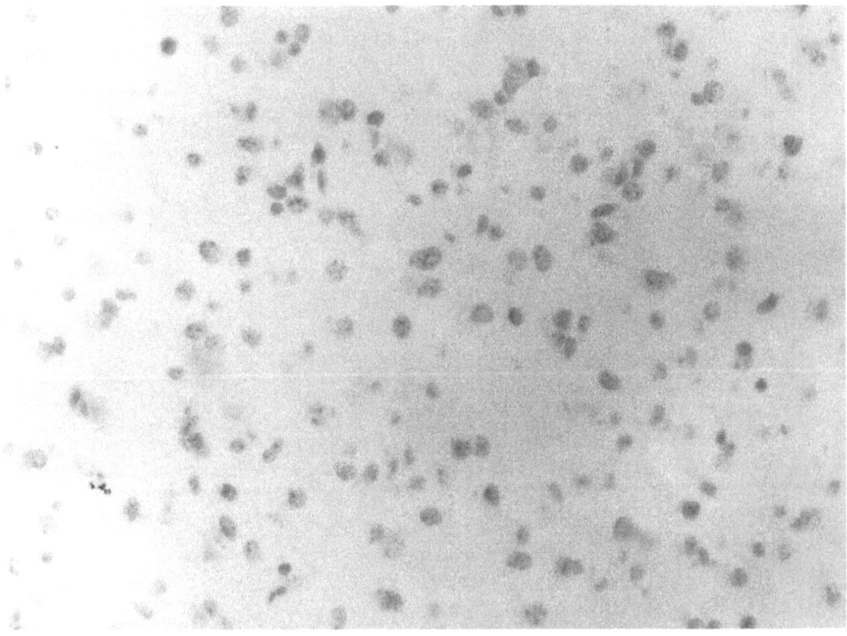

d

Fig. 2. c Positive cytoplasmic and membranous immunoreaction with EGFR antibody E30 in a glioblastoma. **d** No immunoreaction was detected in normal cortex or in the same tumor with nonimmune mouse IgG (data not shown).

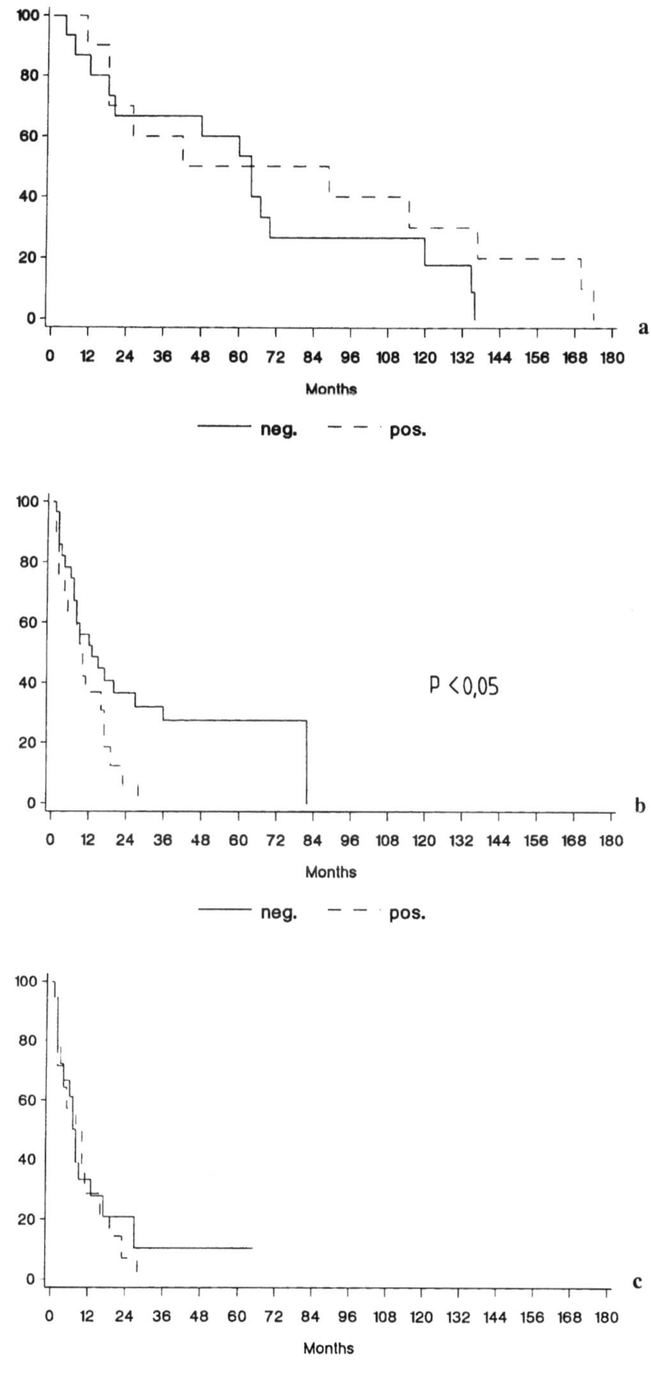

Fig. 3a-c. Kaplan-Meyer survival curves. **a** In low-grade astrocytomas, aberrant expression of p53 (*dotted line*) and no expression of p53 (*continuous line*). **b** In malignant gliomas, EGFR expression (*dotted line*) and no EGFR expression (*continuous line*). **c** EGFR-immunopositive and EGFR-negative tumors are compared for glioblastomas only cortex did not stain. The immunoreactivity appeared to be slightly more pronounced in malignant gliomas than in low-grade gliomas; however, this was not statistically significant. Immunoreactivity was present as intense cytoplasmic staining spread throughout large tumor areas (data not shown). There was some sparing of highly cellular areas in malignant gliomas consisting of small, monomorphic, highly anaplastic tumor cells. Reactive astrocytes at the tumor periphery showed intense staining.

Oncoprotein Expression and Clinical Outcome. In none of the tumor grades nor in the overall group was there a correlation between the presence of p53 expression and survival time. The time between initial surgery and recurrence did not correlate with expression of p53 (Fig. 3a). EGFR expression in malignant gliomas showed a negative correlation with survival (Fig. 3b); however, this result reflected only the fact that grade III gliomas with a substantially longer survival did not overexpress EGFR to the same extent as glioblastomas. Analysis of the grade IV tumors alone failed to demonstrate any correlation between EGFR expression and outcome (Fig. 3c). Aberrant expression of TGF-α, which was present in nearly all tumors, also did not correlate with clinical course.

SSCP Analysis. We carried out SSCP analysis in 20 WHO grade II astrocytomas and nine corresponding malignant recurrent tumors. Exons 5–8 were screened for mutations. With SSCP analysis p53 mutations were detected in 8 of 20 low-grade astrocytomas. In two cases bands representing the wild-type allel were not present, suggesting the loss of the nonmutant allele. (An example is depicted in Fig. 4.) Mutations were present in six of nine malignant recurrent gliomas. In only one case was an abnormal migration pattern in the recurrent glioma not present in the corresponding low-grade initial tumor, a result compatible with clonal expansion in this single case. Two of the low-grade tumors with mutations showed no immunoreactivivity. Three tumors without a detectable mutation showed a positive immunoreaction.

The average survival in astrocytomas WHO grade II with mutant p53 was 94 months and in tumors without detectable p53 mutation 70 months.

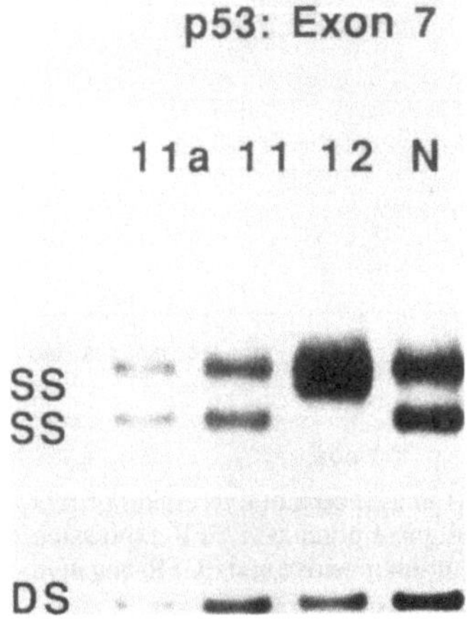

Fig. 4. SSCP of exon 7 of the p53 gene: *SS*, single strands; *DS*, double strands; *N*, normal DNA. A number of tumors are depicted. In case 12 abnormal migration patterns suggest mutation of the gene. No normal bands are detectable. This suggests a loss of the wild-type allele

Discussion

Seventy-two primary and nine corresponding recurrent gliomas were investigated for a possible prognostic relevance of oncoprotein expression and genetic mutation. Overexpression of the EGFR was detected in about half of the glioblastomas and in a third of anaplastic astrocytomas studied. This result is comparable with data from other studies (Libermann 1984, 1985; Reifenberger 1989). EGFR antibody E30 recognizes an extracellular domain of the receptor, which has not been further characterized (Merck, product description). Due to the lack of molecular investigation in this study it cannot be stated whether the whole protein or only a truncated receptor was detected, or whether the overexpressed receptor was responsive to its ligand or not. EGFR overexpression is most likely the result of gene amplification (Libermann 1985), and it is reasonable to assume that both amplification and overexpression play a biological role in glioma development. However, in the present study no prognostic significance independent of tumor grade was found. Additional studies are necessary to determine whether different mutations are associated with varying degrees of tumor cell proliferation.

TGF-α is the main ligand of the EGFR in human tumors (Massegue 1990). In our study there was no statistically significant correlation between TGF-a expression and prognosis or tumor grade.

Mutations in the tumor suppressor gene p53 are of particular interest in human astrocytomas. They have been reported in WHO grade II astrocytomas (v.Deimling 1992) and are of potential importance for malignant progression of gliomas (Sidransky 1992). The optimal therapy for WHO grade II astrocytomas is still undetermined, particularly with respect to the potential use of radiation therapy (Shaw 1990; Cairncross 1990). Therefore, additional prognostic parameters may possibly provide important therapeutic guidelines. In the present study neither the aberrant immunohistochemical expression of p53 nor the presence of a p53 genetic mutation as detected by SSCP analysis showed a correlation with survival time or recurrence-free interval. In contrast, Jaros et al. (1992) reported a correlation between aberrant p53 expression, tumor grade, and poor clinical outcome. One possible explanation of this discrepancy may be the fact that pilocytic astrocytomas (WHO grade I) were included by Jaros et al. but not in our study. In our series, clonal expansion did not play a significant role. In only one of six cases of corresponding primary and recurrent malignant tumor was a mutation present in the recurrent tumor not detectable in the low-grade initial tumor. p53 mutations within different regions of the gene may have a different biological effect, and therefore a small series may not be representative. However, one of the mutant tumors with loss of wild-type allel was the one with longest recurrence free interval of more than 174 months.

In summary, the investigation of some of the best characterized oncoprotein/-gene alterations in astrocytic gliomas revealed no new prognostically relevant information. The studies were carried out in a univariate fashion on a rather limited number of tumors. A multivariate analysis in a larger number of patients must be carried out to confirm these results. In addition, newly discovered genetic alterations in gliomas need to be examined with respect to their prognostic and potential therapeutic relevance.

References

Agosti RM, Leuthold M, Gullick WJ, Yasargil MG, Wiestler OD (1992) Expression of the epidermal growth factor receptor in astrocytic tumors is specifically associated with glioblastoma multiforme. Virchows Arch A Pathol Anat 420:321–325

Banks L, Matlashewski G, Crawford L (1986) Isolation of human-p53-specific monoclonal antibodies and their use in the studies of human p53 expression. Eur J Biochem 159:529–534

Bartek J, Iggo R, Gannon J, Lane DP (1990) Genetic and immunohistochemical analysis of mutant p53 in human breast cancer cell lines. Oncogene 5:893–899

Bartek J, Bartkova J, Vojtesek B, Staskova Z, Lukas J, Rejthar A, Kovarik J, Midgley CA, Gannon JV, Lane DP (1992) Aberrant expression of the p53 oncoprotein is a common feature of a wide spectrum of human malignancies. Oncogene 7:1699–1703

Bigner SH (1991) Chromosomal and molecular alterations in brain tumors. International Workshop on Chromosomes in Solid Tumors, Tucson, 2, 23–27, 91:B18

Bishop JM (1987) The molecular genetics of cancer. Science 235:305–311

Cairncross JG (1990) Low-grade gliomas: To treat or not to treat ? A reply. Arch Neurol 47:1139–1140

Collins VP, James CD (1990) Molecular genetics of primary intracranial tumors. Curr Opin Oncol 2:666 –6721

de Fromentel CC, Soussi T (1992) TP53 tumor suppressor gene: A model for investigating human mutagenesis. Genes Chrom Cancer 4:1–15

Ekstrand AJ, James CD, Cavenee WK, Seliger B, Petterson RF, Collins VP (1991) Genes for Epidermal growth factor receptor, transforming growth factor α, and epidermal growth factor and their expression in human gliomas in vivo. Cancer Res 51:2164–2172

Ekstrand AJ, Sugawa N, James CD, Collins VP (1992) Amplified and rearranged epidermal growth factor receptor genes in human glioblastomas reveal deletions of sequences encoding portions of the N- and/or C-terminal tails. Proc Natl Acad Sci 89:4309–4313

Frankel RH, Bayona W, Koslow M, Newcomb EW (1992) p53 mutations in human malignant gliomas: Comparison of loss of heterocygosity with mutation frequency. Cancer Res 52:1427–1433

Fults D, Brockmeyer D, Tullous MW, Pedone CA, Cawthon RM (1992) p53 mutation and loss of heterocygosity on chromosomes 17 and 10 during human astrocytoma progression. Cancer Res 52:674–679

Humphrey PA, Wong AJ, Vogelstein B, Zalutsky MR, Fuller GN, Archer GE, Friedman HS, Kwatra MM, Bigner SH, Bigner DD (1990) Anti-synthetic peptide antibody reacting at the fusion junction of deletion-mutatnt epidermal growth factor receptors in human glioblastoma. Proc Natl Acad Sci 87:4207–4211

Humphrey PA, Gangarosa LM, Wong AJ, Archer GE, Lund-Johansen M, Bjerkvig R, Laerum O-D, Friedman HS, Bigner DD (1991) Deletion-mutant epidermal growth factor receptor in human gliomas:Effect of type II mutation on receptor function. Biochem Biophys Res Com 178:1413–1420

Hurtt MR, Moossy J, Donovan-Peluso M, Locker J (1992) Amplification of epidermal growth factor receptor gene in gliomas: Histopathology and prognosis. J Neuropath Exp Neurol 51:84–90

Jaros E, Perry RH, Adam L, Kelly PJ, Crawford PJ, Kalbag RM, Mendelow AD, Sengupta RP, Pearson AD (1992) Prognostic implications of p53 protein, epidermal growth factor receptor, and KI-67 labeling in brain tumors. Brit J Cancer 66:373–385

Kleihues P, Burger PC, Scheithauer BW (eds) (1993) Histological typing of tumors of the central nervous system, 2nd edn. Springer, Berlin Heidelberg, New York

Liberman TA, Razon N, Bartal AD, Yarden Y, Schlessinger J, Soreq H (1984) Expression of epidermal growth factor receptors in human brain tumors. Cancer Res 44:753 –760

Libermann TA, Nusbaum HR, Razon N, Kris R, Lax I, Soreq H, Whittle N, Waterfeld MD, Ulrich A, Schlessinger J (1985) Amplification, enhanced expression and possible rearrangement of EGFR gene in primary human brain tumours of glial origin. Nature 313:144–147

Massegue J (1990) Transforming growth factor-α. A model for membrane-anchored growth factors. J Biol Chem 265; 21393–21396

Midgley CA, Fisher CJ, Bartek J, Vojtesek B, Lane DP, Barnes DM (1992) Analysis of p53 expression in human tumours:an antibody raised against human p53 expressed in Eschericia coli. J Cell Sci 101:183–189

Nigro JM, Baker SJ, Preisinger AC, Jessup JM, Hostetter R, Cleary K, Bigner SH, Davidson N, Baylin S, Devilee P, Glover T, Collins FS, Weston A, Modali R, Harris CC, Vogelstein B (1989) Mutations in the p53 gene occur in diverse human tumour types. Nature 342:705–708

Reifenberger G, Prior R, Deckert M, Wechsler W (1989) Epidermal growth factor receptor expression and growth fraction in human tumours of the nervous system. Virchows Archiv A Pathol Anat 414:147–155

Reifenberger G, Vogeley KT, Figge C, Messing M, Roosen N, Patt S, Reiffen K-A, Weber W, Wechsler W (1993) Immunochemical analysis of epidermal growth factor receptor expression in tumors of the nervous system using the new monoclonal antibody E30. Cancer submitted

Schlegel U, Moots PL, Rosenblum MK, Thaler HT, Furneaux HM (1990) Expression of transforming growth factor alpha in human gliomas Oncogene 5:1839–1842

Schlegel U, Rosenfeld MR, Volkenandt M, Rosenblum M, Dalmau J, and Furneaux H (1992) p53 gene mutations in primary lung tumors are conserved in brain metastases. J Neuro-Oncol 14:93–100

Shaw EG (1990) Low-grade gliomas:To treat or not to treat ? A radiation oncologist's viewpoint. Arch Neurol 47:1138–1139

Sidransky D, Mikkelsen T, Schwechheimer K, Rosenblum ML, Cavenee W, Vogelstein B (1992) Clonal expansion of p53 mutant cells is associated with brain tumor progression. Nature 355:846–847

Slamon DJ, Clark GM, Wong SG, Levin WJ, Ullrich A, McGuire WL (1987) Human breast cancer: Correlation of relapse and survival with amplification of the her-2/neu oncogene. Science 235:177–182

Slebos RJC, Kibbelaar RE, Dalesio O, Kooistra A, Stam J, Meijer CJLM, Wagenaar SS, Vanderschueren RGJRA, v.Zandwijk N, Mooi WJ, Bos JL, Rodenhuis S (1990) K-Ras oncogene activation as a prognostic marker in adenocarcinoma of the lung. New Engl J Med 323:561–565

von Deimling A, Eibl RH, Ohgaki H, Louis DN, v. Ammon K, Petersen I, Kleihues P, Chung RY, Wiestler OD, Seizinger BR (1992) p53 mutations are associated with 17p allelic loss in grade II and grad III astrocytoma. Cancer Res 52:2987–2990

Weinberg RA (1991) Tumor suppressor genes. Science 254:1138–1145

Yamazaki H, Fukui Y, Ueyama Y, Tamaoki N, Kawamoto T, Taniguchi S, Shibuya M (1988) Amplifikation of the structurally and functionally altered epidermal growth factor receptor gene (c-erbB) in human brain tumors. Mol Cell Biol 8:1816–1820

Oncogene Transfer into the Brain

O. D. Wiestler[1], O. Brüstle[2], R. H. Eibl[2], H. Radner[2], A. Aguzzi[2], and P. Kleihues[2]

[1]Institut für Neuropathologie, Universitätskliniken Bonn, Sigmund-Freud-Str. 25, 53127 Bonn, Germany
[2]Institut für Neuropathologie, Departement Pathologie, Universitätsspital Zürich, Schmelzbergstr. 12, 8091 Zürich, Switzerland

Introduction

With the spectacular advances in the characterization of genes associated with brain tumors and other neurological disorders, experimental approaches to stably introduce and express foreign genes in vivo have recently evolved as an important tool to study the specific pathogenetic role of candidate genes. A well-characterized and frequently used model are transgenic mice (Wagner 1990; Hanahan 1989; Pattengale et al. 1989). These animals are generated by introduction of DNA constructs into fertilized eggs or into embryonic stem cells. They carry copies of the transgene in all somatic and germ cells and stably transmit the gene to their offspring in a Mendelian fashion. Transcription of the transgene is critically dependent on regulatory sequences. Using specific promoter elements, it is possible to achieve cell- and tissue-specific expression. Cross-breeding of transgenic lines which carry distinct transgenes allows to study the combined effects of the respective genes in vivo.

The transgenic approach is a powerful and efficient experimental model system. Integration of the transgene in every cell of the animal represents an intriguing model for hereditary disorders. During sporadic tumor formation, however, genetically modified preneoplastic or neoplastic cells are confronted and interacting with an environment of unmodified neighboring cells. The requirement of cell-type specific promoter elements for targeted expression of the foreign DNA has also been a limiting factor as suitable promoter sequences are not available for many cell types. This includes various cell types in the brain and precursor cells in developing tissues.

Our laboratory has recently developed an alternative model which employs retrovirus-mediated gene transfer into neural transplants (Aguzzi et al. 1988; Wiestler et al. 1992a; Wiestler et al. 1992b). The rationale is to introduce and express foreign genes in fetal rat brain transplants using as genetic vehicle a replication-defective retroviral vector into which the gene of interest has been inserted. We have extensively employed this transplantation system for studies on the effects of transforming genes in the developing and adult rat brain. While an increasing number of transforming genes and transformation-associated chromosomal loci have been identified in human CNS neoplasms, little information is available on molecular transformation pathways operating in these tumors and on the functions of wild type and mutant proteins encoded by the respective gene.

In this review we focus on five interesting aspects of this work: (a) the cellular tropism of various oncogenes in the CNS, (b) the possibilty to achieve long-term growth factor expression in neural grafts, (c) studies demonstrating a combined and complementary action of transforming genes in the brain, (d) a new model for primitive neuroectodermal tumors, and (e) a potential approach to study neural tumor suppressor genes.

The Transplantation Model

Our experimental procedure combines two established procedures, i.e., transplantation of fetal brain tissue and retrovirus-mediated gene transfer (Fig. 1). Since these transplants develop into highly differentiated CNS tissue, they provide an excellent model for the central nervous system in vivo. Retroviral vectors can efficiently be introduced and expressed in different cell types of neural transplants. Expression of these genes can be driven by constitutively active viral promoters (Fig. 2). Tissue-specific regulatory sequences are therefore not required. In contrast to transgenic animals, stable integration and expression of the retrovirally transmitted genes succeed only in a small fraction of the fetal donor cells. Gene transfer at different stages of embryonic CNS development allows to modulate the target cell population. A potential disadvantage of this approach is the inability of retroviral vectors to stably integrate into the genome of resting cells such as postmitotic neurons.

The constructs used in these studies are based on the Moloney murine leukemia virus genome and contain regulatory long terminal repeat sequences, a retroviral packaging signal, a cDNA for the respective oncogene and a neomycin phosphotransferase (neo) selectable marker gene (Cone and Mulligan 1984; Stuhlmann et al. 1984). Structural genes of the Moloney genome, i.e., *gag, pol,* and *env* have been deleted to render these particles replication-deficient (Mann et al. 1983). This prevents a productive viral infection following intracerebral transplantation of infected fetal donor cells. Rodent fibroblast cell lines which harbor the Moloney *gag-pol* and *env* genes are used as packaging cell lines to provide the replication-deficient retroviral genome with an ecotropic Moloney virus envelope (Markowitz et al. 1988).

Fetal donor cell suspensions are prepared from E12-E14 rat brains, mock-infected or incubated with a retroviral construct and grafted intracerebrally into syngeneic host animals. Two months after stereotaxic implantation, control grafts show the characteristic morphology of fetal brain transplants with an irregular distribution of neurons and glial elements and formation of pseudocortical architectures. Immunohistochemically, neurons in the grafts exhibit a strong expression of neuron-specific enolase, synaptophysin, and neurofilament protein. Astrocytes can be identified with antibodies to glial fibrillary acidic protein and oligodendrocytes with an antiserum to myelin basic protein. These organotypic transplants are, therefore, a suitable model for the in vivo brain.

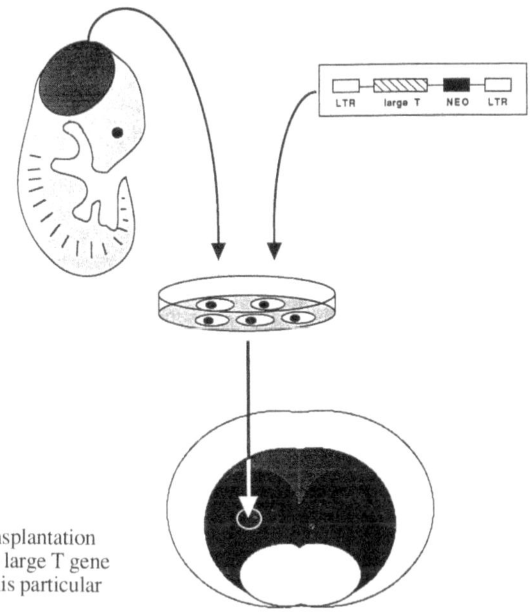

Fig. 1. Schematic illustration of the transplantation model. A retroviral vector encoding the large T gene of SV40 virus (large T) is depicted in this particular example

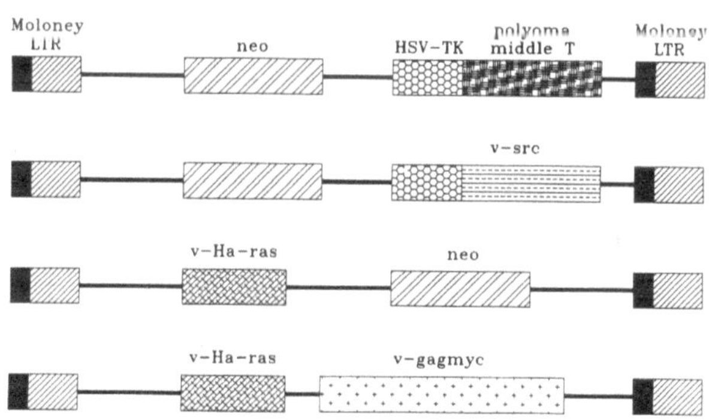

Fig. 2. Structure of retroviral genomes used for oncogene transfer into CNS transplants. The upper three constructs contain both, cDNAs for the respective oncogene and a neomycin phosphotransferase marker gene. The retroviral vector shown at the bottom will coexpress the oncogenes v-Ha-*ras* and v-*gag*/*myc* from the same retroviral genome. *HSV-TK*, Thymidine kinase promoter element derived from Herpes simplex virus

In order to identify target cells for retroviral constructs in CNS transplants, retroviral vectors harboring the *Escherichia coli* β-galactosidase marker gene were incubated with the fetal donor cell population. The expression of this bacterial marker gene can be specifically localized in situ with an X-Gal histochemical staining reaction. By double labeling with antibodies to the neuronal protein synaptophysin or to glial fibrillary acidic protein (GFAP) and X-Gal histochemistry, we could demonstrate expression of the retroviral construct in all major cell types of the graft including neurons, astrocytes and endothelial cells (Wiestler et al. 1992). There was no evidence that integration and expression of retroviral constructs interfere with the development of the transplants. Using retrovirus-mediated gene transfer into neural grafts, it is therefore possible to study putative oncogene effects in neuroectodermal and nonneuroectodermal cells.

Cellular Tropism of Oncogenes in the CNS

Many of the neurotropic oncogenes which we studied in neural grafts have exerted a striking tropism for distinct target cells in the brain. Two examples of genes with target specificity for endothelial cells are the polyoma medium T gene and the K-*fgf* oncogene. Medium T is the transforming gene of the polyoma DNA tumor virus. It encodes a membrane protein which associates with and activates cellular protein-tyrosine kinases including the products of the proto-oncogenes *src*, *yes*, and *fyn* (Grussenmeyer et al. 1985). Since some of these proto-oncogenes are preferentially expressed in the nervous system, medium T was an interesting candidate for a gene with potential neurotropic effects. To our surprise, the great majority of host animals carrying neural grafts exposed to the medium T retroviral vector (Williams et al. 1988) developed fatal intracerebral hemorrhage within the first month following stereotaxic transplantation (Fig. 3). Histopathologically, the transplants exhibited vascular malformations with morphological features of endothelial hemangiomas (Aguzzi et al. 1991). In situ hybridization experiments were carried out to localize transcripts of the medium T gene in the grafts. These reactions demonstrated high levels of medium T RNA in affected endothelia but also in neurons and astrocytes which showed a normal morphology. This indicates that the selective induction of endothelial lesions is the result of a particular susceptibility of developing CNS endothelia for a growth disrupting activity of medium T. Other cell types in the brain appear to tolerate this oncoprotein without morphologically detectable changes. However, in the few host animals which survived for an extended period, occasional

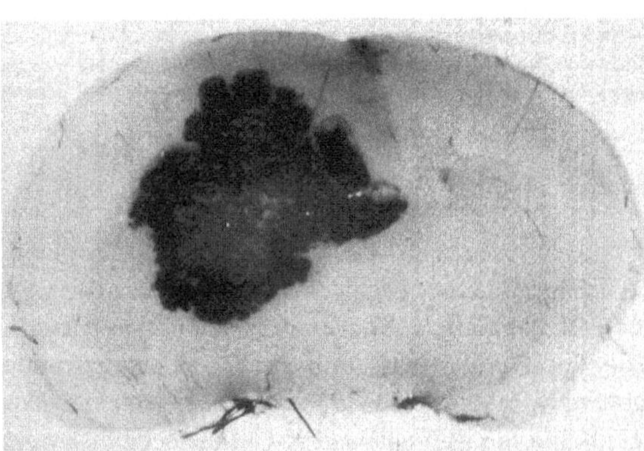

Fig. 3. Hemangioma with fatal intracerebral hemorrhage in a graft harboring the medium T gene of polyoma virus

astrocytomas were observed in the transplant after latency periods of 9–12 months. From this finding it would appear that in addition to interfering with the differentiation of endothelial cells, medium T also has the potential to initiate an early stage of transformation in astrocytes. Taking advantage of the neomycin phosphotransferase selectable marker gene contained in the retroviral construct, we have been able to derive G418-resistant endothelial cell lines from hemangiomas in neural transplants. These cells are currently analysed for blood brain barrier properties.

The K-*fgf*/*hst* oncogene is a member of the fibroblast growth factor family which at present comprises seven genes. K-*fgf* was originally identified by transfection of DNA from Kaposi's sarcoma and gastric carcinomas into NIH-3T3 cells (Delli-Bovi et al. 1987; Sakamoto et al. 1986). It encodes a secretory protein, which, in contrast to other fibroblast growth factors (FGFs), harbors a signal peptide sequence (Marics et al. 1989). At the time when we initiated transplantation experiments with a retroviral vector containing the K-*fgf* cDNA, little was known about potential in vivo effects of this growth factor, and there was no evidence for a neurotropic activity (Talarico and Basilico 1991). Recipient animals harboring neural grafts exposed to K-*fgf* were asymptomatic for observation periods up to 18 months. There was no evidence for tumor development in any of these transplants. However, upon histopathological anaylsis, focal accumulation of proliferated capillaries was seen in all cases (Brüstle et al. 1992). These foci were always confined to the transplanted tissue. The changes were very prominent in two of the grafts and were classified as angiomas in these two animals. We have never observed similar lesions in mock-infected grafts or in neural transplants exposed to other oncogenes. Immunohistochemical reactions with an antiserum to K-FGF and in situ hybridization experiments with an antisense RNA probe complementary to the K-*fgf* sequence demonstrated expression of the gene in a small fraction of perivascular cells adjacent to the proliferated capillaries. These cells showed a glial morphology and most likely represent astrocytes. No signal was observed in endothelia. This pattern of expression suggests a paracrine mechanism of endothelial growth stimulation. K-FGF is produced and secreted by neural cells and exerts a specific effect on neighboring endothelia which presumably carry receptors for this growth factor. These findings raise the intriguing questions if K-*fgf* functions as a physiological growth and differentiation signal in CNS endothelia and if it plays a role in the pathogenesis of CNS vascular malformations.

Long-Term Growth Factor Expression in Neural Transplants

An important finding of the work with K-*fgf* was the long-term expression of the Kaposi's sarcoma-derived fibroblast growth factor (K-FGF) for a period of at least 13 months following transplantation. These results provide strong evidence for long-term expression of a biologically active growth factor in primary neural transplants.

Gene transfer into living organisms represents one of the most promising therapeutic strategies for the treatment of many hereditary and nonhereditary diseases.

Several cell types, i.e., myoblasts, keratinocytes, skin fibroblasts, hepatocytes, lymphocytes, and bone marrow cells have been used as delivery systems for recombinant proteins (Armentano et al. 1990; Barr and Leiden 1991; Flowers et al. 1990; Friedmann 1989; Miller 1990). These cell types offer the advantage that they can be easily isolated from the recipient and – after in vitro transduction – reintroduced into the donor organism. However, in many instances expression of the transmitted genes is not sustained in the grafts in vivo (Miller 1990). Genetically modified cells have also been transplanted into the central nervous system. Most of these studies have employed nonneural donor cells such as fibroblasts (Fisher et al. 1991). Surprisingly, high-level expression of K-*fgf* in the grafts was maintained at the longest posttransplantation interval, i.e., 13 months. Although the number of recombinant cells could not be assessed quantitatively, we would estimate the percentage of K-*fgf* expressing cells at 0.1%–1% of the graft cell population. No neoplastic or preneoplastic lesions were found in any of the grafts. To further investigate the oncogenic potential of the K-*fgf* gene in vivo, we have combined the retroviral vector encoding K-*fgf* with a second transforming agent by transplacentally exposing the fetal donor cells to *N*-ethyl-*N*-nitrosourea (NEU), a powerful neurotropic carcinogen (Burger et al. 1988; Druckrey et al. 1966). It was shown previously that a single transplacental exposure of the donor animals to NEU is not sufficient to induce neoplasms but results in an increased susceptibility of neural grafts to neoplastic transformation by an activated *myc* oncogene (Brüstle et al., 1993). The combination of NEU-pretreatment and retroviral transfer of the K-*fgf* gene failed to induce a neoplastic phenotype in CNS transplants, indicating that integration and expression of K-*fgf* had no significant transforming effect on cells of the central nervous system.

Although our results are at a preliminary stage and have to be complemented by a detailed correlation between the age of the transplant and transgene expression, they provide clear evidence that retrovirus-mediated gene transfer into syngeneic fetal brain transplants represents an efficient approach for introduction and long-term expression of foreign genes in the central nervous system. Stable integration and expression of the retrovirally transmitted genes in a small subset of the donor cell population can be sufficient to induce a trophic effect without causing neoplastic or preneoplastic lesions. In contrast to the high levels of transgene expression which are required for systemic substitution purposes, for example, delivery of recombinant growth hormone from genetically modified myoblast grafts (Dhawan et al. 1991), local expression of secretory proteins in only a small percentage of grafted cells appears to be sufficient to achieve a significant biological effect in neural transplants. Since the high levels of transgene expression observed in neurons and glia were not associated with morphological alterations in the respective cells, Moloney murine leukemia virus (MoMLV) derived retroviral vectors appear to represent a useful vehicle for gene transfer into neural cells. Gene transfer studies with MoMLV-derived retroviruses in nonneural tissues have usually not achieved long-term transgene expression (Gage and Fisher 1991). This may indicate that primary neural cells are a preferred candidate for stable expression of retrovirally transmitted genes.

Cooperation of Transforming Genes in the Brain

The multistep nature of neoplastic transformation strongly suggests the involvement of a number of tumor-associated genes which accomplish distinct stages of this process. In some instances such as human colon cancer or malignant gliomas (see von Deimling et al., this issue), specific combinations of affected oncogenes and tumor-supressor genes have already been identified (Hunter 1991). A paradigm for oncogene complementation are the *ras* and *myc* genes which efficiently cooperate in transforming fibroblasts in vitro and the developing prostate gland in vivo (Thompson et al. 1989; Land et al. 1983). Retrovirus-mediated gene transfer into neural grafts provided us with a potent approach to study the cooperation of these two genes in the brain. For these experiments, we have used retroviral vectos which either encode a solitary v-Ha-*ras* or v-*gag*/*myc* gene or coexpress both genes simultaneously from the same retroviral genome (Wiestler et al. 1992). The *myc* gene did not cause any pathological phenotype in the transplants. Upon transfer of an activated v-Ha-*ras* oncogene, 50% of the grafts developed gliomas after latency periods of 6–9 months indicating that ras may initiate transformation of glial cells which requires additional, spontaneous mutations of cellular genes for macroscopic tumors to develop. In contrast, the ras&myc retroviral vector exhibited a striking tumorigenic potential in fetal brain transplants. Within 2–4 weeks following stereotaxic transplantation, there were multiple malignant tumors present in all recipients with vital grafts. Histopathologically, these neoplasms were classified as poorly differentiated neuroectodermal tumors of glial origin. Many of these tumors exhibited features of human glioblastomas. Aggressive cell lines were readily established from several of these gliomas and expression of both oncogenes was demonstrated in the tumor cells. These findings indicate that ras&myc exert a powerful complementary transforming potential on neuroglial precursor cells in vivo.

In contrast to a variety of human carcinomas, brain tumors do not usually carry activated *ras* oncogenes. We were, therefore, wondering what other genes may cooperate with a *myc* oncogene in transforming cells of the brain. In an attempt to mutationally activate and identify such genes we have modified the transplantation approach by combining two carcinogenic agents, i.e. a neurotropic chemical carcinogen and the v-*gag*/*myc* gene. Using a combination of transplacental carcinogen exposure and retrovirus-mediated oncogene transfer into fetal brain transplants, we have studied complementary transformation by NEU and the v-*myc* oncogene in the nervous system. Previous experiments had demonstrated that both agents will not induce tumors independently. On embryonal day 14 (ED14), pregnant donor animals (F344 rats) received a single intravenous dose of NEU (50 mg/kg). Twenty-four hours later (ED15), the fetal brains were removed, triturated and incubated with a retroviral vector carrying the v-*gag*/*myc* oncogene. Subsequently, these primary cell suspensions were transplanted stereotactically into the caudate-putamen of syngenic adult recipients. Of ten recipients harboring ED15 fetal brain transplants, five developed macroscopic tumors in the grafts after latency periods of 3–6 months. Histopathologically, all neoplasms were classified as malignant, poorly differentiated neuroectodermal tumors. No tumor development was observed in seven recipients harboring ED16 neural grafts. Cell lines were established from two tumors and the 110-kDa gag/myc fusion protein encoded by the retroviral construct was identified in the tumors by Western blotting. Several candidate genes for mutational activation by NEU including the H-*ras*, K-*ras*, and *neu* oncogenes were analyzed for specific point mutations by polymerase chain reaction (PCR) and direct DNA sequencing of the PCR products. However, no mutations were found in any of these genes indicating that NEU-mediated transformation in neural grafts may involve a novel cellular transforming gene. These findings lend further support to the multistep hypothesis of neoplastic transformation in the brain. The tumors induced in this model provide an interesting tool for the identification of cellular genes which cooperate with an activated *myc* oncogene in neurocarcinogenesis.

A Model for Primitive Neuroectodermal Tumors

Primitive neuroectodermal tumors (PNET) are a family of neoplasms which originate from multipotent precusor cells of the central nervous system (Aguzzi et al. 1988). These tumors are predominantly observed in children and young adults. The most common among the PNETs is the cerebellar medulloblastoma. A series of transplantation experiments with a retroviral construct encoding large T antigen, the transforming gene of the SV40 DNA tumor virus has surprisingly yielded an interesting model for PNETs. There is recent evidence that SV40 or a closely related virus which differs from human polyomaviruses JC and BK may have an etiological role in the development of ependymomas and choroid plexus papillomas in childhood (Bergsagel 1992). It has also been shown that expression of SV40 large T antigen under the control of different promoter elements can induce choroid plexus papillomas, retinoblastomas and PNETs of the pineal gland in transgenic mice (Theuring et al. 1990; Brinster et al. 1984). In CNS transplants carrying a retroviral vector with the cDNA for SV40 large T, PNETs developed in 75% of the grafts (Fig. 4). There was a median latency period of 9 months indicating that spontaneous mutations of cellular genes are required to complement the effect of large T. With the exception of a single well differentiated astrocytoma, only PNETs were observed in neural grafts exposed to large T. Histopathologically, these neoplasms were indistinguishable from human medulloblastoms. They also exhibited a characteristic immunohistochemical differentiation profile of PNETs, i.e., focal expression of synaptophysin and GFAP as evidence for both neuronal and glial differentiation pathways. Large T antigen was identified in these tumors immunohistochemically with a monoclonal antibody to large T protein and by PCR-mediated DNA amplification and sequence analysis of a 272-bp fragment of the large T gene. Several cell lines were derived from these PNETs. Upon intracerebral injection into syngeneic hosts, these cell lines gave rise to PNETs with identical morphological properties compared to the original neoplasms. Some of these PNETs displayed a striking migratory capacity which resulted in an extensive infiltration into both hemispheres of the adjacent host brain. The tumors may, therefore, represent an interesting model to study mechanisms of tumor cell infiltration in the brain.

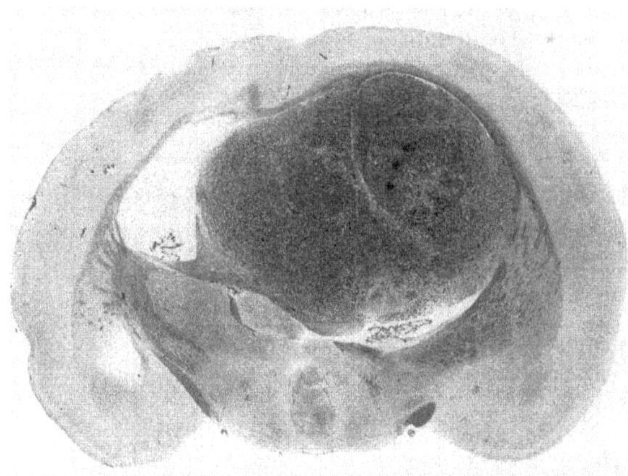

Fig. 4. Large solid tumor mass originating from a transplant exposed to the large T gene of SV40 virus. Histopathologically, this neoplasm exhibited characteristic features of a primitive neuroectodermal tumor

An intriguing property of the large T gene is the transformation mechanism employed by large T antigen. It encodes a nuclear phosphoprotein with specific DNA binding activity and a striking potential for complex formation with cellular proteins (Ludlow et al. 1989; DeCaprio et al. 1988). Among the nuclear proteins interacting with large T are the products of cellular tumor suppressor genes including p53 and RB-1 as well as heat shock proteins. Similar protein-protein complexes have also been reported in cell lines harboring the adenovirus E1A and E1B (Whyte et al. 1989) and the papilloma virus E7 genes (Dyson et al. 1989). This indicates that complex formation with and inactivation of tumor suppressor proteins may constitute an important mode of transformation by DNA tumor viruses. Due to this unique property of large T antigen, the PNETs induced in neural grafts and the cell lines derived from these tumors are an interesting model system to study complex formation of the large T polypeptide with cellular proteins in neoplasms originating in the grafts. Some of these proteins may be encoded by tumor suppressor genes with a particular tropism for cells of the nervous system.

Perspectives

The data summarized in this review demonstrate the potential of retrovirus-mediated gene transfer into brain transplants as an experimental approach to characterize in vivo functions of neurotropic genes and to study pathogenic mechanisms of neurological disorders. We have, so far, mainly focussed on tumor-associated genes (Table 1). However, neural grafts may also be employed to examine the pathogenesis of nonneoplastic disorders of the brain such as Alzheimer's disease or HIV-associated encephalopathies. Retroviral constructs with cDNAs for HIV-encoded structural and regulatory genes or wild-type and mutant forms of the A4 amyloid precursor gene are available for such experiments.

A drawback of the current model is the limited time period during which primary neural donor cells can be manipulated in vitro. Attempts will, therefore, be made to

Table 1. Survey of neuropathological phenotypes observed in neural transplants following retrovirus-mediated transfer of oncogene cDNAs.

Oncogene	Phenotype	Latency
medium T	Hemangiomas	2–6 weeks
medium T	Anaplastic gliomas	9–15 months
v-src	Gliomas, sarcomas	3–6 months
K-fgf/hst	Capillary proliferation Capillary angiomas	6–12 months
SV40 large T	PNET	5–9 months
v-Ha-ras	Anaplastic gliomas	4–6 months
v-myc *v-Ha-ras & v-myc*	PNET (rare) Anaplastic gliomas	2–8 weeks
v-Ha-ras & v-myc *Newborn host*	Hemangioendotheliomas PNET, leukemias	4–8 weeks
v-myc + ENU	Anaplastic gliomas	3–5 months

For a detailed description, see Wiestler et al. 1992a.

use pluripotent neural precursors as alternative donor cells. This would allow to introduce multiple genetic alterations and to achieve targeted gene disruption in neural cells. The extraordinary potential of the homologous recombination technique for specific mutagenesis of cellular genes has already been shown in analogous experiments with embryonic stem cells in chimeric and transgenic mice (Wright and Hogan 1991). Experimental and clinical neurobiology will particularly benefit from such studies.

References

Aguzzi A, Wiestler OD, Kleihues P (1988) Differentiation in the medulloblastoma: an immunohistochemical evaluation of 247 cases from the therapy trial SIOP/GPO MED 84. Verh Dtsch Ges Path 72:284–287

Aguzzi A, Kleihues P, Heckl K, Wiestler OD (1991) Cell type-specific tumor induction in neural transplants by retrovirus-mediated oncogene transfer. Oncogene 6:113–118

Armentano D, Thompson AR, Darlington G, Woo SLC (1990) Expression of human factor IX in rabbit hepatocytes by retrovirus-mediated gene transfer: potential for gene therapy of hemophilia B. Proc Natl Acad Sci USA 87:6141–6145

Barr E, Leiden JM (1991) Systemic delivery of recombinant proteins by genetically modified myoblasts. Science 254:1507–1509

Bergsagel DJ, Finegold MJ, Butel S, Kupsky WJ, Garcea RL (1992) DNA sequences similar to those of simian virus 40 in ependymomas and choroid plexus tumors of childhood. N Engl J Med 326:988–993

Brinster RL, Chen HY, Messing A, van Dyke T, Levine AJ, Palmiter R (1984) Transgenic mice harboring SV40 T antigen genes develop characteristic brain tumors. Cell 37:367–379

Brüstle O, Aguzzi A, Talarico D, Basilico C, Kleihues P, Wiestler OD (1992) Angiogenic activity of the K-fgf/hst oncogene in neural transplants. Oncogene 7:1177–1183

Brüstle O, Petersen I, Radner H, Höll T, Plate KH, Kleihues P, Wiestler OD (1993) Complementary tumor induction in neural grafts exposed to *N*-ethyl-*N*-nitrosourea and an activated *myc* gene. Carcinogenesis 14:1715–1718

Burger PC, Shibata T, Aguzzi, A, Kleihues P (1988) Selective induction by N-nitrosoethylurea of oligodendrogliomas in fetal forebrain transplants. Cancer Res 48:2871–2875
Cone RD, Mulligan RC (1984) High efficiency gene transfer into mammalian cells: generation of helper-free recombinant retrovirus with broad mammalian host range. Proc Natl Acad Sci USA 81:6349–6353
DeCaprio JA, Ludlow JW, Figge J, Shew J-Y, Huang C-M, Lee W-H, Marsilio E, Paucha E, Livingston DM (1988) SV40 large tumor antigen forms a specific complex with the product of the retinoblastoma susceptibility gene. Cell 54:275–283
Delli-Bovi P, Curatola AM, Kern FG, Greco A, Ittmann M, Basilico C (1987) An oncogene isolated by transfection of Kaposi's sarcoma DNA encodes a growth factor that is a member of the FGF family. Cell 50:729–737
Dhawan J, Pan LC, Pavlath GK, Travis MA, Lanctot AM, Blau HM (1991) Systemic delivery of human growth hormone by injection of genetically engineered myoblasts. Science 254:1509–1512
Druckrey H, Ivankovic S, Preussmann R (1966) Teratogenic and carcinogenic effects in the offspring after a single injection of ethylnitrosourea to pregnant rats. Nature 210:1378–1379
Dyson N, Howley PM, Münger K, Harlow E (1989) The human papilloma virus-16 E7 oncoprotein is able to bind to the retinoblastoma gene product. Science 243:934–937
Fisher LJ, Jinnah HA, Kale LC, Higgins GA, Gage FH (1991) Survival and function of intrastriatally grafted primary fibroblasts genetically modified to produce L-Dopa. Neuron 6:371–380
Flowers MED, Stockschlaeder MAR, Schuening FG, Niederwieser D, Hackman R, Miller AD, Storb R (1990) Long-term transplantation of canine keratinocytes made resistant to G418 through retrovirus-mediated gene transfer. Proc Natl Acad Sci USA 87:2349–2353
Friedmann T (1989) Progress toward human gene therapy. Science 244:1275–1281
Gage FH, Fisher, LJ (1991) Intracerebral grafting: a tool for the neurobiologist. Neuron 6:1–12
Grussenmeyer T, Scheidtmann KH, Hutchinson MA, Eckhart W, Walter G (1985) Complexes of polyoma virus medium T antigen and cellular proteins. Proc Natl Acad Sci USA 82:7952–7954
Hanahan D (1989) Transgenic mice as probes into complex systems. Science 246:1265–1275
Hunter T (1991) Cooperation between oncogenes. Cell 64:249–270
Land H, Parada LF, Weinberg RA (1983) Tumorigenic conversion of primary embryo fibroblasts requires at least two cooperating oncogenes. Nature 304:596–602
Ludlow JW, DeCaprio JA, Huang C-M, Lee W-H, Paucha E, Livingston DM (1989) SV40 large T antigen binds preferentially to an underphosphorylated member of the retinoblastoma susceptibility gene product family. Cell 56:57–65
Mann R, Mulligan RC, Baltimore D (1983) Construction of a retrovirus packaging mutant and its use to produce helper-free defective retrovirus. Cell 33:153–159
Marics I, Adelaide J, Raybaud F, Mattei M-G, Coulier F, Planche J, de Lapeyriere O, Birnbaum D (1989) Characterization of the HST-related FGF.6 gene, a new member of the fibroblast growth factor family. Oncogene 4:335–340
Markowitz D, Goff S, Bank A (1988) A safe packaging line for gene transfer: separating viral genes on two different plasmids. J Virol 62:1120–1124
Miller AD (1990) Progress toward human gene therapy. Blood 76:271–278
Pattengale PK, Stewart TA, Leder A, Sinn E, Muller W, Tepler I, Schmidt E, Leder P (1989) Animal models of human disease. Pathology and molecular biology of spontaneous neoplasms occuring in transgenic mice carrying and expressing activated cellular oncogenes. Am J Pathol 135:39–61
Sakamoto H, Mori M, Taira M, Yoshida T, Matsukawa S, Shimizu K, Sekiguchi M, Terada M, Sugimura T (1986) Transforming gene from human stomach cancers and a noncancerous portion of stomach mucosa. Proc Natl Acad Sci USA. 83:3997–4001
Stuhlmann H, Cone R, Mulligan RC, Jaenisch R (1984) Introduction of a selectable gene into different animal tissue by a retrovirus recombinant vector. Proc Natl Acad Sci USA 81:7151–7155
Talarico D, Basilico C (1991) The K-fgf/hst oncogene induces transformation through an autocrine mechanism that requires extracellular stimulation of the mitogenic pathway. Mol Cell Biol 11:1138–1145
Theuring F, Götz W, Balling R, Korf H-W, Schulze F, Herken R, Gruss P (1990) Tumorigenesis and eye abnormalities in transgenic mice expressing MSV-SV40 large T-antigen. Oncogene 5:225-232
Thompson TC, Southgate J, Kitchener G, Land H (1989) Multistage carcinogenesis induced by ras and myc oncogenes in a reconstituted organ. Cell 56:917–930

Wagner EF (1990) On transfering genes into stem cells and mice. EMBO J 9:3025–3032
Whyte P, Williamson NM, Harlow E (1989) Cellular targets for transformation by the adenovirus E1A proteins. Cell 56:67–75
Wiestler OD, Aguzzi A, Schneemann M, Eibl R, von Deimling A , Kleihues P (1992) Oncogene complementation in fetal brain transplants. Cancer Res 52:3760–3767
Wiestler OD, Brüstle O, Eibl RH, Radner H, Aguzzi A, Kleihues P (1992a) Retrovirus-mediated oncogene transfer into neural transplants. Brain Pathol 2:47–59
Wiestler OD, Brüstle O, Eibl RH, Radner H, von Deimling A, Plate K, Aguzzi A, Kleihues P (1992b) A new approach to the molecular basis of neoplastic transformation in the brain. Neuropathol Appl Neurobiol 18:443–453
Williams RL, Courtneidge SA, Wagner EF (1988) Embryonic lethalities and endothelial tumors in chimeric mice expressing polyoma middle T oncogene. Cell 52:121–131
Wright C, Hogan B (1991) Another hit for gene targeting. Nature 350:458–459

The O-2A Lineage: From Rats to Humans

M. Noble

Ludwig Institute for Cancer Research, 91 Riding House St., London, W1P 8BT, UK

The O-2A^{perinatal} Progenitor

One aspect of our research programme has been to develop an analysis of precursor division and differentiation sufficiently detailed to allow growth of purified precursor cells in a manner compatible with subsequent transplantation of these cells into demyelinated lesions of the adult CNS. Accomplishment of this goal has required identification of the precursor cells for oligodendrocytes, elucidation of the cellular and molecular interactions which regulate the differentiation of these precursors and development of strategies for growing highly enriched precursor populations in a manner suitable for use in transplantation experiments.

The first step in our studies on oligodendrocyte development was the discovery that cultures derived from white matter tracts of the CNS contain two distinct astrocyte populations, termed type 1 and type 2 astrocytes (Raff et al. 1983a). These two cell types could be readily distinguished from each other on the basis of morphology, antigenic phenotype and response to growth factors. Most importantly, we found that optic nerves of perinatal rats contained a population of glial precursors which did not express glial fibrillary acidic protein (GFAP) at the time of isolation, but which could be induced to become GFAP$^+$ by growth in tissue culture.

Shortly after the identification of type 2 astrocytes we discovered that the precursor cells which we had shown can become type 2 astrocytes in vitro could also be induced to differentiate into oligodendrocytes (Raff et al. 1983b). Oligodendrocytic differentiation of these cells occurred when progenitors were grown in chemically defined medium and did not require the presence of inducing factors. In contrast, astrocytic differentiation required the presence of appropriate inducing factors, at least one of which is found in fetal sera of a number of different species (Raff et al. 1983b,c).

Initial studies on oligodendrocytic differentiation of oligodendrocyte-type 2 astrocyte (O-2A) progenitors isolated from optic nerves of perinatal rats presented the paradox that the cells we were studying were isolated at a time of maximal division of this lineage in vivo (Skoff et al. 1976a,b), yet cells did not divide in tissue culture. Resolution of this paradox began with the discovery that cortical astrocytes promote O-2A^{perinatal} progenitor division in vitro (Noble and Murray 1984). The astrocytes used in these studies expressed a similar phenotype to that of type 1 astrocytes of the optic nerve, which are the first identifiable glial cells to appear in the nerve (Miller et al. 1985). The similarity of these two populations led us to suggest that these astrocytes are responsible for supplying the mitogen(s) required to keep O-2A progenitors in division. Moreover, populations of O-2A^{perinatal} progenitors grown in the presence of purified cortical astrocytes were capable of undergoing extended division while also continuing to generate more oligodendrocytes (Noble and Murray 1984), a pattern of behaviour similar to that occurring in vivo. Thus, the failure of O-2A^{perinatal} progenitors to divide in our initial in vitro studies was due to the lack of necessary mitogens, which appeared to be supplied by another glial cell type. The discovery that purified cortical astrocytes can promote O-2A^{perinatal} progenitor division also helped to explain why these cells continue to divide in vivo even after the axons of the optic nerve were severed (David et al. 1984).

Further studies demonstrated that purified cortical astrocytes also promote the correctly timed differentiation in vitro of O-2A^{perinatal} progenitors isolated from optic nerves of embryonic rats (Raff et al. 1985). The mechanism by which this timing is controlled remains a mystery, although all evidence to date indicates that it is the O-2A^{perinatal} progenitors themselves which are measuring elapsed time (Temple and Raff 1986; Raff et al. 1988). A potential linkage between the measurement of elapsed time by dividing cells and the control of differentiation has also been observed for fibroblasts and haematopoetic stem cells (for review, see Groves et al. 1991). In the case of O-2A^{perinatal} progenitors, it appears that this biological clock causes clonally related dividing progenitors to differentiate synchronously into oligodendrocytes within a limited number of cell divisions (Temple and Raff 1986; Raff et al. 1988; Wren et al. 1992). However, it is not yet known whether the mechanism which underlies this synchronous differentiation of clones of dividing cells is also responsible for the first appearance of oligodendrocytes in the rat optic nerve at the day of birth in vivo, or the equivalent time in vitro.

The effects of purified cortical astrocytes, and of type 1 astrocytes from the optic nerve, on O-2A^{perinatal} progenitor division in vitro appear to be mediated by platelet-derived growth factor (PDGF; Noble et al. 1988; Raff et al. 1988; Richardson et al. 1988; Pringle et al. 1989). O-2A^{perinatal}progenitors exposed to either PDGF or astrocyte-conditioned medium exhibited a bipolar morphology, migrated extensively (with an average migration rate of 21.4 1.6 mm/h) and divided with an average cell cycle length of 18 h. PDGF was also as potent as type 1 astrocytes at promoting the correctly timed differentiation in vitro of embryonic O-2A progenitors into oligodendrocytes (Raff et al. 1988). Moreover, antibodies to PDGF blocked the mitogenic effect of type 1 astrocytes on embryonic O-2A progenitor cells, causing these cells to cease division and to differentiate prematurely even when growing on monolayers of type 1 astrocytes. Thus, this single mitogen was able to elicit a complex behavioural phenotype from O-2A^{perinatal} progenitors which included normal functioning of the cellular mechanisms involved in the measurement of elapsed time. It is interesting that recent studies have indicated that neurons, which also promote division of O-2A^{perinatal} progenitors in vitro (Gard and Pfeiffer 1990;

Hunter and Bottenstein 1991), may also be a source of PDGF. Indeed, the results of in situ labelling of sections of normal adult CNS with PDGF cDNA probes suggests that neurons are the major producers of this mitogen in adult tissue (Sasahara et al. 1991; Yeh et al. 1991). However, the specific contributions of either neuronal or astrocytic production of PDGF to the development of the O-2A lineage in vivo is not yet known.

O-2A progenitors can also express a variety of developmental programmes other than the one elicited by exposure to PDGF (Bögler et al. 1990). For example, O-2A^{perinatal} progenitors induced to divide by basic fibroblast growth factor (bFGF) were multipolar and showed little migratory behaviour. In addition, cells induced to divide by bFGF had a cell-cycle length of 45 12 h, in contrast with the 18 4 h cell cycle length elicited by exposure to PDGF. These results indicate that PDGF and bFGF function in the O-2A lineage as modulators of differentiation as well as functioning as promoters of cell division. PDGF and bFGF also differ in their effects on oligodendrocytes themselves, in that only bFGF is able to promote division of these cells (Eccleston and Silberberg 1985; Saneto and de Vellis 1985; Bögler et al. 1990). Moreover, bFGF can inhibit the differentiation of purified O-2A^{perinatal} progenitors (McKinnon et al. 1990; Mayer et al. 1993), an inhibition which can be overridden by a factor (or factors) secreted by astrocytes (Mayer et al. 1993), and also by ciliary neurotrophic factor (CNTF) and leukaemia inhibitory factor (Mayer et al., 1994).

The most intriguing result of our studies with PDGF and bFGF was the discovery that O-2A^{perinatal} progenitors exposed simultaneously to these two mitogens continued to divide without differentiating into oligodendrocytes (Bögler et al. 1990). For example, cultures of optic nerves of 19-day-old rat embryos began to generate oligodendrocytes after 2 days when established in the presence of PDGF alone (Raff et al. 1988; Bögler et al. 1990), yet remained oligodendrocyte-free even after 10 days of growth in the presence of PDGF + bFGF (Bögler et al. 1990). Further experimentation has demonstrated that O-2A^{perinatal} progenitors can be continually grown for many months in vitro so long as cells are continuously exposed to both of these mitogens (S.C. Barnett and MN, unpublished observations). O-2A^{perinatal} progenitors grown in this manner retain the ability to undergo oligodendrocytic differentiation when removed from the presence of both mitogens.

The discovery that cooperation between growth factors can cause prolonged self-renewal of precursors revealed a previously unknown means of regulating self-renewal in a precursor population. Such cooperation may, however, represent a more general phenomenon, as indicated by the importance of growth factor cooperation in promoting the extended division in vitro of haematopoetic stem cells (Cross and Dexter 1991) and primordial germ cells (Matsoi et al. 1992).

The ability to specifically expand populations of O-2A^{perinatal} progenitors in vitro has allowed us finally to achieve our goal of using such populations to repair demyelinated lesions in vivo. In collaboration with W. Blakemore, J. Crang and R. Franklin (University of Cambridge) we have injected various preparations of highly enriched O-2A^{perinatal} progenitor populations into demyelinated lesions of the rat spinal cord. In particular, purified populations of O-2A^{perinatal} progenitors expanded in vitro for 3 weeks were able to remyelinate more than 90% of the denuded axons in a lesion site following transplantation (Groves et al., 1993).

The O-2A^{adult} Progenitor

To attempt to gain insights into the cellular mechanisms underlying repair of demyelinated lesions in the adult animal, we also initiated studies on O-2A progenitors of the adult CNS. In our initial studies, which were again focused on the rat optic nerve, we found that O-2A progenitors isolated from adult animals differed from their perinatal counterparts in several ways. O-2A^{adult} progenitors have a unipolar morphology in vitro (Wolswijk and Noble 1989), whereas O-2A^{perinatal} progenitors are usually bipolar (Small et al. 1987; Wolswijk and Noble 1989). In addition, O-2A^{adult} progenitors have a longer average cell-cycle time in vitro than O-2A^{perinatal} progenitors (65 ± 18 versus 18 ± 4 h; Noble et al. 1988; Wolswijk and Noble 1989), migrate more slowly (4.3 ± 0.7 versus 21.4 ± 1.6 mm/h; Small et al. 1987; Wolswijk and Noble 1989) and take longer to differentiate (5 days versus 2 days for 50% differentiation; Wolswijk and Noble 1989). Furthermore, O-2A^{adult} progenitors stimulated to divide by type 1 astrocytes are $O4^+$ while dividing O-2A^{perinatal} progenitors are $O4^-$ (Wolswijk and Noble 1989; I. Sommer and MN, unpublished observations).

The discovery of an adult-specific glial precursor population raised a series of questions which were addressed in our subsequent studies. These questions were: (a) When do O-2A^{adult} progenitors first appear? (b) What is the developmental origin of these cells? (c) How is a population of O-2A progenitors maintained in the optic nerve of adult animals? (d) What are the molecular mechanisms responsible for the differences in behaviour between O-2A^{perinatal} progenitors and O-2A^{adult} progenitors?

O-2A^{adult} progenitor-like cells can be identified in rat optic nerve cultures from as early as 7 days after birth, while such cells do not appear to be present in optic nerve cultures isolated from newborn animals (Wolswijk et al. 1990). O-2A^{adult} progenitors become the dominant progenitor population in the optic nerve by 1 month after birth. However, replacement of the *perinatal* progenitor population by the *adult* one occurs gradually, and both O-2A^{perinatal} and O-2A^{adult} progenitors can be isolated from optic nerves during the period between 7 days and 1 month after birth.

The source of O-2A^{adult} progenitors during development appears to be a subpopulation of O-2A^{perinatal} progenitors (Wren et al. 1992). This hypothesis is supported by time-lapse microcinematographic observations of cultures of dividing progenitors isolated from optic nerves of 3-week old rats. In these experiments, we observed families of cells in which the founder member expressed characteristics of O-2A^{perinatal} progenitors and initially gave rise to further cells with the characteristics of O-2A^{perinatal} progenitors (i.e. bipolar morphology, rapid rates of migration and division), but subsequent progeny in the family expressed the characteristics of O-2A^{adult} progenitors (i.e. unipolar morphology, slow rates of division and migration). In addition, continued passaging of *perinatal* progenitors on monolayers of purified cortical astrocytes was associated with the generation of *adult* progenitor-like cells and loss of *perinatal*-progenitor-like cells, a transition superficially similar to that which appears to occur in vivo (Wolswijk et al. 1990).

In contrast to the events thought to be involved in the initial appearance of O-2A^{adult} progenitors, we think that maintenance of these cells in the adult optic nerve may be the result of asymmetric division and differentiation of O-2A^{adult} progenitors themselves (Wren et al. 1992). Analysis of the composition of individual colonies derived from O-2A^{adult} progenitors, grown at clonal densities, indicates that these cells can produce colonies containing both oligodendrocytes and dividing progenitor cells. Such a colony composition is strikingly different from that observed in colonies derived from O-2A^{perinatal} progenitors, in which the generation of oligodendrocytes is associated with cessation of progenitor division and initiation of differentiation in all members of a clonal family (Temple and Raff 1986; Wren et al. 1992).

The capacity of O-2A^{adult} progenitors to undergo assymmetric division and differentiation is consistent with the hypothesis that these cells are stem cells (Wren et al. 1992). O-2A^{adult} progenitors also express other properties of stem cells, such as long cell-cycle times (Wolswijk and Noble 1989; Wolswijk et al. 1991; Wren et al. 1992). The composition of clonal colonies of O-2A^{adult} progenitors growing in vitro on purified cortical astrocytes for 25 days also suggests that some of these cells may be able to also exist in a near-quiescent state, with cell-cycle lengths in excess of 150 h, without differentiating (Wren et al. 1992). Moreover, O-2A^{adult} progenitors seem to be capable of undergoing prolonged self-renewal, at least in vitro (Wren et al. 1992). Finally, these cells have the important quality of being maintained in the optic nerve throughout life (Wolswijk and Noble 1989; Wolswijk et al. 1990). Thus, at this stage of our research, we would suggest that it is most appropriate to regard O-2A^{adult} progenitors as stem cells (i.e. cells which are capable of functioning as a self-renewing population throughout life) and to regard O-2A^{perinatal} progenitors as true progenitor cells (i.e. cells which are programmed to differentiate within a limited time-span).

The derivation of O-2A^{adult} progenitors from O-2A^{perinatal} progenitors has interesting implications in respect to the possible developmental origin of stem cell populations. The results of our studies suggest that precursor cells with properties appropriate for early development can give rise not only to terminally differentiated end-stage cells, but also to a second generation of precursors with properties appropriate for later developmental periods (see discussions in Wolswijk and Noble 1989; Noble et al. 1991). In the O-2A lineage, it is this second group of precursors which represents the self-renewing stem cells. Whether the ancestral relationship between stem cells and pre-stem cells in other lineages is similar to that seen in the O-2A lineage is not yet known.

We have only recently begun to investigate the molecular mechanisms which allow O-2A^{perinatal} and O-2A^{adult} progenitors to express their different behaviours and know very little about the physiological alterations which underlie the differences between these cells. We have seen that O-2A^{perinatal} and O-2A^{adult} progenitors express their characteristic properties when grown on the same monolayer of purified cortical astrocytes (Wolswijk et al. 1990). We have also found that both types of progenitors can be isolated from optic nerves of perinatal rats of between 7 days and 1 month of age, suggesting that these populations also co-exist in vivo. Moreover, we have found that the specific properties of O-2A*adult* progenitors are elicited by growth in the presence of PDGF (Wolswijk et al. 1991), just as exposure of O-2A*perinatal* progenitors cells to PDGF is associated with expression of the specific properties which characterize these cells (Noble et al. 1988). Thus, these two cell types respond to a single signalling molecule by expressing different behaviours. Taken together, these results indicate that the differences between the O-2A*adult* and O-2A*perinatal* progenitors are intrinsic to the cells themselves and are not likely to be due to, for example, changes in the microenvironments found in the perinatal versus adult CNS or due to responsiveness to different growth factors found within the same environment.

O-2A Lineage Cells and Repair of Demyelinating Damage in Multiple Sclerosis

It has been of continued interest to find striking similarities between the properties of O-2Aadult progenitors cells and certain features of multiple sclerosis. We originally suggested that the slow division rate of O-2A*adult* progenitors induced to divide by type 1 astrocytes or PDGF might limit the ability of these cells to participate in lesion repair (Wolswijk and Noble 1989; Noble et al. 1991). In addition, we found that O-2A*adult* progenitors and immature oligodendrocytes bind and activate complement in the apparent absence of specific antibody, thus leading to their own destruction (Wren and Noble 1989; see also Scolding et al. 1989). This property was not shared by O-2A*perinatal* progenitors or other glial cells. Both of these properties are consistent with observations that repair of demyelinating lesions in children may occur more effectively than in adults (Kriss et al. 1988; for discussion of these issues see also Wren and Noble 1989; Compston et al. 1991).

One of our most exciting recent findings concerning O-2A*adult* progenitors is the discovery that simultaneous exposure of these cells to PDGF + bFGF converts many of them to a rapidly dividing and highly motile phenotype (Wolswijk and Noble 1992). The potential relevance of such findings to the repair of lesions in vivo is indicated by the increased production of FGFs and PDGF in CNS lesions (Logan 1988; Nietro-Sampedro et al. 1988; Lotan and Schwarz 1992) and indications that repair of virally-induced demyelination in vivo appears to be preceded by increases in the numbers of O-2A*adult* progenitor-like cells (Godfraind et al. 1989). It is particularly intriguing that our studies also suggest that the ability of O-2A*adult* progenitors to maintain a rapidly dividing phenotype is not maintained beyond a small number of divisions, suggesting intrinsic limitations may exist in the extent to which these cells are capable of contributing to myelin repair (Wolswijk and Noble 1992). Such a possibility is reminiscent of claims that multiple sclerosis lesions are initially repaired but eventually become permanently demyelinated.

The Human O-2A Lineage

Our confidence in the potential relevance of our work on rodent tissues to the analysis of human oligodendrocytes and their precursors has been recently increased by the results of experiments on cells derived from human gliomas. Specifically, by growing human glioma specimens in a variety of conditions we have been able to isolate a population of cells which are clearly derived from human O-2A progenitors (work in progress). These cells express antigens characteristic of the O-2A lineage of the rat (and are HNK-1$^+$, A2B5$^+$ and GD3$^+$) can differentiate into astrocytes when grown in medium containing fetal calf serum and can generate both more progenitor-like cells and O4$^+$GalC$^+$ oligodendrocytes when grown in chemically defined medium conditioned by purified rat cortical astrocytes. Even more striking are our observations that these Hu-O-2A(Gb1) cells express a ^{1}H-labelled nuclear magnetic resonance (^{1}H-NMR) spectrum which is essentially identical to that otherwise uniquely expressed by O-2A^{perinatal} progenitors derived from rat tissues (see Urenjak et al. 1992a, b for ^{1}H-NMR characterization of normal glial cells).

The properties expressed by Hu-O-2A(Gb1) cells increase our confidence in the relevance of our rodent studies for several reasons. First, the phenotypic characteristics of the Hu-O-2A(Gb1) cells are remarkably similar to those of O-2A^{perinatal} progenitors. Second, the similarity in ^{1}H-NMR profiles between these cells and their rodent relatives is particularly dramatic in light of our findings that all of the major cell types of the CNS can be unambiguously distinguished from each other by their ^{1}H-NMR profiles (Urenjak et al. 1992b). Moreover, no other glioma-derived cells express a similar ^{1}H-NMR spectrum, just as no other glioma-derived cells that we have examined express the antigenic characteristics of an O-2A progenitor or the capacity to differentiate into oligodendrocytes. Finally, the cell-cell interaction which promotes division of Hu-O-2A(Gb1) cells is the same as that for O-2A progenitors of the rat, in that division of Hu-O-2A(Gb1) cells in vitro is specifically promoted by factor(s) secreted by purified cortical astrocytes.

It is critical to stress that the Hu-O-2A(Gb1) cells do not have the characteristics of fully transformed cells. Hu-O-2A(Gb1) cells grow as substrate-adherent cells which are absolutely dependent upon exogenous growth factors for their division. Moreover, as mentioned, Hu-O-2A(Gb1) cells can yield O4$^+$GalC$^+$ oligodendrocytes when grown in appropriate conditions.

References

Bögler O, Wren D, Barnett SC, Land H, Noble M (1990) Cooperation between two growth factors promotes extended self-renewal and inhibits differentiation of O-2A progenitor cells. Proc Natl Acad Sci USA 87:6368–6372

Compston DAS, Scolding NJ, Wren DR, Noble M (1991) The pathogenesis of demyelinating disease: insights from cell biology. Trends Neurosci 14:175–182

Crang AJ, Franklin JRM, Blakemore WF, Noble M, Barnett SC, Groves A, Trotter J, Schachner M (1992) The differentiation of glial cell progenitor populations following transplantation into non-repairing CNS glial lesions in adult animals. J Neuroimmunol 40:243–254

Cross M, Dexter TM (1991) Growth factors in development transformation and tumorigenesis. Cell 64:271–280
David S, Miller RH, Patel R, Raff MC (1984) Effects of neonatal transection on glial cell development in the rat optic nerve: Evidence thta the oligodendrocyte-type 2 astrocyte cell lineage depends on axons for its survival. J Neurocytol 13:961–974
Eccleston A, Silberberg DR (1985) Fibroblast growth factor is a mitogen for oligodendrocytes in vitro. Dev Brain Res 21:315–318
Fulton BP, Burne JF, Raff MC (1991) Glial cells in the rat optic nerve: The search for the type 2 astrocytes. Ann NY Acad Sci 633:27–34
Gard AL, Pfeiffer SE (1990) Two proliferative stages of the oligodendrocyte lineage: (A2B5+O4- and O4+GalC-) under different mitogenic control. Neuron 5:615–625
Godfraind C, Friedrich VL, Holmes KV, Dubois-Dalcq M (1989) In vivo analysis of glial cell phenotypes during a viral demyelinating disease in mice. J Cell Biol 109:2405–2416
Groves A, Bögler O, Jat P, Noble M (1991) The cellular measurement of time. Curr Opin Cell Biol 3:224–229
Groves AK, Barnett SC, Franklin RJM, Crong AJ, Mayer M, Blakemore WF, Noble M (1993) Repair of demyelinated lesions by transplantation of purified O-2A progenitor cells. Nature 362:453–455
Hunter SF, Bottenstein JE (1991) O-2A glial progenitors from mature brain respond to CNS neuronal cell line-derived growth factors. J Neurosci Res 28:574–582
Kriss A, Francis DA, Cuendet F, Halliday AM, Taylor DS, Wilson J, Keast-Butler J, Batchelor JR, McDonald WI (1988) Recovery after optic neuritis in childhood. J Neurol Neurosurg Psychiatr 51:1253–1258
Logan A (1988) Elevation of acidic fibroblast growth factors in lesioned rat brain. Mol Cell Endocrinol, 58:275–278
Lotan M, Schwarz M (1992) Postinjury changes in platelet derived growth factor-like activity in fish and rat optic nerves: possible implications in regeneration. J Neurochem 58:1637–1642
Matsoi Y, Zsebo K, Hogan BL (1992) Derivation of pluri potential embryonic stem cells from murine primordial gem cells in culture. Cell 70:841–847
Mayer M, Noble M (1992) The inhibition of oligodendrocytic differentiation of O-2A progenitors caused by basic fibroblast growth factor is overridden by astrocytes. Glia 8:12–19
Mayer M, Bhakoo K, Noble M (1994) Ciliary neurotrophic factor and leukemia inhibitory factor promote the generation, survival and maturation of oligo dendrocytes in vitro. Development (in press)
McKinnon RD, Matsui T, Dubois-Dalcq M, Aaronson SA (1990) FGF modulates the PDGF-driven pathway of oligodendrocyte development. Neuron 5:603–614
Miller RH, David S, Patel ER, Raff MC (1985) A quantitative immunohistochemical study of macroglial cell development in the rat optic nerve: In vivo evidence for two distinct astrocyte lineages. Dev Biol 111:35–43
Nietro-Sampedro M, Lim R, Hicklin DJ, Cotman CW (1988) Early release of glia maturation factor, acidic fibroblast growth factor after rat brain injury. Neurosci Lett 86:361–365
Noble M (1991) Points of controversy in the O-2A lineage: Clocks and type-2 astrocytes. Glia 4:157–164
Noble M, Murray K (1984) Purified astrocytes promote the division of a bipotential glial progenitor cell. EMBO Jl 3:2243–2247
Noble M, Murray K, Stroobant P, Waterfield M, Riddle P (1988) Platelet-derived growth factor promotes division and motility and inhibits premature differentiation of the oligodendrocyte-type-2 astrocyte progenitor cell. Nature 333:560–562
Noble M, Ataliotis P, Barnett SC, Bevan K, Bögler O, Wolswijk PG, Wren D (1991) Development differentiation and neoplasia in glial cells of the central nervous system Ann NYAS 633:35–47
Pringle N, Collarini EJ, Mosley MJ, Heldin C-H, Westermark B, Richardson WD (1989) PDGF A chain homodimers drive proliferation of bipotential: (O-2A) glial progenitor cells in the developing rat optic nerve EMBO J 8:1049–1056
Raff MC (1989) Glial cell diversification in the rat optic nerve. Science 243:1450–1455
Raff MC, Abney ER, Cohen J, Lindsay R, Noble M (1983a) Two types of astrocytes in cultures of developing rat white matter: differences in morphology surface properties and growth characteristics. J Neurosci 3:1289–1300
Raff MC, Miller RH, Noble M (1983b) A glial progenitor cell that develops in vitro into an astrocyte or an oligodendrocyte depending on the culture medium. Nature 303:390–396

Raff MC, Miller RH, Noble M (1983c) Glial cell lineages in the rat optic nerve. Cold Spring Harbor Symp Quant Biol 48:569–572
Raff MC, Abney ER, Fok-Seang J (1985) Reconstitution of a developmental clock in vitro: A critical role for astrocytes in the timing of oligodendrocyte differentiation. Cell 42:61–69
Raff MC, Lillien LE, Richardson WD, Burne JF, Noble MD (1988) Platelet-derived growth factor from astrocytes drives the clock that times oligodendrocyte development in culture. Nature 333:562–565
Richardson WD, Pringle N, Mosley MJ, Westermark B, Dubois-Dalcq M (1988) A role for platelet-derived growth factor in normal gliogenesis in the central nervous system. Cell 53:309–319
Richardson WD, Raff M, Noble M (1991) The oligodendrocyte-type-2 astrocyte cell lineage. Semin Neurosci 2:445–454
Saneto RP, DeVellis J (1985) Characterization of cultured rat oligodendrocytes proliferating in a serum-free chemically defined medium. Proc Natl Acad Sci USA 82:3509–3513
Sasahara M, Fries JWU, Raines EW, Gown AM, Westrum LE, Frosch MP, Bonthron DT, Ross R, Collins T (1991) PDGF B-chain in neurons of the central nervous system posterior pituitary and in a transgenic model. Cell 64:217–227
Scolding NJ, Morgan BP, Houston A, Campbell AK, Linington C, Compston DAS (1989) Normal rat serum cytotoxicity against syngeneic oligodendrocytes. J Neurol Sci 89:289–300
Skoff RP, Price DL, Stocks A (1976a) Electron microscopic autoradiographic studies of gliogenesis in rat optic nerve 1 Cell proliferation. J Comp Anat 169:291–311
Skoff RP, Price DL, Stocks A (1976b) Electron microscopic autoradiographic studies of gliogenesis in rat optic nerve 2 Time of origin. J Comp Anat 169:313–323
Skoff RP, Knapp PE (1991) Division of astroblasts and oligodendroblasts in postnatal rodent brain: Evidence for separate astrocyte and oligodendrocyte lineages Glia 4:165–174
Small R, Riddle P, Noble M (1987) Evidence for migration of oligodendrocyte-type-2 astrocyte progenitor cells into the developing rat optic nerve. Nature 328:155–157
Temple S, Raff MC (1986) Clonal analysis of oligodendrocyte development in culture: Evidence for a developmental clock that counts cell divisions. Cell 44:773–779
Urenjak J, Williams S, Gadian D, Noble M (1992) Specific expression of N-acetyl-aspartate in neurones O-2A progenitors and immature oligodendrocytes in vitro. J Neurochem 59:55–61
Urenjak J, Williams S, Gadian D, Noble M (1992) Proton nuclear magnetic resonance spectroscopy unambiguously identifies different neural cell types. J Neurosci 13:981–989
Vaysse PJ-J, Goldman JE (1990) A clonal analysis of glial lineages in neonatal forebrain development in vitro. Neuron 5:227–235
Wolswijk G, Noble M (1989) Identification of an adult-specific glial progenitor cell Development. 105:387–400
Wolswijk G, Riddle P, Noble M (1990) Co-existence of perinatal and adult forms of a glial progenitor cell during development of the rat optic nerve. Development 109:691–698
Wolswijk G, Riddle P, Noble M (1991) Platelet-derived growth factor is mitogenic for O-2A^{adult} progenitor cells. Glia 4:495–503
Wolswijk G, Noble M (1992) Cooperation between PDGF and FGF converts slowly dividing O-2A^{adult} progenitor cells to rapidly dividing cells with characteristics of their perinatal counterparts. J Cell Biol 118:889–900
Wren D, Noble M (1989) Oligodendrocytes and oligodendrocyte-type-2 astrocyte progenitor cells of adult rats are specifically susceptible to the lytic effects of complement in absence of antibody. Proc Natl Acad Sci USA 86:9025–9029
Wren D, Wolswijk G, Noble M (1992) In vitro analysis of origin and maintenance of O-2A^{adult} progenitor cells. J Cell Biol 116:167–176
Yeh J-J, Ruit KG, Wang Y-X, Parks WC, Snider WD, Deuel TF (1991) PDGF A-chain is expressed by mammalian neurons during development and in maturity. Cell 64:209–219

The Anti-Hu Syndrome: A Model Paraneoplastic Disorder

J. B. Posner

Memorial Sloan-Kettering Cancer Center, 1275 York Avenue, New York, NY 10021, USA

Introduction

In 1948 Derek Denny-Brown, one of the major figures in twentieth century neurology, published a paper describing two patients with a rapidly developing sensory neuropathy [1]. The pathological abnormalities included an inflammatory degeneration of neurons in the dorsal root ganglia and small cell lung cancer that had not metastasized to the nervous system. Although paraneoplastic syndromes affecting the nervous system had been described in occasional case reports as far back as the last century [2,3], and although a subacutely developing sensory neuropathy associated with occult cancer had also been described previously [4], Denny-Brown's careful clinical and pathological description was a major contribution, generating interest in these rare but physiologically interesting nervous system disorders. (This despite an almost certainly incorrect hypothesis that the tumor and the nervous system were competing for an essential substrate; he believed it to be pantothenic acid.)

Paraneoplastic syndromes can be defined as disorders occurring in patients with identifiable or occult cancer that affect organs or tissues remote from the site of the cancer and are not ascribable to invasion of the involved organism by cancer. When the nervous system is affected, paraneoplastic syndromes have also been called "remote effects" of cancer on the nervous system [5]. The term paraneoplastic syndrome applied to nervous system disorders associated with cancer was probably first used by Guichard in 1949, shortly following Denny-Brown's paper [6]. Popularized by him in a 1956 paper, the term was used to refer to polyneuritis associated with an underlying cancer [7]. In the 1950s and 1960s a spate of publications, particularly from the United Kingdom, popularized the notion of paraneoplastic syndromes and culminated in a symposium volume published in 1965 entitled *The Remote Effects of Cancer on the Nervous System* [5]. The interest generated in those years continues until today.

Cancer arising outside the nervous system can secondarily affect the nervous system in one of two ways. Tumor can either metastasize to brain, spinal cord, leptomeninges, or nerve plexuses, causing symptoms by compression, invasion or destruction, or the tumor can cause its nervous system symptoms indirectly (nonmetastatic complications of cancer) by infection, vascular disorders, metabolic and nutritional abnormalities or by cancer side effects of therapy. The neurological complications of cancer include the following:

Direct Neoplastic Effects (metastatic)
- Brain (usually parenchymal tumors)
- Spinal cord (usually compression)
- Peripheral and cranial nerves
- Leptomeningeal

Indirect (not metastatic or paraneoplastic complications)
- Metabolic
- Nutritional
- Infections
- Vascular disorders
- Complications of cancer therapy
- Paraneoplastic or "remote effects"

Strictly speaking, all of these nonmetastatic disorders are "paraneoplastic," but when the neurologist uses this term, he is referring to a much rarer group of disorders in which small, sometimes microscopic, cancers are specifically associated with destructive lesions of the central nervous system, usually affecting neurons rather than other cells or cell processes. Paraneoplastic syndromes can affect any portion of the central or peripheral nervous system [8], often producing characteristic disorders such as blindness from photoreceptor degeneration, memory loss and behavioral disturbances from limbic encephalitis, ataxia from Purkinje cell degeneration, quadriplegia or paraplegia from transverse myelopathy, and subacute sensory neuropathy (actually neuronopathy since the site of pathology is in the cell body as described by Denny-Brown [1]). More peripherally, the Lambert-Eaton myasthenic syndrome (a result of an antibody against calcium channels which complexes calcium channels at the neuromuscular junction and prevents release of acetylcholine) and dermatomyositis are also rather characteristic paraneoplastic syndromes. Other, less characteristic syndromes include sensorimotor peripheral neuropathy and proximal muscle weakness. Together, these patients are said to be suffering from neuromyopathy associated with cancer [9]. However, many of these symptoms may be a result of malnutrition and cachexia associated with cancer [10] although some appear to be pure paraneoplastic syndromes.

Paraneoplastic syndromes are not common. Even if one includes rather noncharacteristic syndromes of neuromyopathy, clinically evident paraneoplastic syndromes affect no more than 5%–6% of patients with cancer [11]. When one restricts oneself to more characteristic syndromes, (e.g. cerebellar degeneration, opsoclonus), the incidence is even lower. Characteristic syndromes were reported by the London group to occur in less than 1% of 1476 patients with cancer [11]. Except for the Lambert-Eaton myasthenic syndrome, where the incidence in patients with small cell cancer may be as high as 2%–3% [12], characteristic paraneoplastic syndromes occur with a frequency of considerably less than 1%. Their rarity in patients with cancer often leads oncologists to doubt their existence. For example, a gynecological oncologist may see 500 patients with ovarian cancer without encountering one with paraneoplastic cerebellar degeneration [13]. However, for the neurologist the situation is different: If the question is "How many patients with subacutely developing cerebellar degeneration in middle age have ovarian cancer?" rather than "How many patients with ovarian cancer have cerebellar degeneration?" the incidence figures change dramatically [13]. Recent estimates show that fully one-half of women with such a clinical syndrome have breast or gynecological cancer as its underlying cause. Estimates for the other characteristic syndromes are similar, from a not statistically significant 2% for patients with motor neuron disease to a high of 60% for patients with the Lambert-Eaton myasthenic syndrome. The estimated incidence of neurological symptoms associated with cancer is: Lambert-Eaton myasthenic syndrome, 60%; subacute cerebellar degeneration, 50%; subacute sensory neuronopathy, 20%; opsoclonus-myoclonus (children), 50%; opsoclonus-myoclonus (adults), 20%; sensorimotor peripheral neuropathy 10%; encephalomyelitis, 10%; dermatomyositis, 10%.

The wide variety of clinical paraneoplastic syndromes and the extensive literature on the topic make it impossible to review them all. Therefore, this review concentrates on one syndrome, that described by Denny-Brown, as a paradigm of most or all of the characteristic paraneoplastic syndromes.

History

The syndrome described by Denny-Brown in 1948 we now call the anti-Hu syndrome [14]. The syndrome is defined as sensory neuronopathy with or without encephalomyelitis associated with a specific autoantibody in serum and CSF called anti-Hu. Most often the patients are discovered to be suffering from small cell lung cancer.

In 1954 Henson et al. [15], examining the pathological findings in other patients, reported that in addition to the dorsal root ganglionitis there were inflammatory infiltrates and some cellular destruction in brainstem and spinal cord. Henson and colleagues [16] subsequently proposed the term "encephalomyelitis with carcinoma" many years later. In 1960 Brierley et al. [17] described a clinical and pathological syndrome that they called "subacute encephalitis...mainly affecting the limbic areas." This disorder was characterized by inflammatory infiltrates in limbic systems associated with an amnestic psychosis. Although they noted that at autopsy, two of their patients had small cell cancer of the lung, they believed it to be a coincidence and not related to the underlying disease. (In 1968 Corsellis and colleagues[18] recognized the association of limbic encephalitis and cancer.) The next year, Russell [19], referring to some of the cases of Henson et al., suggested that the inflammatory infiltrates need not be caused by a micro-organism such as a virus, as was believed at that time, but could represent an immune reaction. In 1965 Wilkinson and Zeromski [20], looking at the serum in a group of patients with paraneoplastic syndromes, described the presence in low titer of an antibody that reacted with guinea pig neurons. They described the antibody as reacting with the cytoplasm of neurons. Careful inspection of the photographs published reveals that the reaction was, in fact, nuclear. In 1982 Henson and Urich [21] reported that 89 patients in the literature had clinical signs of damage to different parts of the nervous system and postmortem findings of inflammation within the brain, brainstem, spinal cord, posterior root ganglia, and nerve roots associated with cancer. In 20, the disorder was restricted to dorsal root ganglia (sensory neuronopathy). Sixty-nine suffered from lung cancer; most cases were of small cell lung cancer. In 1985 and 1986 Graus and colleagues [22, 23] reported first two and then four patients with either encephalomyelitis or a pure sensory neuropathy associated with cancer. They found a high titer autoantibody in the serum that reacted with the nuclei of neurons throughout the nervous system. Graus et al. called the antibody anti-Hu after the first two letters of the last name of the index patient. Because of the clinical description by Wilkinson of cytoplasmic antibodies, the authors did not recognize that they were probably seeing the same antibody by a better technique that Wilkinson had described 20 years before.

Since 1985 the laboratory at Memorial Sloan-Kettering Cancer Center has collected over 70 serum or spinal fluid specimens containing high-titer anti-Hu antibodies [14]. These patients all have neurological disability which we have called the anti-Hu syndrome, clinically characterized by subacute sensory neuropathy and/or encephalomyelopathy. The encephalomyelopathy is characterized by one or usually more of the following findings: clinical and/or pathological involvement of limbic structures of the brain, cerebellum, brainstem, spinal cord, or autonomic neurons in spinal cord, or sympathetic ganglia. It is the clinical and pathological findings in this study that forms the basis of this review.

The Anti-Hu Antibody

The anti-Hu syndrome is defined by an antibody found at high titer in serum and cerebral spinal fluid (CSF) that reacts specifically with neurons of the central and peripheral nervous systems. The antibody does not react with non-neuronal structures in the central or peripheral nervous systems, nor does it react with other tissues outside the nervous system with the exception of some cells in the adrenal medulla and some cells, probably neurons, in the bronchial mucosa. Some cells in the anterior pituitary are also positive. The serum does react with several cancers, specifically all small cell lung cancers, and a substantial proportion of neuroblastomas as well as a few other tumors [24]. The antibody is not found in the serum of normal individuals, the serum of most patients with cancer who do not have paraneoplastic syndromes, or the serum of patients who have paraneoplastic syndromes other than encephalomyelitis or sensory neuronopathy. The antibody, however, is found at low titer in about 10% of patients with small cell lung cancer who do not have a paraneoplastic syndrome [25]. Evidence suggests that these patients differ significantly from patients with small cell lung cancer who do not harbor measurable titers of the antibody in that patients possessing the antibody have limited rather than extensive disease. Because these data were collected from consecutive patients being treated for lung cancer, the lesser disease in the antibody-positive patient is not accounted for by neurological symptoms which bring the patient to see a physician when the cancer was smaller. Instead, the data suggest that there is some association between the presence of the antibody and indolent growth of the cancer. A similar phenomenon has also been reported in the opsoclonus-myoclonus syndrome of infants and children associated with neuroblastoma [26]. However, in this disorder no antibody has been found [27].

The anti-Hu antibody is present in both serum and CSF. When the relative specific activity of the antibody in CSF is compared with that in serum from simultaneously drawn samples, the reactivity in the CSF is higher than that in the serum [28]. The implication is that the antibody is being synthesized in the central nervous system, probably by B cells within the brain itself. Selective transport of specific immunoglobulin across the blood-brain barrier seems a less likely explanation.

The antibody in CSF is more difficult to remove by plasma exchange than that in serum. Plasma exchanges were able to lower the serum titer of the antibody to 20% of its resting value but did not change the CSF titer at all [28]. If removing the antibody is clinically desirable, either more plasma exchange or another mechanism is then required.

The antibody can be identified by the antigen not only by immunohistochemistry but also by Western blot [23]. Extracts of cortical neurons from small cell lung cancer electrophoresed on polyacrylamide gels, then transferred to nitrocellulose and reacted with anti-Hu positive sera, give positive bands that are found with relative molecular weights between 35 and 40 kDa. Those bands are not found with normal sera nor are the bands found when anti-Hu sera is blotted against normal tissues with the exception of several tumors.

Clinical Findings in Anti-Hu Syndrome

Dalmau has reviewed the clinical findings in 71 patients with the anti-Hu syndrome as defined by the presence of high titers of the anti-Hu autoantibody in serum [14]. Fifty-five (77%) of these patients had small cell lung cancer but in only two of them was the cancer extensive (i.e. metastatic outside the lung and mediastinum). Other cancers (prostate, neuroblastoma, sarcoma) were rarely associated with the syndrome. When tumor from those patients was available, it invariably contained the Hu antigen. In nine patients no tumor has yet been found, including two who were examined at autopsy. (It is well known that tumors associated with paraneoplastic syndromes are often quite small. They frequently elude detection on clinical examination and imaging techniques in life and they may elude detection even after death. In one patient with a paraneoplastic syndrome, a careful search of the lungs revealed only one 4 mm focus of carcinoma [29], a finding that would have been missed had the pathologist not believed that a cancer had to be present and conducted an assiduous search. It is likely that in other patients the cancer has either been missed or an autoimmune mechanism destroyed the cancer. However, this point remains moot.)

In most paraneoplastic syndromes, the neurological disorder generally precedes the discovery of the cancer. In some patients symptoms precede any clinical or laboratory evidence of tumor. In a minority of patients, the tumor has been identified and may be under treatment at the time that the paraneoplastic syndrome develops. In a few patients with other paraneoplastic syndromes not associated with small cell lung cancer, the paraneoplastic syndrome may appear when the tumor recurs after initial successful treatment.

In over half of the patients with the anti-Hu syndrome, the clinical onset includes sensory symptoms, with a rapidly developing sensory loss in the hands and feet. In some patients the symptoms begin asymmetrically and may remain so throughout the illness. In a few patients the sensory loss begins in the trunk or face, and the extremities are initially spared. In the typical patient, after a few weeks or months, the sensory loss involves all four extremities.

In somewhat less than half of the patients, the presenting symptoms are nonsensory. These symptoms include: (a) limbic encephalopathy characterized by memory loss, behavioral changes, and sometimes complex partial seizures; (b) cerebellar signs including ataxia, dysarthria, and nystagmus not significantly different from another well-known paraneoplastic syndrome called paraneoplastic cerebellar degeneration [13]; (c) myelopathy including focal or generalized motor weakness or autoimmune failure; (d) brainstem signs including nystagmus, dysarthria, dysphagia, deafness, and sometimes extrapyramidal syndromes; (e) autonomic nervous system signs with postural hypotension, obstipation, etc. Although often unifocal at onset, by the time a few weeks to months have passed, most patients have evidence of symptoms in more than one area of the central or peripheral nervous system. Only a quarter of Dalmau's 71 patients remained unifocal throughout their course. When symptoms remain unifocal they usually are, as Denny-Brown described, those of sensory neuropathy. Other unifocal symptoms include limbic encephalopathy without evidence of motor or sensory system involvement and brainstem encephalitis.

When the symptoms are multifocal, about half of the patients have evidence of two of the above areas of the nervous system involved, and the others have three or more areas involved.

It is the rapid evolution of the neurological symptoms which helps identify the disorder as paraneoplastic rather than one of the more common multisystem degenerative disorders of middle age. This finding is true not only of the anti-Hu syndrome, but of most paraneoplastic syndromes in general. Characteristically, the symptoms begin relatively suddenly; the patient may actually be able to report the day of onset. They evolve rapidly. In a few patients, the symptoms have reached their maximum in several days. In others, they increase over several weeks to a few months and then cease getting worse. In a small minority of patients, symptoms may continue to worsen over many months to a year or more, or may worsen in an intermittent fashion.

The neurological symptoms are usually severe, disabling, and sometimes lethal. At its peak, the sensory neuropathy may be so severe that the patient is unable to stand or walk, sit without support, or feed herself even though motor function may be normal. In patients with limbic encephalitis, the loss of memory may be so severe that it mimics Korsakoff's syndrome. In patients with autonomic dysfunction, blood pressure, cardiac and respiratory status may be impaired sufficiently to cause early death. The median survival of Dalmau's patients with the anti-Hu syndrome was 7 months, actually less than the current median survival of the general population of patients with small cell lung cancer. However, the patients did not die as a direct result of their cancer since in all but two the disease remained limited at the time of death. Instead, they usually died of cardiovascular collapse, a direct result of their autonomic dysfunction.

Laboratory Data

The CSF is usually marked by a modest pleocytosis of 20–50 cells, especially if the patient is examined during the first several weeks of the illness. Thereafter the fluid may be acellular. In most patients the total protein is slightly elevated, although generally less than 100 mg/dl. There is an increase in IgG and evidence of intrathecal IgG synthesis [28]. When oligoclonal bands are searched for, the results are often positive. If the anti-Hu antibody is present in the serum, it also is in the CSF as well. Results of computed tomography and magnetic resonance imaging are generally normal. However, in a few patients, abnormalities have been identified in the medial temporal lobe of patients suffering from limbic encephalitis [30]. The abnormalities usually consist of a nonenhancing hypodensity on computed tomography or a nonenhancing hyperdensity on T2-weighted magnetic resonance images. Occasionally there is contrast enhancement in the medial temporal lobes early in the illness, which disappears as the illness progresses.

Treatment

A few patients with paraneoplastic syndromes have been reported to respond with improvement in their neurological state when the underlying tumor was successfully treated, or when the patient was treated with one or more immunosuppressive agents. Plasmapheresis has been reported to be effective in occasional patients as has immunosuppressive chemotherapy using agents directed at both the tumor and the immune system (e.g., cyclophosphamide). Spontaneous remissions have also been occasionally reported. Our own experience has been less happy [14]. Of 22 patients treated with corticosteroids, only two appeared to respond. No patients treated with plasma exchange or other immune suppressing agents have had a response. Instead, after several weeks to months, most patients stabilized. Stabilization tends to occur regardless of whether the patient is severely disabled or only moderately disabled. Those who are moderately disabled may continue to function, and treatment of the underlying tumor is usually more successful than one might expect from reading the literature concerning the treatment of small cell lung cancer. Those who are severely affected may die whether or not the underlying tumor is treated.

Pathological Abnormalities

At autopsy the tumor is usually a small cell lung cancer, 1 cm or so in diameter in the lung and microscopic in a few mediastinal lymph nodes. Frequently, the primary tumor cannot be found, and tumor is found only in the mediastinal lymph nodes. In the few patients who had cancers other than small cell lung cancer, the tumors were, likewise, small and nonmetastatic. The brain, brainstem, and cerebellum usually appear normal on microscopic inspection. In some spinal cords one can identify pallor of myelin in the posterior columns and/or atrophy of dorsal root ganglia. We have not found gross abnormalities in the limbic system although one might expect to see atrophy and, perhaps, gross gliosis of medial temporal lobes in some patients.

The microscopic pathology of the anti-Hu syndrome consists of three findings [32]. The first is neuronal loss which may affect any neuron in the central or peripheral nervous system, including myenteric plexus. The second is gliosis, usually at the site of the major neural loss and often associated with the formation of microglial nodules. The third finding is inflammation. Perivascular lymphocytic infiltration with T and B cells is found throughout the nervous system, and parenchymal infiltration, usually exclusively with T cells, is often found at sites of major neuronal and glial abnormality.

In the typical patient, large and small neurons in the dorsal root ganglia have disappeared. The sites of neuronal loss are marked either by inflammatory infiltrates with T cells or by nodules of Nagotte. There is secondary demyelination and axonal loss in the sensory nerves extending distally toward the periphery and proximally into the spinal cord involving the posterior columns. The spinal cord may be normal save for involvement of the posterior columns, or one might find more widespread damage to the spinal cord including loss of anterior horn cells and loss of axons in the lateral columns. Inflammatory infiltrates and cellular loss in the brainstem are common as well. In some patients there may be diffuse loss of Purkinje cells of the cerebellum similar to anti-Yo positive paraneoplastic cerebellar degeneration, but in one of our patients that loss was accompanied by T cell infiltrates at the site of the absent Purkinje cells, a finding not previously described in paraneoplastic cerebellar degeneration. Neuronal drop-out, gliosis, and inflammation occur in the brain as well, particularly in the limbic system, but at times in basal ganglion and cerebral cortex.

In general, there is a gross correlation between the site of major clinical findings and the pathology [32]. There are, however, exceptions. In one of our patients, sensory examination and deep tendon reflexes were reported to be normal 6 weeks before his death. Despite that, examination of many dorsal root ganglia revealed virtually no intact neurons and gross inflammatory infiltrates where neurons had formerly been. In another patient with such severe limbic encephalopathy that she was unable to care for herself because of memory and behavioral disturbances, autopsy revealed inflammation and gliosis of the limbic system, but the neurons of the hippocampus appeared strikingly well preserved. This was particularly striking because the patient died of cardiorespiratory collapse and remained essentially brain dead on a respirator for a week. Unequivocal ischemic changes were found in other neurons but seemed to spare those neurons which were putatively the site of the patient's clinical symptomatology.

Immunopathology

There is no difference in the appearance of tumor cells between anti-Hu patients and those who do not harbor the autoantibody. However, in addition to the fact that the tumors are often smaller and have not metastasized outside the thorax, there are other changes suggesting an immune response against the tumor. In this and other paraneoplastic syndromes, inflammatory infiltration has been reported to a greater degree than in patients with similar tumors but without paraneoplastic syndromes [33]. The inflammatory infiltrate seems to consist of T cells, B cells, natural killer cells, and macrophages. In addition, preliminary evidence suggests that MHC class 1 antigens are expressed on the surface of the tumor cells of those patients with the anti-Hu syndrome to a greater extent than can be found in patients with the anti-Hu negative small cell lung cancer.

Szabo and colleagues, using a biotinylated fusion protein cloned from a small cell lung cancer library (see below), have demonstrated that lymphocytes, both T cells and B cells, in the tumor of anti-Hu positive patients recognize the Hu antigen [34].

The inflammatory infiltrates in the central nervous system consist of a mixture of B and T cells (largely T) in the perivascular spaces and exclusively T cells in the parenchyma, with a preponderance of CD4 in some and CD8 in others[35], similar to that which one finds in other autoimmune disorders associated with inflammatory infiltrates in the central nervous system (e.g., multiple sclerosis). As in the tumor, biotinylated fusion protein identifies lymphocytes within the central nervous system of both T and B variety [34].

Perhaps the most striking immunopathological finding in the anti-Hu syndrome is the presence of IgG in the central nervous system. There are clinical reports of IgG and other plasma proteins being found within neurons in the central nervous system, particularly within neurons such as Purkinje cells and anterior horn cells, when the nervous system is examined at autopsy. In the hands of some investigators, proteins have been found in neurons regardless of the cause of death [36]. Others have reported IgG in neurons of the nervous system only in a particular disease. For example, Engelhardt and Appel reported IgG in anterior horn cells of patients dying of amyotrophic lateral sclerosis but not in patients dying of other diseases, even in a patient who had had ischemic damage to the spinal cord [37].

In the experimental situation, Fabian and Petroff [38] have reported that when rabbit IgG is injected intraperitoneally in rats, IgG can be found in neurons throughout the central nervous system, particularly in Purkinje cells and anterior horn cells. Injection of IgG into the subarachnoid space in experimental animals has been reported to be taken up by Purkinje cells. Graus has reported the injection of anti-Yo antibody (an autoantibody associated with paraneoplastic cerebellar degeneration and gynecological cancer) to be taken up selectively by Purkinje cells [39].

Our own autopsy experience has been different. We have not encountered identifiable IgG in the neurons of patients who die of cancer even when they have suffered severe anoxia prior to death. However, in all of the patients with the anti-Hu syndrome whom we have studied at autopsy, IgG can be found in neurons, not only the cytoplasm but the nucleus as well, sparing the nucleolus [32]. The IgG staining looks identical to the indirect immunoperoxidase reaction for the presence of the antigen, save for the fact that the anti-IgG stain often reacts with the neuropil and with glial cells, a finding one does not encounter when one attempts to identify the antigen.

The IgG found in the brains of patients with the anti-Hu syndrome is probably mostly anti-Hu antibody, as indicated by the fact that if one elutes the IgG from the brain and reacts it with cortical neuronal preparations on western blot, one finds the typical 35 to 40-kDa banding pattern of Hu. Furthermore, when identical amounts of IgG are applied to the nitrocellulose strips, the signal is stronger from brain than it is from either serum or CSF, indicating a higher relative specific activity of anti-Hu within the brain parenchyma when compared with serum or CSF. The same finding is true when IgG is eluted from the small cell lung cancers of anti-Hu positive patients. No such staining can be identified nor can antibody be eluted from the small cell lung cancers of patients who are not anti-Hu positive.

The anti-Hu antibody found in the nervous system of patients who die of the anti-Hu syndrome is not evenly distributed. Although the antigen can be found in all neurons, the antibody is found only in some neurons varying from patient to patient. For example, in one patient, no identifiable IgG could be found in the cerebellum despite the fact that the antigen is present in all cerebellar neurons. In general, there is a rough correlation between sites of major IgG deposition and the clinical and pathological abnormalities. That correlation suggests that the antibody may play a role in the pathogenesis of the disease.

The possibility that the IgG reached the nervous system in the agonal or early postmortem period is ruled out by the fact that identical IgG deposits within neurons have been found on biopsy of a patient with anti-Hu positive limbic encephalitis associated with small cell lung cancer. Similar biopsy from two patients with limbic encephalitis who were not anti-Hu positive (one with Hodgkin's disease and another with testicular cancer) failed to reveal IgG in neurons of the limbic system although inflammatory infiltrates were easily identified in perivascular spaces and in the parenchyma.

How the antibody enters the cell and how, once in the cell, it enters the nucleus is not understood. However, if the observations are accurate, the binding of the antibody to the antigen may inhibit its function and ultimately lead to the death of the cells. Alternately, the antibody may play no significant role in the pathogenesis of the disorder. The presence of T cells in the central nervous system and, in particular, the presence of T cells at the site of major neuronal pathology, suggests the possibility of a T cell attack on neurons. Because neurons are not believed to express MHC antigens on their surface, and these antigens are believed required for T cell recognition and cytotoxic attack, the problem of pathogenesis remains moot and will probably do so until an animal model of this paraneoplastic syndrome is developed. Our own attempts to produce an animal model by injection of antibody have failed to even identify the antibody within the central nervous system. Graus has identified antibody within Purkinje cells of the nervous system using the anti-Yo antibody injected intrathecally, but he detected no clinical or pathological changes in these animals [39]. The availability of fusion protein allows one to immunize the animals with antigen and, if this antigen plays a role in the pathogenesis of the disorder, one should be able to reproduce the disease.

Molecular Biology

Autoantibodies circulating in the serum of our patients with anti-Hu positive paraneoplastic syndromes make excellent probes to search expression libraries in order to locate the antigen identified by the anti-Hu antibody. Szabo and colleagues have cloned a gene from both a small cell lung cancer expression library and a brain expression library [34]. The gene codes for a protein that is recognized by all anti-Hu positive sera but by no normal sera nor sera of any patient with other autoimmune disease or other circulating autoantibodies. The gene codes for protein were approximately 35 kDa. The concensus sequence of the protein contains three RNA binding sites. The protein termed HuD is highly homologous with a *Drosophila* protein called ELAV, required for the normal development of the *Drosophila* nervous system. Muresu and colleagues[40] have mapped the gene to the short arm of chromosome 1. The gene appears to be alternately spliced with three transcripts present. The three transcripts are identical in brain and small cell lung cancer; the quantity of each is different in small cell lung cancer than in brain.

A second protein, HuC, has also been cloned from a brain library. The protein is highly homologous with HuD but is enclosed by a different gene, suggesting that there may be a family of Hu antigens that occur in different quantities or at different times in the developing nervous system.

Marusich and Weston[41] have reported that the Hu antigen is the earliest identifiable marker of neuronal development in the quail. Appearing when E2 neuroblasts have become committed neurons, Hu appears before any other neuronal markers are unequivocally positive. Similar findings in the mouse have been identified by Manley et al.(unpublished data) and by Graus [42].

Conclusions

The anti-Hu antibody is present in a subset of patients with small cell lung cancer. When present at high titer it is associated with a variety of neurological disorders including encephalomyelitis and sensory neuropathy, probably best called the anti-Hu syndrome. The presence of the anti-Hu antibody in the serum of a patient strongly suggests that the patient is suffering from small cell lung cancer or, more rarely, some other small cell tumor whether or not he has a paraneoplastic disorder. It also strongly suggests that if the patient has neurological disability, it is paraneoplastic in origin and associated with small cell lung cancer. Thus, the anti-Hu antibody, as with other antibodies that have been identified in patients with paraneoplastic syndromes, makes an excellent marker which not only strongly suggests that the patient's neurological disorder is paraneoplastic, but also suggests to the physician that a careful search for an underlying tumor should be undertaken.

In addition, autoantibodies in patients with paraneoplastic syndromes, which are relatively specific for tumor and central nervous system, make excellent probes for the cloning of proteins that may be of neurobiological interest. The fact that the antibodies identify antigens shared between nervous system and cancers suggests that the antigens may play a role in cellular growth, development and differentiation.

At the present time, the pathogenesis of central nervous system paraneoplastic disorders remains obscure. Unlike the Lambert-Eaton myasthenic syndrome in which the circulating IgG has been demonstrated to cause the clinical and electrophysiological symptoms, it is entirely unclear whether the autoantibodies in the anti-Hu syndrome and other central nervous system paraneoplastic syndromes play a role in clinical and pathological changes. However, the identification of the anti-Hu antibody within the neurons and within the nuclei of central nervous system suggests such a role.

References

1. Denny-Brown D (1948) Primary sensory neuropathy with muscular changes associated with carcinoma. J Neurol Neurosurg Psychiatr 11:73–81
2. Oppenheim H (1888) Uber hirnsymptome bein carcinomatose ohne nachweisbare veranderungen im gehirn. Charite-Ann 13:335–344
3. Oppenheim H (1899) Weiterer beitrag zur lehre von der acuten, nichteitrigen encephalitis und der poliencephalomyelitis. Z Nervenheilkd 15:1–27
4. Wyburn-Mason R (1948) Bronchial carcinoma presenting as polyneuritis. Lancet i:203–206
5. Brain L, Norris F (eds) (1965) The remote effects of cancer on the nervous system. Contemporary Neurology Symposia, vol 1. Grune and Stratton, New York
6. Guichard A, Vignon G (1949) La polyradiculonevrite cancereuse metastatique. J Med Lyon 5 (March):197–207
7. Guichard MMA, Cabanne F, Tommasi M, Fayolle J (1956) Polynevrites chez les cancereux et polynevrites paraneoplasiques. Lyon Med 41:309–329
8. Posner JB (1992) Pathogenesis of central nervous system paraneoplastic syndromes. Rev Neurol 148:505–512
9. Posner JB (1991) Paraneoplastic syndromes. Neurol Clin 9:919–936
10. Hawley RJ, Cohen MH, Saini N, et al.(1980) The carcinomatous neuromyopathy of oat cell lung cancer. Ann Neurol 7:65–72
11. Croft PB, Wilkinson M (1965) The incidence of carcinomatous neuromyopathy in patients with various types of carcinoma. Brain 88:427–434
12. Erlington GM, Murray NMF, Spiro SG, Newsom-Davis J (1991) Neurological paraneoplastic syndromes in patients with small cell lung cancer. A prospective survey of 150 patients. J Neurol Neurosurg Psychiat 54:764–767
13. Peterson K, Rosenblum MK, Kotanides H, Posner JB (1992) Paraneoplastic cerebellar degeneration: I. A clinical analysis of 55 anti-Yo antibody positive patients. Neurology 42:1938–1943
14. Dalmau J, Graus F, Rosenblum MK, Posner JB (1992) Anti-Hu associated paraneoplastic encephalomyelitis/sensory neuronopathy: A clinical study of 71 patients. Medicine 71:59–72
15. Henson RA, Russell DS, Wilkinson M (1954) Carcinomatous neuropathy and myopathy. A clinical and pathological study. Brain 77:82–121
16. Henson RA, Hoffman HL, Urich H (1965) Encephalomyelitis with carcinoma. Brain 88:449–464

17. Brierley JB, Corsellis JAN, Hierons R, Nevin S (1960) Subacute encephalitis of later adult life. Mainly affecting the limbic areas. Brain 83:357–368
18. Corsellis JAN, Goldberg GJ, Norton AR (1968) "Limbic encephalitis" and its association with carcinoma. Brain 91:481–496
19. Russell DS (1961) In: van Bogaert L, Radermecker J, Hozay J, Lowenthal A (eds) Encephalitides. Elsevier, Amsterdam, pp 131–135
20. Wilkinson PC, Zeromski J (1965) Immunofluorescent detection of antibodies against neurons in sensory carcinomatous neuropathy. Brain 88:529–538
21. Henson RA, Urich H (1982) Cancer and the nervous system. Blackwell Scientific, London
22. Graus F, Cordon-Cardo, Posner JB (1985) Neuronal antinuclear antibody in sensory neuronopathy from lung cancer. Neurology 35:538–543
23. Graus F, Elkon KB, Cordon-Cardo C, Posner JB (1986) Sensory neuronopathy and small cell lung cancer: An antineuronal antibody that also reacts with the tumor. Am J Med 80:45–52
24. Dalmau J, Furneaux HM, Cordon-Cardo C, Posner JB (1992) The expression of the Hu (paraneoplastic encephalomyelitis/sensory neuronopathy) antigen in human normal and tumor tissues. Am J Pathol 141:881–886
25. Dalmau J, Furneaux HM, Gralla RJ, Kris MG, Posner JB (1990) Detection of the anti-Hu antibody in the serum of patients with small cell lung cancer – a quantitative Western blot analysis. Ann Neurol 27:544–552
26. Altman AJ, Bachner RL (1976) Favorable prognosis for survival in children with coincident opso-myoclonus and neuroblastoma. Cancer 37:846–852
27. Luque FA, Furneaux HM, Ferziger R, Rosenblum MK, Wray SH, Schold SC, Glantz MJ, Jaeckle KA, Biran H, Lesser M, Paulsen WA, River ME, Posner JB (1991) Anti-Ri: an antibody 29 associated with paraneoplastic opsoclonus and breast cancer. Ann Neurol 29:241–251
28. Furneaux HM, Reich L, Posner JB (1990) Autoantibody synthesis in the central nervous system of patients with paraneoplastic syndromes. Neurology 40:1085–1091
29. Anderson NE, Budde-Steffen C, Wiley RG, Thurman L, Nadeau SE, Posner JB (1988) A variant of the anti-Purkinje cell antibody in a patient with paraneoplastic cerebellar degeneration. Neurology 38:1018–1026
30. Dirr LY, Elster AD, Donofrio PD, Smith M (1990) Evolution of brain MRI abnormalities in limbic encephalitis. Neurology 40:1304–1306
31. Graus F, Vega F, Delattre JY, Bonaventura I, Rene R, Arbaiza D, Tolosa E (1992) Plasmapheresis and antineoplastic treatment in CNS paraneoplastic syndromes with antineuronal autoantibodies. Neurology 42:536–540
32. Dalmau J, Furneaux HM, Rosenblum MK, Graus F, Posner JB (1991) Detection of the anti-Hu antibody in specific regions of the nervous system and tumor from patients with paraneoplastic encephalomyelitis/sensory neuronopathy. Neurology 41:1757–1764
33. Hetzel DJ, Stanhope R, O'Neil BP, Lennon VA (1990) Gynecologic cancer in patients with subacute cerebellar degeneration predicted by anti-Purkinje cell antibodies and limited in metastatic volume. Mayo Clin Proc 65:1558–1563
34. Szabo A, Dalmau J, Manley G, Rosenfeld M, Wong E, Henson J, Posner JB, Furneaux HM (1991) HuD a paraneoplastic encephalomyelitis antigen contains RNA binding domains and is homologous to elav and sex-lethal. Cell 67:325–333
35. Graus F, Ribalta T, Campo E, Monforte R, Urbano A, Rozman C (1990) Immunohistochemical analysis of the immune reaction in the nervous system in paraneoplastic encephalomyelitis. Neurology 40:219–222
36. Liu HM, Atack JR, Rapoport SI (1989) Immunohistochemical localization of intracellular plasma proteins in the human central nervous system. Acta Neuropathol 78:16–21
37. Engelhardt JI, Appel SH (1990) IgG reactivity in the spinal cord and motor cortex in amyotrophic lateral sclerosis. Arch Neurol 47:1210–121
38. Fabian RH, Petroff G (1987) Intraneuronal IgG in the central nervous system: Uptake by retrograde axonal transport. Neurology 37:1780–1784
39. Graus F, Illa I, Agusti M, Ribalta T, Cruz-Sanchez F, Juarez C (1991) Effect of intraventricular injection of an anti-Purkinje cell antibody (anti-Yo) in a guinea pig model. J Neurol Sci 106:82–87
40. Muresu R, Baldini A, Gress T, Posner JP, Furneaux HM, Siniscalco M HuD (1994) Mapping of the gene coding for a paraneoplastic encephalomyelitis antigen (HuD) to human chromosome site 1p34. Genet 65:171–178

41. Marusich MF, Weston JA (1992) Identification of early neurogenic cells in the neural crest lineage. Dev Biol 149:295–306
42. Graus F, Ferrer I (1990) Analysis of a neuronal antigen (Hu) expression in the developing rat brain detected by autoantibodies from patients with paraneoplastic encephalomyelitis. Neurosci Letters 112:14–18

Radiosurgery/Stereotactic External Beam Radiotherapy for Malignant Brain Tumours: The Royal Marsden Hospital Experience

M. Brada and R. Laing

Neuro-oncology Unit, and Academic Unit of Radiotherapy and Oncology, Institute of Cancer Research, and Royal Marsden Hospital, Downs Road, Sutton, Surrey SM2 5PT, UK

Introduction

Stereotactic external beam radiotherapy (SRT), often described as radiosurgery, is a method of delivering highly localized irradiation using either dedicated or conventional radiotherapy equipment. As a high-precision technique it requires accurate localization of tumour, improved patient immobilization and means of delivering focused radiation.

Neurosurgical technology with stereotactic frame and localization devices adapted for radiotherapy enables firm patient fixation and localization of tumour in three-dimensional space defined by stereotactic coordinates. Increasing the number of beams of external irradiation focuses radiation within the treated volume at the intersection of the beams with a higher dose differential between target and surrounding normal tissue. Historically this was carried out with multiple fixed orthovoltage beams and subsequently with multiple fixed Co^{60} sources (Leksell 1951). Currently available commercial equipment described as gamma knife contains over 200 collimated Co^{60} sources arranged in hemispheric distribution and focused onto a central point.

Moving the radiation source in an arc is equivalent to multiple fixed beams. Arrangement of multiple non-coplanar arcs or multiple non-coplanar beams achieve a localized dose distribution equivalent and in many ways superior to the gamma knife. Relatively simple adaptation of modern isocentrically mounted linear accelerator enables such high-precision focused irradiation and is often described as X-knife.

SRT was initially developed for the treatment of acoustic neuromas and arteriovenous malformations. As single-fraction radiosurgery, it has become accepted as the treatment of choice for small, inoperable arteriovenous malformations. The rationale for SRT in brain tumours has been based on the assumption that intracranial tumours are localized, and that increasing the dose of radiation improves tumour control. Higher dose to the tumour without increased normal tissue toxicity is enabled by steeper dose differential between tumour and surrounding normal tissue. In many instances these assumptions have not been proven, but SRT has been accepted as a practical treatment method and has been tested empirically.

Localized irradiation has been used in the form of interstitial radiotherapy inserting radiation sources directly into the tumour (see M.G. Malkin, this volume). The results provide a guide to potential effectiveness of SRT, which offers similar dose distribution and is a non-invasive alternative to interstitial radiotherapy; it has therefore been exploited in the treatment of brain tumours. A major advance in SRT has come from the development of relocatable stereotactic frames. These allow for fractionated SRT with potential biological advantages in the treatment of brain tumours and a closer radiobiological resemblance to low-dose brachytherapy.

In the following discussion we describe the development of a fractionated SRT technique at the Royal Marsden Hospital and the initial clinical experience in the treatment of brain tumours. The technique is currently limited to tumours less than 5 cm in diameter and is ideally suited to spherical lesions. This is not a common clinical situation, and further development of conformal radiotherapy technology may allow treatment of larger and irregular tumours. Present restriction of the technique to small volumes coupled with excitement about seemingly revolutionary treatment has frequently led to indiscriminate use of SRT based solely on tumour size. This approach using unconventional fractionation schedules with unknown long-term effects may lead to higher toxicity without demonstrable clinical benefits. The results of clinical studies evaluating the role of SRT should therefore be carefully compared to the results of conventional therapy in terms of tumour control, survival, and toxicity to avoid inappropriate use of this new technology.

Technique of Stereotactic Radiotherapy

Technical Aspects

There are four requirements for SRT which are common to all the available systems: precise patient fixation, accurate delineation of the target, localization of the target in space coupled with three-dimensional treatment planning, and most importantly a means of focused radiation delivery. The gamma knife and linear accelerator based SRT systems share the requirements for SRT, but they differ in the details of use and flexibility.

The commercially available gamma unit consists of 201 Co^{60} sources distributed radially over a hemisphere (Walton and Bomford 1987). The sources are individually collimated to a single isocentre, and final collimation is achieved by a Tungsten helmet serving as a secondary collimator. The diameter of a single isocentre treatment ranges from 4 to 18 mm. Lesions with a diameter larger than 2 cm must be treated with multiple isocentres. Patients are immobilized in a Leksell frame which locates by insertion of pins into the outer table of the skull. With present technology fractionation is possible only with the frame being retained in position over extended time. The mechanical accuracy of the system is very high as there are no moving parts during irradiation. The position of the isocentre is accurate to 0.1 mm (Walton and Bomford 1987).

Modern isocentrically mounted linear accelerators of various energies in use for conventional radiotherapy can be adapted for stereotactic treatment. The highly localized irradiation can be produced by non-coplanar arcs of rotation or multiple fixed non-coplanar beams around single or multiple isocentres (Hartmann et al.1985; Thomson et al.1990; Graham et al.1991a). The resulting dose distribution outside the target volume for targets of 2 cm is equivalent to that obtained with the gamma unit (Podgorsak et al.1989). There is no maximum size for a single isocentre treatment. However the amount of normal tissue sparing is dependent on the size of target. There is a relative sparing of normal tissue when compared to conventional treatment with target sizes up to 5 cm in diameter (Graham et al.1991a). Because the majority of tumours can be covered with a single isocentre the planning is achieved with a dose homogeneity that is similar to conventional radiotherapy with a dose gradient of less than 10% across the target. The mechanical accuracy of linac-based systems is in the range of 0.5–1 mm (Lutz et al.1988).

There are a number of commercially available fixation devices adapted from neurosurgery that are based on the Brown-Roberts-Wells (BRW) fiducial system and most locate with a series of pins inserted into the skull. New stereotactic frames have been developed that are non-invasive . They can be relocated with high precision (Gill et al.1991; Graham et al.1991b; Hariz et al.1990) and allow planning and treatment to be spread over a number of days.

While the gamma knife system has an apparent advantage in mechanical accuracy the greatest inaccuracy comes from the delineation of intracranial lesions which is inherent to both systems. The gamma unit carries a high capital cost and a subsequent cost of source replacement. Linear accelerator based systems are cheaper, and they utilize available equipment in everyday use in most radiotherapy centres. The ease with which larger tumours can be treated, improved target dose homogeneity and the possibility of fractionation, give linear accelerator SRT systems an overall advantage when considering SRT for the treatment of brain tumours.

Optimization of SRT

Both linac-based systems and the gamma knife deliver dose to a spherical volume, and there is no apparent difference between the two methods of radiation delivery for small spherical lesions (Podgorsak et al.1989). For linear accelerator systems there is no significant effect on the dose distribution at megavoltage energies between 4 and 24 MV (Serago et al.1992). The volume of normal tissue outside the target treated to more than 50% of the prescribed dose is not further reduced by increasing the arc number above 4 (Graham et al.1991a; Serago et al.1992). It is therefore unlikely that the toxicity of treatment as determined by the amount of normal tissue treated can be improved by increasing the treatment complexity using a large number of arcs.

The treatment of irregular volumes such as that encountered with gliomas poses a greater problem. If the target is encompassed by a spherical isodose, normal tissue will be incorporated in the high dose volume. Some beam shaping is possible with the gamma unit by selective blocking of the secondary collimator ports (Flickinger et al.1990a, 1990b). However, the majority of tumours measure more than 2 cm in diameter, and multiple isocentres are needed. Although complex three-dimensional volumes can be covered, this is at the price of dose inhomogeneity across the target, and such techniques may predispose to increased late radiation damage (Nedzi et al.1991). Tumours with a diameter greater than 5 cm and nonspherical tumours may be best treated with linear accelerator using static non-coplanar beams, which can be individually shaped to minimize the amount of normal tissue treated (Laing et al. 1993a). The ultimate optimization may be achieved by dynamic adjustment of shaped fields with multileaf collimators during arcing to conform to the shape of the tumour (Leavitt et al.1991). At present this technology is not commercially available, and the additional benefit of dynamic over static conformal therapy is not known and unlikely to be large.

The Royal Marsden Hospital Technique

Fractionated SRT has been in clinical use at the Royal Marsden Hospital since 1989 and has become a part of the routine clinical workload of the Department. Patients are immobilized in the Gill-Thomas relocatable stereotactic frame (Radionics, Burlington MA; Graham et al.1991b; Gill et al.1991). A dental impression of the upper and lower teeth is made with an acrylic compound that hardens in ultra-violet light (Light-Don/U), keyed onto a perspex bite block, and this achieves accuracy of relocation. Individually moulded headrest made from rubberized putty and a set of straps over the vertex stabilize the frame in position. Relocation accuracy, which is 1 mm or smaller (usually $\leqq$ 0.5 mm; Graham et al.1991b), depends on the precision of the dental impression, which is operator dependent, and the quality of the patients dentition. The frame is secured to the treatment and computed tomography (CT) couch by way of an adjustable support bracket. Patient tolerance of the frame is satisfactory for up to 1 h, and fractionated regimes lasting up to 6 weeks (Laing et al. 1993b).

All tumours were localized by CT scanning in the stereotactic frame with 4-mm slices through the entire head, followed by 2-mm slices through the tumour with a fiducial marker system fitted to the frame. The tumour margins and sensitive structures were defined, and the target isocentre was located with the beams-eye view option of the planning system (Target, IGE). All patients were treated with single isocentre plans using three to five non-coplanar arcs of rotations or six non-coplanar fixed fields depending on the size and site of the tumour. Circular tertiary collimators ranged from 10 to 55 mm in diameter at the isocentre. Before treatment the plan was verified by a further CT scan through the isocentre of the volume.

Treatment was carried out on a Philips SL75/5 linear accelerator. Prior to each treatment a quality assurance procedure was performed to check the accuracy of isocentric positioning. Treatment was carried out by rotation of fixed isocentre fields defined by marks on a localization box attached to the frame. A 3 arc treatment to deliver 5 Gy to a 90% isodose takes approximately 30 min of machine time, which includes pre-treatment checks and patient positioning.

Studies in High-Grade Glioma

Stereotactic radiotherapy has been introduced into the treatment of gliomas largely because of the poor results of conventional therapy (Shapiro 1986; Brada 1989). The case for the potential benefit of SRT as a method of delivery of high-dose localized irradiation rests on the assumption that gliomas are localized tumours, and that increasing dose of radiation improves tumour control (Brada 1989).

Although some low-grade gliomas, particularly pilocytic astrocytomas, are well defined localized tumours, the evidence for localized nature of other gliomas is not convincing. On histological examination gliomas appear infiltrating with tumour cells well beyond the putative margin seen on CT or magnetic resonance imaging (Daumas-Duport et al.1987; Burger et al.1988). However, the majority of tumours recur locally as an extension of the residual mass or in its vicinity (Hochberg and Pruitt 1980; Wallner et al.1989). This may reflect a statistical phenomenon with recurrence at the site of the highest tumour cell density. Nevertheless even with more widespread tumour infiltration improvement in the control of the major tumour mass may lead to prolonged tumour control even though permanent eradication may not be possible.

There is evidence for dose-response relationship between 45 and 60 Gy using conventional external beam radiotherapy to large treatment volumes (Bleehen and Stenning 1991; Walker et al.1979). Increasing dose of radiation beyond 60 Gy using standard radiotherapy does not improve survival further (Chang et al.1983). It is possible that 60 Gy is the optimal dose in terms of therapeutic ratio of tumour control and normal tissue toxicity in the treatment of large target volumes. Increasing the dose differential between tumour and normal tissue and the use of conformal technique of irradiation may allow a higher tumour dose without increased normal tissue toxicity. It is assumed that such higher dose localized to the tumour may improve tumour control and survival further.

Some information on the potential benefit of SRT comes from the results of brachytherapy. In phase II studies, patients with high-grade glioma treated with interstitial radiotherapy to doses ranging from 50 to 120 Gy reach a median survival of 53 weeks for glioblastoma multiformae and 86 weeks for anaplastic astrocytoma (Leibel et al.1989). It is not clear if such good results are entirely or partly due to patient selection (Florell et al.1992) and the role of interstitial radiotherapy boost is currently being studied in randomized trials. Despite the apparent early success most patients treated with interstitial radiotherapy fail, and the majority suffer recurrence adjacent to the high dose region (Loeffler et al.1990). This confirms the suspicion of the more widespread infiltrative nature of gliomas.

At the Royal Marsden Hospital we embarked on phase I and II studies of fractionated stereotactic radiotherapy in patients with recurrent high-grade glioma as a non-invasive out-patient based alternative to interstitial irradiation (Laing et al. 1993c). Between January 1989 and March 1992 a total of 25 patients were treated. All had small tumours (maximum 6 cm diameter, median volume 25 cm^3), good performance status (Karnofsky score above 50, median 70) and were relatively young (median age of 34 years, range 14–56 years). All had high-grade gliomas

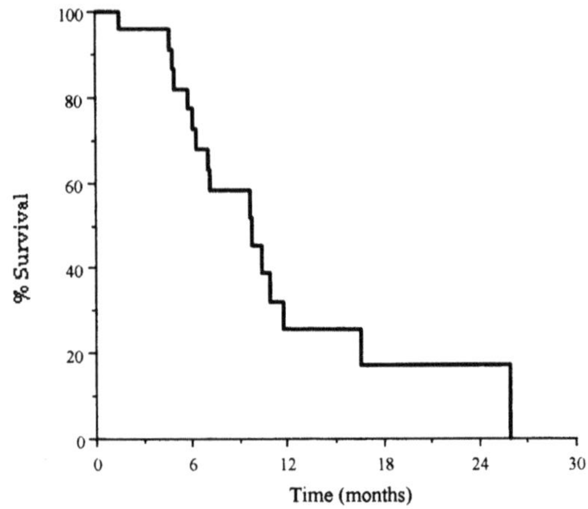

Fig. 1. Actuarial survival of 25 patients with recurrent high-grade glioma treated with fractionated SRT (from the date of SRT)

recurrent after initial surgery and full dose conventional radiotherapy. At the time of relapse prior to SRT six patients had partial tumour excision, three had biopsy and eight had progressive disease on salvage chemotherapy. Patients were treated with fractionated stereotactic radiotherapy on a dose escalation protocol of 20–50 Gy at 5 Gy per fraction. Ten patients received doses of 35 Gy or less, and 15 received doses of 40 Gy or more. At the time of analysis patients were followed up for 1.5–25 months (median 9 months).

The overall survival is shown in Fig. 1. Sixteen patients died from progressive glioma, and the median survival was 10 months. No specific prognostic factors for survival were identified, but this is largely due to the small sample size. The treatment was well tolerated, and in patients without disability it was carried out without the need for hospital admission. However, fractionated SRT for recurrence was not without toxicity. Five patients developed neurological deterioration 4–6 months after treatment, which responded to steroids and was not apparently associated with tumour progression. It is assumed that the steroid-dependent neurological deterioration represents late radiation damage, and this was confirmed in three patients by low uptake of 18-fluorodeoxyglucose on positron emission tomography.

There are a number of variables which determine the risk of radiation damage in patients with recurrent glioma receiving re-irradiation. These include both initial patient and treatment characteristics as well as parameters at the time of recurrence. The patients studied were heterogeneous in terms of initial radiotherapy volume, disease-free interval and detailed histology. At the time of recurrence the size of irradiated volume and the dose of SRT varied (according to the dose escalation protocol), and both may be important additional determinants of late damage. The relationship between target volume, SRT dose and toxicity for patients surviving a minimum of 6 months suggests higher risk of damage in patients with larger target volume and in those receiving doses over 40 Gy.

Apart from assessing SRT in terms of the ability to control tumour progression the treatment administered to patients with poor prognosis recurrent disease must be effective as palliation. Patients with brain tumour frequently have a neurological deficit, and the palliative effect should be assessed either as improvement or as maintenance of neurological function. The assessment of functional status was performed using a modified Barthel index of activities of daily living. At 3 months 77% and at 6 months 67% of survivors either improved or remained functionally unchanged. Deterioration occurred in five patients as a result of radiation damage and in most instances was reversible with corticosteroids. In other patients deterioration was a hallmark of tumour progression.

Single-fraction SRT has been employed in selected patients with recurrent high-grade glioma. Preliminary data suggest reasonable tumour control although the toxicity of this approach has not been reported (Loeffler and Alexander 1991).

SRT may serve as a means of delivering high-dose boost to primary tumour following conventional surgery and radiotherapy, which can be considered akin to interstitial radiotherapy boost. If the randomized trials currently underway show benefit for interstitial boost, it may be possible to extrapolate the results to other means of delivering localized radiation, and certainly fractionated SRT would offer biologically and physically equivalent form of localized irradiation which is entirely non-invasive. Ideally the role of SRT boost should also be tested in randomized studies. It is possible that fractionated SRT may become the treatment of choice as a boost following conventional treatment of high-grade glioma.

SRT cannot at present be considered as an alternative to conventional surgery and radiotherapy in the primary treatment of high-grade gliomas. Selected patients with high-grade tumours have been treated with radiosurgery alone at other centres with high morbidity and unsatisfactory survival results (Sturm, personal communication).

The currently used protocol at the Royal Marsden Hospital is to treat patients with recurrent high-grade gliomas less than 5 cm in diameter with fractionated SRT to doses of 30–35 Gy at 5 Gy per fraction on a daily schedule. The future of fractionated SRT undoubtedly lies in the use of this technique as a non-invasive alternative to interstitial irradiation in the treatment of primary or recurrent gliomas.

Brain Metastases

The development of brain metastases usually heralds the terminal phase of malignant disease with a median survival of 3–6 months (Borgelt et al.1980). Whilst whole brain radiotherapy (WBRT) has a place in the palliation of symptoms, the majority of patients die with uncontrolled disease (Kurtz et al.1981). This scenario may be different with solitary metastases where the term radical palliation may be appropriate. In the absence of other systemic disease radical local treatment may achieve long-term survival (Galicich et al.1980; Sarma and Weilbaecher 1986; Salerno et al.1978). Surgical excision in combination with WBRT prolongs survival, although the median survival is only 40 weeks (Patchell et al.1990), reflecting the poor overall prognosis of patients with metastatic disease. While boosting a

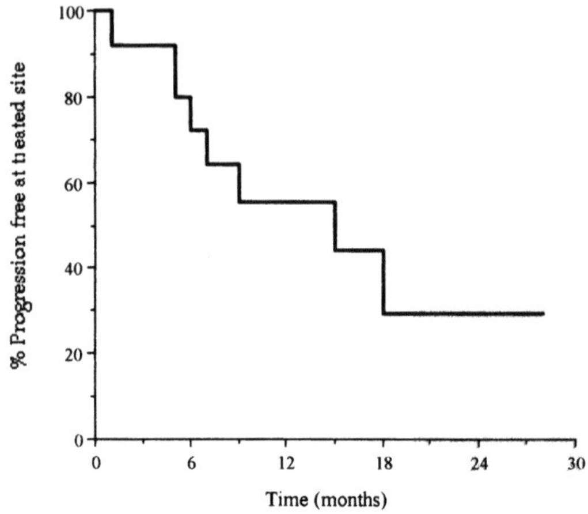

Fig. 2. Actuarial progression free survival of 32 brain metastases (28 patients) at the treated site

solitary metastasis with conventional radiotherapy does not appear to alter survival (Hoskin et al.1990), single fraction radiosurgery or fractionated stereotactic radiotherapy may offer the same local control as excision avoiding the toxicity of surgical intervention (Laing et al. 1993d).

At the Royal Marsden Hospital we treated 28 selected patients with 33 brain metastases with SRT. All had good performance status (Karnofsky score 70) and primary tumour and systemic disease were under control. Initially 10 patients received an SRT boost after WBRT (30 Gy in ten fractions) with 5 Gy daily fractions prescribed to the 90% isodose that surrounded the tumour with a 2 mm margin. The SRT dose ranged from 10 to 30 Gy. Eighteen patients (21 metastases) received 20 Gy in two fractions 4 days apart, 11 after WBRT and 7 without previous radiotherapy.

Radiological evidence of complete or partial response was observed in 50% of those with follow-up scans, at a median interval of 24 weeks from SRT. No neurological deterioration attributable to radiation damage has been observed.

Radiological or clinical evidence of relapse at the treated site occurred in nine lesions. The actuarial median progression-free survival at the treated site was 15 months (Fig. 2). The overall median survival from time of SRT was 17 months.

Similar results have been reported with radiosurgery with either gamma knife (Coffey et al.1991) or linac based systems (Sturm et al.1991; Loeffler et al.1990; Adler et al.1992; Fuller et al.1992; Caron et al.1992; Table 1). Direct comparison of results from different institutions is difficult because of differing patient selection criteria and the technique, including dose and dose prescription. Most studies report crude rather than actuarial control rates. However, the reported local control is almost universally high and comparable with the results for WBRT and excision surgery (Patchell et al.1990).

Table 1. Reported results of SRT/radiosurgery in the treatment of cerebral metastases

Reference	Number of patients	Number of metastases	SRT Dose (Gy) Range (median)	Prescribed to isodose	Fractionation*	Local Control (%)	Median PFS*** (months)
Loeffler et al. '90	18	21	9–25 (15)	70–90%	S	90% **	N/A
Caron et al. '92	9	11	20–25 (20)	90%	S	88% **	N/A
Fuller et al. '92	27	47	16–35 (24.6)	80%	S	88%	N/A
Coffey et al. '91	32	34	16–20	50–90%	S	92%	N/A
Sturm et al. '91	30		15–50 (22)	80%	S	89%	N/A
Present series	28	33	10–20	90%	F	70%	15

* S Single fraction.
F Fractionated.
** including patients failing in the immediate margin.
*** PFS acturial progression free survival at the treated site.

There are unresolved questions regarding the dose and fractionation of SRT and the role of WBRT in the management of solitary metastases. The doses used for SRT of cerebral metastases have varied (Table 1), and the studies included patients treated with SRT alone, patients relapsing after WBRT and those receiving SRT boost after WBRT. In addition the studies included a wide range of histologies reflecting the range of tumours metastasizing to the brain. Fractionated regimes used at Royal Marsden Hospital can be compared with single fraction radiosurgery by using the linear quadratic formula (Brenner et al.1991), and 20 Gy in two fractions is similar in terms of tumour control to a 16 Gy single fraction. Currently the optimum dose and fractionation are not defined. In the absence of randomized trials the low toxicity and acceptable tumour control of single fraction of 16 Gy or two fractions of 10 Gy (total 20 Gy) encourage us to continue this policy.

In a palliative treatment the number of hospital visits and treatments should be minimized. Providing the toxicity is minimal, single fraction SRT particularly in patients who are expected to have poor prognosis may be appropriate. However, when large lesions are treated, the volume of normal tissue included within the high-dose regions is large, and a fractionated regime may have a theoretical advantage. This may also be important when combining SRT with WBRT and in patients with relatively long survival.

It has been assumed that the presence of an apparently solitary metastasis is the hallmark of more extensive disease in the brain. WBRT has therefore been added to surgery or radiosurgery. Retrospective studies comparing the role of WBRT following surgery give conflicting results, claiming either no improvement in the control of intracranial disease and survival (Dosoretz et al.1980) or better results with WBRT after surgery (Smalley et al.1987) or stereotactic radiotherapy (Fuller et al.1992). However these studies have the pitfalls of retrospective analysis and report on small numbers of patients and the role of WBRT remains undefined. The Royal Marsden Hospital policy is to treat solitary metastases, confirmed by magnetic resonance imaging, with SRT alone and reserve WBRT for the time of relapse. This policy provides the simplest non-invasive radical palliation and avoids significant alopecia associated with WBRT.

In summary we conclude that fractionated stereotactic radiotherapy is an effective, well-tolerated and non-invasive form of intensive local treatment of solitary brain metastases and seems equivalent in efficacy to local neurosurgical excision. For these reasons stereotactic radiotherapy is likely to become the treatment of choice for patients with solitary brain metastases.

Potential Role in Other Brain Tumours

SRT has been employed in a range of intracranial tumours where the rationale for its application has largely rested on the size of the lesion. Among more benign of the brain tumours particular attention has focused on the treatment of acoustic neuromas (Leksell 1987; Flickinger et al.1991). At present the role of SRT remains controversial as it is not without toxicity, and long-term results are not yet available (Brada 1991). Other tumours considered suitable for SRT include pituitary adenoma and craniopharyngioma. On present evidence standard treatment with conservative surgery and conventional fractionated radiotherapy is highly effective and carries little toxicity (Brada et al.1993, Rajan et al. 1993). The use of SRT, particularly as single-fraction radiosurgery may carry higher morbidity with unknown effectiveness in terms of long-term tumour control. At present it is not justified to use it in the primary treatment, and SRT should be reserved for the few selected patients with recurrent disease. However, SRT technology offers the potential for high-precision conformal treatment, and this should be exploited in fractionated radiotherapy for all small intracranial lesions considered suitable for radiotherapy.

Cranial germ cell tumours (GCT) are usually localized to the pineal region and at first sight appear at least technically suitable for SRT. However, they are malignant infiltrative tumours with potential for CSF seeding. Cranial germinomas which are histologically identical to testicular seminoma are highly sensitive to radiation and following conventional wide-field irradiation the cure rate is near 100% with little long-term toxicity (Dearnaley et al.1990). In patients with isolated pineal GCT it is therefore hard to justify the use of SRT simply on the basis that such technique is available and possible to administer. Patients with recurrent GCT, usually after inappropriate treatment in inexperienced hands, fare badly with salvage therapy, and new treatment approaches which increase the risk of geographical miss because of too localized treatment are barely ethically justifiable. The current new treatment approaches in cranial germinoma include the use of primary chemotherapy. The excellent responses achieved allow for lower dose of radiation. In this context a fractionated localized boost may be appropriate to small residual lesions but does not resolve the problem of the risk of CSF dissemination (Brada and Rajan 1990).

The results of treatment of cranial non-seminomatous GCT (teratomas) with conventional external beam radiotherapy are unsatisfactory. Chemotherapy is highly effective in testicular teratoma and has therefore been exploited in cranial tumours. The addition of chemotherapy in cranial teratomas results in responses and probably an improvement in survival although the rarity of these tumours precludes a definite statement about the long-term outcome. As in teratomas of testicular origins, residual masses may remain after treatment and SRT may become a non-invasive alternative to potentially hazardous attempts at surgical excision to reduce the risk of local recurrence.

Medulloblastomas are highly chemosensitive and radiosensitive tumours yet despite increasingly aggressive treatment 30%–40% of patients fail, and the majority do so at the primary site in the posterior fossa (Tait et al.1990; Evans et al.1990). Patients at particular risk are those with residual disease after surgery. The dose that can be delivered by conventional radiotherapy is limited by the risk of radiation damage to the brain stem. SRT may therefore theoretically have a role as a means of delivering a radiation boost avoiding sensitive local structures. This hypothesis has not yet been tested in practice as the current treatment approaches largely include the use of intensive chemotherapy regimens.

The Royal Marsden Hospital experience in medulloblastoma is limited to patients with recurrent disease in the posterior fossa who are either chemoresistant or in second relapse. All three patients treated with fractionated SRT achieved excellent local control with neurological improvement and returned to normal life, but two patients suffered a relapse a year later outside the irradiated volume.

In conclusion, in medulloblastoma SRT may have a role as an additional treatment to improve the control of disease at the primary site, and its deployment depends on the success of current chemotherapy regimens. It can also be employed as an additional treatment to chemotherapy in patients with recurrent disease confined to the posterior fossa.

Summary and Conclusions

SRT is a high-precision technique of radiotherapy which delivers focused irradiation to small target volumes. In the context of external beam radiotherapy it can be described as stereotactically guided conformal radiotherapy. As the technique originated from neurosurgical technology, it has initially been limited to single fraction treatment. However, with the use of relocatable fixation devices the way ahead particularly in its application in the treatment of brain tumours is in fractionated SRT.

Currently, single fraction SRT/radiosurgery is of proven value only in the treatment of small inoperable arteriovenous malformations. It is being exploited in the management of brain tumours but so far remains an experimental treatment. We have demonstrated that fractionated SRT in patients with gliomas is a non-invasive equivalent to brachytherapy and in patients with solitary metastases a non-invasive alternative to surgical excision. However, the treatment is not without side effects, and the long-term effectiveness and toxicity of SRT, particularly with the use of unconventional fractionation, is not defined.

The future use of SRT in the treatment of brain tumours should not be guided simply by the technical possibilities but by a rational appraisal of all treatment options to achieve the best disease control, survival and toxicity. Although there is potential for benefit in a number of small tumours, SRT cannot at present be recommended as the primary treatment in any tumour. In addition, its use should be discouraged in the treatment of unbiopsied brain lesions and as the major form of treatment of pineal germinomas. The technology of stereotactic radiotherapy is evolving, and it is likely that SRT will be integrated into conventional radiotherapy practice to become simply a high-precision technique of radiotherapy delivery in everyday use.

Acknowledgements. The authors are grateful to Mr A P Warrington, Physicist at The Royal Marsden Hospital who enabled the SRT technique to be introduced and to all the Radiotherapy Department, and the Neuro-oncology Unit staff for their enthusiastic cooperation. Mrs Sally Crowley kindly helped in the preparation of this manuscript. The SRT programme is funded in part by grants from the Julian Bloom Research Fund, Cancer Research Campaign and the Royal Marsden Hospital.

References

Adler J, Cox R, Kaplan I, Martin D (1992) Stereotactic radiosurgical treatment of brain metastases. J Neurosurg 76:444–449
Bleehen N, Stenning S (1991) A Medical Research Council trial of two radiotherapy doses in the treatment of grades 3 and 4 astrocytoma. Br J Cancer 64:769–774
Borgelt B, Gelber R, Kramer S et al.(1980) The palliation of brain metastases: Final results of the first two studies by the Radiation Therapy Oncology Group. Int J Radiat Oncol Biol Phys 6:1–9
Brada M (1989) Back to the future – radiotherapy in high grade gliomas. Br J Cancer 60:1–4
Brada M (1991) Radiosurgery for brain tumours. Eur J Cancer 12:1545–1548
Brada M, Rajan B (1990) Spinal seeding in cranial germinoma. Br J Cancer 61:339–340
Brada M, Rajan B, Traish D, Ashley S, Nussey S, Uttley D (1993) Long term efficacy of conservative surgery and radiotherapy in the control of pituitary adenoma. Clin Endocrinol 38:571–578
Brenner D, Martel M, Hall E (1991) Fractionated regimens for stereotactic radiotherapy of recurrent tumors in the brain. Int J Radiat Oncol Biol Phys 21:819–824
Burger P, Heinz E, Shibata T, Kleihues P (1988) Topographic anatomy and CT correlations in the untreated glioblastoma multiforme. J Neurosurg 68:698
Caron J, Souhami L, Podgorsak E (1992) Dynamic stereotactic radiosurgery in the palliative treatment of cerebral metastatic tumors. J Neuro-oncol 12:173–179
Chang C, Horton J, Schoenfeld D et al (1983) Comparison of postoperative radiotherapy and combined postoperative radiotherapy and chemotherapy in the multidisciplinary management of malignant gliomas. Cancer 52:997–1007
Coffey R, Flickinger J, Lunsford L, Bissonette D (1991) Solitary brain metastasis: Radiosurgery in lieu of microsurgery in 32 patients. Acta Neurochirurgica 52:90–92
Daumas-Duport C, Scheithauer B. W, Kelly P. J (1987) A histologic and cytologic method for the spatial definition of gliomas. Mayo Clin Proc 62:435–449
Dearnaley D, A'Hern R, Whittaker S, Bloom H (1990) Pineal and CNS germ cell tumours: Royal Marsden Hospital experience 1962–1987. Int J Radiat Oncol Biol Phys 18:773–781
Dosoretz D, Blitzer P, Russell A, Wang C (1980) Management of solitary metastasis to the brain: The role of elective brain irradiation following complete surgical resection. Int J Radiat Oncol Biol Phys 6:1727–1730

Evans A, Jenkin D, Sposto R, et al (1990) Results of a prospective randomised trial of radiation therapy with and without CCNU, Vincristine and Prednisone. J Neurosurg 72:572–582
Flickinger J, Lunsford L, Wu A, Maitz A, Kalend A (1990a) Treatment planning for gamma knife radiosurgery with multiple isocenters. Int J Radiat Oncol Biol Phys 18:1495–1501
Flickinger J, Maitz A, Kalend A, Lunsford LD, Wu A (1990b) Treatment volume shaping with selective beam blocking using the Leksell gamma unit. Int J Radiat Oncol Biol Phys 19:783–789
Flickinger J, Lunsford, L, Coffey R et al (1991) Radiosurgery of acoustic neurinomas. Cancer 67:345–352
Florell R, Macdonald D, Irish W et al (1992) Selection bias, survival, and brachytherapy for glioma. J Neurosurg 76:179–183
Fuller B, Kaplan I, Adler J, Cox R, Bagshaw M (1992) Stereotaxic radiosurgery for brain metastases: The importance of adjuvant whole brain irradiation. Int J Radiat Oncol Biol Phys 23:413–418
Galicich, J, Sundaresan N, Arbit E, Passe S (1980) Surgical treatment of single brain metastasis: Factors associated with survival. Cancer 45:381–386
Gill S, Thomas D, Warrington A, Brada M (1991) Relocatable frame for stereotactic external beam radiotherapy. Int J Radiat Oncol Biol Phys 20:599–603
Graham J, Nahum A, Brada M (1991a) A comparison of techniques for stereotactic radiotherapy by linear accelerator based on 3-dimensional dose distributions. Radiother Oncol 23:29–35
Graham J, Warrington A, Gill S, Brada M (1991b) A non-invasive, relocatable stereotactic frame for fractionated radiotherapy and multiple imaging. Radiother Oncol 21:60–62
Hariz M, Henriksson R, Löfroth P-O, Laitinen L, Säterborg N-E (1990) A non-invasive method for fractionated stereotactic irradiation of brain tumors with linear accelerator. Radiother Oncol 17:57–72
Hartmann G, Schlegel W, Sturm V, Kober B, Pastyr O, Lorenz W (1985) Cerebral radiation surgery using moving field irradiation at a linear accelerator facility. Int J Radiat Oncol Biol Phys 11:1185–1192
Hochberg F, Pruitt A (1980) Assumptions in the radiotherapy of glioblastoma. Neurology 30:907
Hoskin P, Crow J, Ford H (1990) The influence of extent and local management of the outcome of radiotherapy for brain metastases. Int J Radiat Oncol Biol Phys 19:111–115
Kurtz J, Gelber R, Brady L, Carella R, Cooper J (1981) The palliation of brain metastases in a favourable patient population: a randomized clinical trial by the Radiation Therapy Oncology Group. Int J Radiat Oncol Biol Phys 7:891–895
Laing RW, Bentley RE, Nahum AE, Warrington AP, Brada M (1993a) Stereotactic radiotherapy of irregular targets: a comparison between static conformal beams and non-coplanar arcs. Radiother Oncolo 28(3):241–246
Laing RW, Thompson V, Warrington AP, Brada M (1993b) Feasibility of patients immobilization for conventional cranial irradiation with a relocatable stereotactic frame. Br J Radiol 66:1020–1024
Laing RW, Warrington AP, Graham J, Britton J, Hines F, Brada M (1993c) Efficacy and toxicity of fractionated stereotactic radiotherapy in the treatment of recurrent gliomas (phase I/II study). Radiother Oncol 27(1):22–39
Laing RW, Warrington AP, Hines F, Graham JD, Brada M (1993d) Fractionated stereotactic external beam radiotherapy in the management of brain metastases. Eur J Cancer 29A(10):1387–1391
Leavitt D, Gibbs F, Heilbrun M, Moeller J, Takach G (1991) Dynamic field shaping to optomize stereotactic radiosurgery. Int J Radiat Oncol Biol Phys 21:1247–1255
Leibel S, Gutin P, Wara W et al (1989) Survival and quality of life after interstitial implication of removable high-activity Iodine-125 sources for the treatment of patients with recurrent malignant gliomas. Int J Radiat Oncol Biol Phys 17:1129–1139
Leksell D G (1987) Stereotactic radiosurgery – present status and future trends. Neurol Res 9:60–68
Leksell L (1951) The stereotactic method and radiosurgery of the brain. Acta Chir Scand 102:316–319
Loeffler J, Alexander III E (1991) Stereotactic radiosurgery for malignant gliomas. In: Second International Neuro-oncology Conference, Royal Marsden Hospital, March 25–26, 1991, London
Loeffler J, Kooy H, Wen P, et al (1990) The treatment of recurrent brain metastases with stereotactic radiosurgery. J Clin Oncol 8:576–582
Loeffler J, Alexander EI, Wen P (1990) Results of stereotactic brachytherapy used as the initial management of patients with glioblastomas. J Natl Cancer Inst 82:1918–1921
Lutz W, Winston K, Maleki N (1988) A system for stereotactic radiosurgery with a linear accelerator. Int J Radiat Oncol Biol Phys 14(2):373–381

Nedzi L, Kooy H, Alexander EI, Gelman R, Loeffler J (1991) Variables associated with the development of complications from radiosurgery of intracranial tumors. Int J Radiat Oncol Biol Phys 21:591–599

Patchell R, Tibbs P, Walsh J et al (1990) A randomized trial of surgery in the treatment of single metastases to the brain. N Engl J Med 322:494–500

Podgorsak EB, Pike G, Olivier A, Pla M, Souhami L (1989) Radiosurgery with high energy photon beams: a comparison among techniques. Int J Radiat Oncol Biol Phys 16:857–865

Rajan B, Ashley S, Gorman C, Jose CC, Horwich A, Bloom HJG, Marsh H, Brada M (1993) Craniopharyngioma – long term results following limited surgery and radiotherapy. Radiother Oncol 26:1–10

Salerno T, Munro D, Little J (1978) Surgical treatment of bronchgenic carcinoma with a brain metastis. J Neurosurg 48 350–354

Sarma D, Weilbaecher T (1986) Long-term survival after brain metastasis from lung cancer. Cancer 58 1363–1370

Serago C, Houdek P, Bauer-Kirpes B et al (1992) Stereotactic radiosurgery: Dose-volume analysis of linear accelerator techniques. Med Phys 19:181–185

Shapiro WR (1986) Therapy of adult malignant brain tumours: what have the clinical trials taught us? Semin Oncol 13:38

Smalley S, Schray M, Laws E, O'Fallon J (1987) Adjuvant radiation therapy after surgical resection of solitary brain metastasis: association with patterm of failure and survival. Int J Radiat Oncol Biol Phys 13:1611–1616

Sturm V, Kimmig B, Engenhardt R et al (1991) Radiosurgical treatment of cerebral metastases. Stereotact Funct Neurosurg 57:7–10

Tait D, Thornton-Jones H, Bloom H, Lemerle J, Morris-Jones P (1990) Adjuvant chemotherapy for medulloblastoma: the first multi-centre control trial of the International Society of Paediatric Oncology (SIOP I) Eur J Cancer 26(4):464–469

Thomson E, Gill S, Doughty D (1990) Stereotactic multiple arc radiotherapy. Br J Radiol 63:745–751

Walker K, Galicich J, Krol G, Arbit E, Malkin M (1979) Patterns of failure following treatment for glioblastoma multiforme and anaplastic astrocytoma. Int J Radiat Oncol Biol Phys 5:1725

Wallner KE, Galicich JH, Krol G, Arbit E, Malkin MG (1989) Patterns of failure following treatment for glioblastoma multiforme and anaplastic astrocytoma. Int J Radiat Oncol Biol Phys 16:1405–1409

Walton L, Bomford C (1987) The Sheffield stereotactic radiosurgery unit: physical characteristics and principles of operation. Br J Radiol 60:897–906

Interstitial Implant Radiosurgery of Brain Tumors: Radiobiology, Indications, and Results

C. B. Ostertag

Abteilung Stereotaktische Neurochirurgie, Neurochirurgische Universitätsklinik, Hugstetter Str. 55, 79106 Freiburg, Germany

History

The discovery of radium by Marie and Pierre Curie in 1898 was followed promptly by the clinical application of this radioisotope in the treatment of various cancers. Alexander Graham Bell suggested in 1903: "There is no reason why a tiny fragment of radium sealed-up in a fine glass tube should not be inserted into the very heart of the cancer, thus acting directly on the diseased material" [2]. This statement accurately describes the irradiation technique that was later known as brachytherapy (greek for radiation therapy in short range, as opposed to teletherapy). The technique is based on the principle of selectively irradiating a tumour while protecting the healthy surrounding brain from radiation energy. The amount of radiation reaching normal tissue varies inversely with the square of the distance from the implanted radioactive source.

Brachytherapy was widely used after World War I. Free-hand implanted radiation sources were used for parenchymal brain tumours as early as 1914 [5]. Hirsch extensively applied and emphasized the use of radium treatment to prevent regrowth and to destroy and to shrink remnants of pituitary tumours not radically removed [10]. Talairach in 1953 was the first to implant radioactive sources (gold-198 grains) stereotactically into brain tumours [30]. The confusing terminology used (brachytherapy, curietherapy, brachycurietherapy, interstitial radiotherapy) gives the impression, however, that the biological basis was not fully understood. Information for clinical dosimetry was based on experiences with radium and with fractionated radiation therapy which have been extrapolated correctly or incorrectly. It remained largely undecided whether the method had to be considered a form of radiation therapy or of radiosurgery, i.e.,, whether the effect in tissue was based on a differential effect between normal and neoplastic cells or simply had a necrotizing effect.

Radiobiology of Interstitial Radiosurgery

The purpose of interstitial implant radiosurgery is to deliver a focal necrotizing dose of radiation to a predefined volume of neoplastic tissue without affecting surroun-

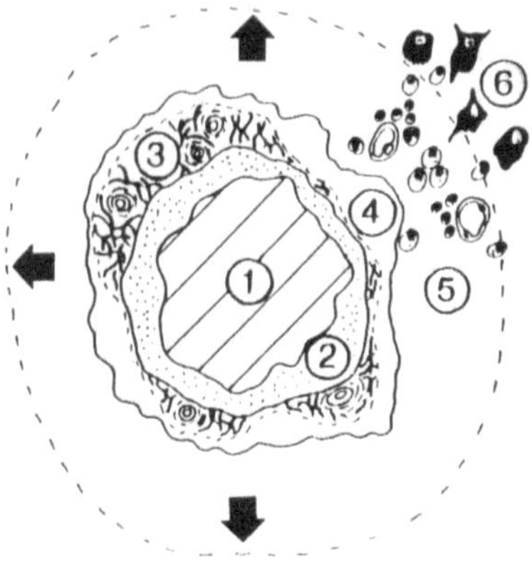

Fig. 1. Schematic illustration of morphological changes to radioactive sources (^{125}I, ^{192}Ir, ^{198}Au) in the brain. The radionecrosis evolves from the centre into the periphery (*arrows*). *Dotted line*, final size of radionecrosis in the brain. *1*, Central coagulation necrosis; *2*, calcified rim of necrosis; *3*, perinecrotic zone of gliosis with fibrinoid vessel wall necrosis; *4*, spongiform "lucent" zone; *5*, zone of organization with macrophages, capillary proliferation, perivascular inflammatory infiltrates; *6*, reactive gliosis and demyelination.

ding normal brain. According to this definition of radiosurgery given by Larsson, the implantation of radioactive sources is but one method of radiosurgery [15]. We here prefer the term interstitial radiosurgery (IRS) instead of brachytherapy because it more accurately describes the radiobiological rationale. Characteristics of radiation toxicity seem to be identical whether cobalt-60 gamma knife, a linear accelerator, heavy charged particles or interstitial radioactive implants are used [17].

Prerequisite for radiosurgery is a precise knowledge of the relationship between the radiation dose, the volume treated and the subsequent response of normal tissue surrounding the lesion. In order to formulate a biological basis for the clinical dosimetry of IRS we have studied sequentially the morphological and physiological effects caused by radio-emitters with different energies and different dose rates in an animal model. Experimental dose effects on the brain (beagle) caused by the photon emitter iodine-125 (half-life 60.2 days, 0.028–0.035 MeV), iridium-192 (half-life 74.2 days, 0.30–0.61 MeV), gold-198 (half-life 2.7 days, 0.41 MeV) were examined consecutively over 5–365 days. Permanent low-activity, low-dose rate implants were compared over time with temporary high-activity, high-dose rate implants, the two delivering the same accumulated total radiation dose. The implants were either permanent (lost implants) or temporary removable implants. The dosimetry for permanent low-dose rate and for temporary high-dose rate implants was calculated such that a 26 000 (10 000) cGy isodose was achieved at a 5 (10) mm distance from the source.

The procedures for implantation, tissue perfusion, histological and immunohistological staining are described elsewhere [12, 19, 21]. Isodose distribution and accumulated tissue dosage were calculated on the assumption of a point source of irradiation. For a detailed description of quantitative measurement of capillary transfer rates, i.e., quantitative autoradiographic and computed tomographic (CT) methods employed in the different experimental series see [6, 7, 32].

There were characteristic morphological responses to all three radiation sources in the brain (Fig. 1). Within 25 days coagulation necrosis developed in the immediate vicinity of the radioactive source, which later increased in size and became progressively mineralized. Vessels within the developing radionecrosis showed the typical hyaloid vessel wall degeneration. Vessels outside the radionecrosis, however, even within a distance of 1 mm, appeared normal. A reactive gliosis with a dense fibrillary network of glial fibrillary acidic protein (GFAP) positive astrocytes was found around the radionecrosis in the surrounding white matter. GFAP-positive astrocytes in later stages were also found in the contralateral hemisphere as a reaction to vasogenic edema which spread via the corpus callosum. Demyelination was always restricted to the ipsilateral centrum semiovale without affecting the internal capsule or the contralateral hemisphere. The neurons next to but not incorporated in the radionecrosis, however, appeared to be morphologically intact even at a distance of 0.2 mm. A remarkable factor was the time course of the lesion growth. Whereas the size of the radiolesion resulting from low-dose rate permanent implants had not reached its maximum until after 70 days, the radionecrosis after high-dose rate temporary implants showed its maximum size after 25 days, after which the lesion decreased relatively quickly in comparison with the radionecrosis induced by permanent implants.

A high dose delivered over a short period caused a larger volume, thus resulting in an increased capillary surface of impaired endothelial cells with the inevitably induced vasogenic edema. Under low doses and long-term exposure small necroses were produced along with moderate, but long-lasting vasogenic edema. When temporary implants were used, lively macrophage acitivity set in after the emitter had been removed, and the zone of necrotic tissue then decreased. The extent of demyelination in the white substance was directly related to the intensity of the vasogenic edema. The glial reaction and demyelination clearly exceeded the physical penetration depth of the gamma radiation, at least that of ^{125}I photon radiation and were therefore considered secondary effects. The effects of scattering and attenuation in tissue vary considerably for the three isotopes used in the experiment. The specific dose rate factor, i.e., the dose rate per unit activity, divided by the geometrical attenuation is not a constant with distance, particularly not for ^{125}I [1, 14, 29]. The volume of radionecroses in normal brain tissue depends on the total dose, the dose rate and energy of the implanted radioactive source. In neoplastic tissue, however, other factors such as neovascularization and susceptibility of tumour cells to radiation are other contributing factors. In a previous experiment we had studied the necrotizing effect of ^{125}I seeds in neoplastic tissue [22]. Avian sarcoma virus induced dog brain tumours were chosen to serve as a primary model for human brain tumours. The response of neoplastic tissue to interstitial irradiation in terms of the volume of necrosis was threee to five times greater than ^{125}I radionecroses in normal brain tissue. The necrobiotic characteristics, however, were similar.

A constant finding was the presence of perifocal edema, which extended into the white matter of the entire ipsilateral hemishere. The temporary, geographically confined opening of the blood-brain barrier is considered a specific side effect of radiosurgery in the brain [4, 31]. The amount of blood-borne fluids that cross the blood-brain barrier depends on the total surface area of the irradiated defective capillaries. Experimental and clinical results from blood to tissue transport studies are usually exressed in terms of a transfer constant K_1, which characterizes the unidirectional transfer across capillaries [7]. Using [^{14}C]α-aminoisobutyric acid autoradiography it could be shown that in comparison with normal brain the layer of irradiated brain tissue on the surface of a necrosis volume develops higher capillary permeability (up to 7.7 times higher) and maintains this over a period of several months after low-dose rate permanent interstitial irradiation [6]. More recently, quantitative computer tomographic methods as described by Groothuis et al. [7] were used, which allow consecutive quantitative in vivo measurements of individual animals. The values for K_1 after temporary interstitial high-dose rate irradiation exceeded those found after low-dose rate permanent irradiation for all three gamma emitters. With ^{198}Au implants, whether permanent or temporary, the highest K_1 values were found. K_1 values for ^{192}Ir temporary implant were slightly lower. All of the experimental animals showed nodular lesions (in the early stages) or ring-shaped lesions of the capillary function in standard computed tomography by the time the first examination was carried out. The capillary permeability in a localized zone surrounding the implant was temporarily 10–40 times higher than that in normal brain tissue. The vascular volume did not differ from normal brain tissue. Whereas after permanent interstitial irradiation the impaired capillary permeability (K_1) remained rather constant over a period of up to 1 year, the capillary permeability after temporary irradiation had a peak after the maximum volume of radionecrosis had developed and after that gradually returned to normal [32].

Based on experimental findings and clinical observations a biological dosimetry has evolved which prefers ^{125}I temporary seeds with a dose rate of 10 cGy/h and a cumulative reference dose on the tumour margin of 60 Gy. The clinical results so far obtained demonstrate that toxic vasogenic edema no longer poses a serious problem. Stereotactic interstitial implant radiosurgery in our hands has replaced open surgery for a variety of brain tumours.

Clinical Interstitial Radiosurgery

Cerebral Gliomas

Cerebral gliomas have variable topographic patterns. The administration of a local therapy must recognize the morphological findings of the individual case. We therefore selected only a small subgroup of gliomas, mostly low-grade gliomas, for IRS which were circumscribed tumours with only limited spread of tumour cells into the periphery [23]. These were only 24% of the total group of all gliomas which were diagnosed at this institution during the same time. Patients with Karnofsky performance rating (KR) of at least 70 with circumscribed unifocal differentiated gliomas of WHO grade I, WHO grade II, circumscribed anaplastic WHO grade III gliomas, and glioblastomas in inaccessible, i.e., deep-seated, or in functionally critical locations in the brain were treated if the lesions could be located on either CT or magnetic resonance imaging (MRI) and with the help of serial stereotactic biopsies. The diameter of most of the lesions on contrast-enhanced CT was less than 4 cm. Diffusely infiltrative tumours crossing the midline with involvement of the corpus callosum, highly malignant, non-definable tumours, and multifocal tumours were excluded because of their invasiveness. Also excluded were patients with a rapidly deteriorating neurological status (KR < 70) or a major mass effect with immanent brain herniation.

Sources and Dosimetry

Exclusively ^{125}I seeds were used (model 6702, Amersham Buchler). The clinical dosimetry for ^{125}I implants was determined on the basis of the physical and biological properties: ^{125}I emits primarily low-energy X-ray radiation of 27–35 KeV. According to several investigators, the relative biological efficiency is in the range of 1.2–1.4 [1]. The specific dose-rate factor used for dosimetry was 1.32 cGy/h and mCi at 1 cm in tissue [29]. Interstitial irradiation was carried out using either permanent (lost) ^{125}I implants (1979–1985) or temporary (removable) im-plants since 1985. For clinical use the calculated accumulated dose ranged between 3000 and 7000 cGy (mean 6000 cGy). This dose was calculated to accumulate at the outer rim of a tumour as defined by contrast enhancement of the CT scan and serial biopsy within 90 days when permanent implants were carried out [dose rate (DR) < 5 cGy/h]. Temporary ^{125}I seed implants, which we have been using since 1985, were left in place for 20–30 days to deliver a tumour destructive dose with the preferred DR of approximately 10 cGy/h. The dose variation was not dependent upon tumour type but upon individual tumour response as observed by CT follow-up examinations. Due to the seed configuration (a titanium rod with welded ends), the dose distribution is unisotropic, which makes calibration difficult [14]. The unisotropic dose distribution, however, is more or less irrelevant for the biological effect, as has been demonstrated experimentally. After the seeds had been implanted, the CT images with marker and implants were digitized with a computer and superimposed with isodose contours.

Patients selected for IRS underwent a stereotactic diagnostic procedure including CT and cerebral angiography under stereotactic conditions [25] and serial biopsies in one or more tracts to establish a morphological diagnosis containing information on invasiveness, composition (solid, cystic or necrotic), vascularity and grading according to the WHO classification. A titanium ball (diameter 0.5 mm) was left in what was considered the centre of the target volume as a marker. In patients with an unequivocal intraoperative tissue diagnosis the implantation of the ^{125}I seeds was carried out in one procedure. If there was still doubt regarding the diagnosis and grading, a second procedure was performed. A modified Riechert stereotactic system was used for the diagnostic and interstitial irradiation procedure. The patients were kept under local anaesthesia with a mild sedative (midazolam). A modified CT table was used for CT scanning, angiography, and operation. The coordinates of the centre of the target volume were derived directly from the CT image (Somatom High Q, Siemens, Erlangen).

The target coordinates chosen for interstitial implants were usually in the centre of the tumour volume or along a suitable axis through the tumour. In the rare case multiple targets and tracts were chosen. The number and activities of the ^{125}I seeds were selected according to the tumour shape and volume with special reference to the anatomical site. Radiation protection regulations limit the level of radiation upon discharge from hospital to less than 1 μSv per hour at a distance of 1 m. Consecutive CT follow-up scans were performed to control seed position 1 day, 6 weeks, and then 3 months following implantation. The patients were closely followed by neurological examination, including KR value, and the findings were compared with those of previous examinations. Neurological examination and tumour response as verified by rating CT and/or MRI were used to evaluate patients at 3- to 6-month intervals.

Response to Treatment

The present series includes 539 patients habouring primary or residual cerebral gliomas. Of these, 54 patients had previously undergone partial resection of their tumour or had suffered local recurrence after resection; 23 had received radiation therapy before biopsy and IRS. All patients presented with progressive neurological deficits or showed evidence of CT/MRI-confirmed tumour growth or both. The majority of the tumours (60.5%) were located in the cerebral hemispheres, 39.4% in the basal nuclei-thalamus and other midline structures. Of the 539 patients, 143 were aged 17 years or younger.

Pilocytic astrocytomas were found in 106 patients. The majority (n = 76) were under 18 years of age. Nonhemispheric tumours were found in the basal ganglia (38%) and in the diencephalon or mesencephalon (50%). Mean treatment volume was 17.4 15.5 ml. Neurological status at follow-up examinations (median follow-up period 4.7 years) revealed an improvement in neurological function in 32 patients (30%), no change in 46 (43%) patients, and a worsening of preoperatively established deficit in 28 patients (27%). The 5-year survival rate in patients aged under 18 years was 86%, as opposed to 58% in patients 18 years of age or older. The patients with lobar tumours (n = 8) had the best survival with a 5-year rate of 90%.

The histological diagnosis of an *astrocytoma* WHO grade II was made in 251 patients. Of this group 41 patients (16.3%) were under 18 years of age. Nonlobar astrocytomas were detected in the basal ganglia (13.1%) and in the diencephalon or mesencephalon in 68 patients (27.5%).

Lobar astrocytomas were mostly found in the frontotemporal region (152 patients; 60.6%; Fig. 2). A total of 176 lesions were found in functionally critical cortical areas of the hemispheres (70%). The mean treatment volume was 21.2 17.5 ml. Follow up examinations (mean 3.5 years) revealed an improvement in 95 patients (38%), stabilization of the disease in 87 patients (35%) and progressive worsening in 69 patients (27%). Additional subsequent external beam radiotherapy because of uncontrolled infiltrative tumour growth was instituted in 24 patients. Expanding tumour cysts were observed in 15 patients 2–10 months after implantation, which required internal or external drainage using a Rickham reservoir. The 5-year survival rate was 65%, after which the survival curve leveled off around this percentage (8-year survival rate 64%). Stereotactic biopsy revealed in 73 patients

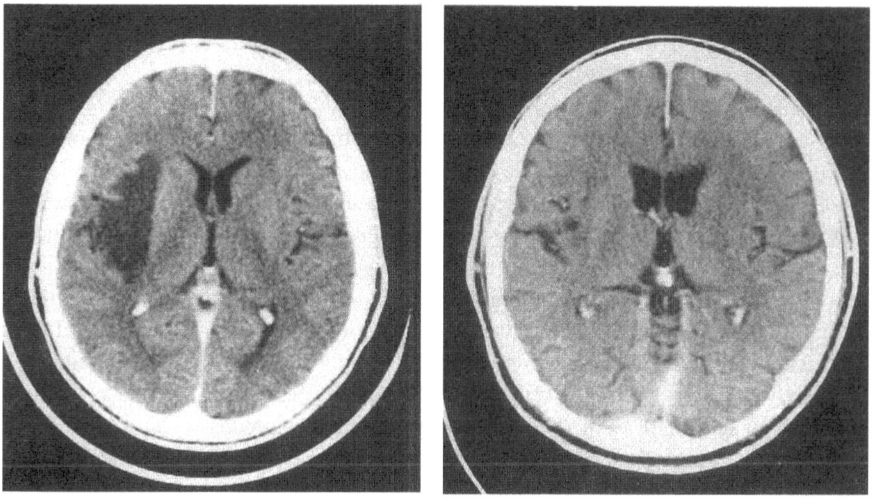

a b

Fig. 2. a Intersitial radiosurgery (two ^{125}I seeds) for fibrillary astrocytoma (WHO grade II) in the right insula (58-year-old man). CT demonstrates a hypodense circumscribed tumor, which was verified as fibrillary astrocytoma by a serial stereotactic biopsy. **b** CT control 2 years after IRS revealed a persistent shrinkage of the tumor without side effects

oligoastrocytomas (44 patients) or *oligodendrogliomas* (29 patients). The mean treatment volume was 17.1 10.5 ml and 24.9 ml, respectively. The follow-up examination (mean follow-up period 3.0 and 3.4 years) revealed improvement in 40 patients (55%), stabilization of the disease in 21 patients (29%), and a progressive worsening due to uncontrolled tumour growth in 12 cases (16%). In patients with oligodendrogliomas the 5-year survival rate was 58% as opposed to 80% in patients with oligoastrocytomas .

Fewer patients were selected for IRS habouring *anaplastic astrocytomas WHO grade III* (75 patients) and *glioblastomas* (34 patients). The mean treatment volume was 31.7 ml (anaplastic astrocytomas) and 41 ml (glioblastomas). Nonlobar anaplastic astrocytomas were found in the basal ganglia in 26 patients and in the diencephalon or mesencephalon in 8 patients. Nonlobar glioblastomas were detected in the brainstem in 8 patients. The Kaplan-Meier curves showed a 1-year survival rate of 49% and a 2-year survival rate of 36% in patients with anaplastic astrocytomas. The median survival time was 8 months (median follow-up 0.8 years). Patients with glioblastomas had a median follow-up period of .55 years with a 1-year survival rate of 48% and a 2-year-survival rate of 16%. The median survival was 6 months. Twenty-eight patients received additional conventional beam radiotherapy at the time of tumour progression.

Operative morbidity in this series of gliomas was 3.9%. There were no deaths as a result of the operative procedure of stereotactic diagnostic biopsy, implantation, and removal of the ^{125}I seeds. Follow-up examinations revealed functional defects in the vicinity of the implant in 17 cases (3.1%), particularly in the hypothalamus and midbrain-thalamus, which was interpreted as a local adverse effect of irradiation. No patient required reoperation due to radionecrosis.

Cerebral Metastases

Patient Selection

Surgical resection of brain metastases is performed in only a small fraction of cases (7%–17%) [11]. Statistically, however, there is no doubt that patients survive longer with a better quality of life after resection of a brain metastasis [24]. Brain metastases are mostly circumscribed, spherical volumes which exert mass effect by producing vasogenic edema. Even in patients with a known primary the presence of a single lesion in the brain does not establish that lesion as a metastasis [24]. The diagnosis of cerebral metastasis was confirmed by CT-guided biopsy in 410 patients. IRS or IRS combined with whole brain radiation therapy (WBRT) were performed in 81 patients (20%) with circumscribed mostly solitary spherical metastases with a diameter of less than 5 cm. The following treatment regimens were used: (a) IRS alone with a tumour dose of 60 Gy ($n = 22$); (b) IRS and WBRT with a local tumour dose of 60 Gy and subsequent radiotherapy with 40 Gy (5 2 Gy/week; $n = 38$); (c) IRS alone as treatment for recurrent disease confirmed by biopsy after previous operation and WBRT (tumour dose 60 Gy; $n = 21$) [13].

Sources and Dosimetry

Exclusively ^{125}I seeds were used as temporary implants. For clinical use the calculated dose ranged between 60 and 100 Gy. This dose was calculated to accumulate at the outer rim of the tumour as defined by contrast enhancement of the CT/MRI scan and serial biopsy. In 18 patients two seed implantations were carried out at the same time because of the presence of more than one confirmed cerebral metastasis. For further details see Sect. 3.1.2.

Response to Treatment

The present series including 81 patients, most with single metastases, had a mean follow up period of 17 months. The median survival time was 17 months after IRS and WBRT, 12 months after IRS, and 7.7 months after WBRT. The median survival after local treatment of recurrent disease was 6 months with a total median survival of 17 months. Twelve patients with a metastasis of a malignant melanoma had a median survival of 16 months after IRS or IRS+WBRT, 15 patients with hypernephroma metastases suvived 18.5 months. Prognostically favourable factors in the multivariate analysis after IRS and IRS+WBRT were a latency period of over 1 year (time interval between diagnosis of primary tumour and cerebral metastasis; p), a solitary cerebral metastasis (p), a KR higher than 70 (p) and absence of disseminated disease (p). The prognosis for lung cancer was worse than for other primary tumours (p). IRS+WBRT was not superior to IRS alone in the multivariate model. No patients died from the locally irradiated metastasis. The implanted metastasis could be

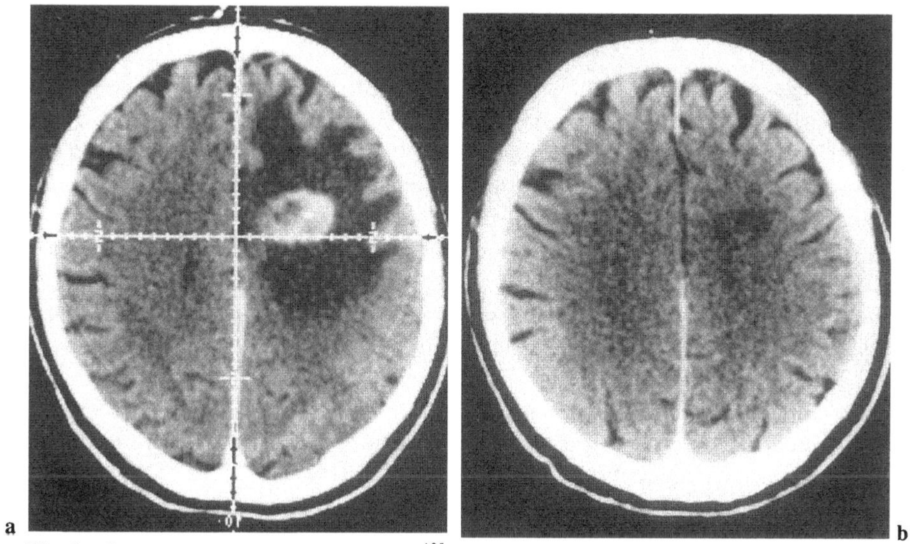

Fig. 3. a Interstitial radiosurgery (temporary ^{125}I seed implant) for a solitary brain metastasis of a non-small-cell lung cancer. Note the solid tumor which is surrounded by an extensive vasogenic edema. b CT control 5 months later demonstrates the complete disappearance of both the solid tumor and the perifocal edema

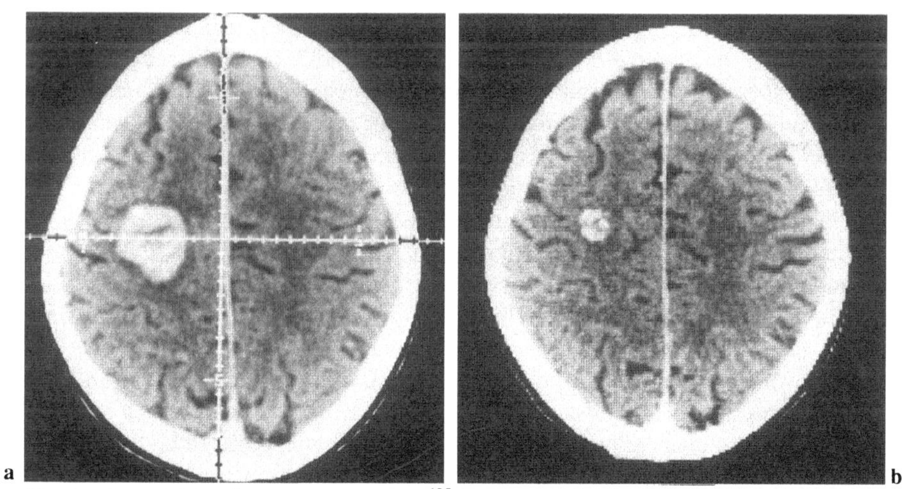

Fig. 4. a Interstitial radiosurgery (temporary ^{125}I seed implant) for a solitary brain metastasis of an ovarian carcinoma. b CT control 4 months after treatment reveals a shrinkage and calcification of the lesion

radiosurgically controlled in every case (in eight patients not until reimplantation with a total tumour dose of 100 Gy; Figs.3, 4). No patient experienced a radionecrosis with mass effect requiring operative treatment. In ten patients receiving IRS alone WBRT was performed after a latency period (median 6 months) when multiple cerebral metastases became evident.

Conclusion

Growth characteristics, mitotic activity, and vascularity of both gliomas and metastases in the brain are the major factors determining the biological effect of therapeutic radiation [28]. In external beam radiotherapy the tolerance of the healthy brain is critical. It presupposes a difference in radiosensitivity between tumour and brain, referred to as therapeutic ratio. There is no doubt that external beam irradiation is effective for highly proliferating tumours such as glioblastomas and some metastases [26]. However, whether it is as effective for low-grade gliomas with a very low proliferation capacity and no neovascularization and a variety of radioresistant metastases is another matter. In the latter cases it would seem to be more effective to remove as much tumour as possible. If, however, there is no harmless way of surgical removal, as is the case with gliomas or metastases in the basal ganglia, brain stem or in functionally critical cortical areas, stereotactic IRS is considered to be a less invasive treatment modality.

The subgroup of patients with low-grade cerebral gliomas in our series had a better or similar survival index when compared with data from the literature [3, 8, 16, 18, 27, 33]. The patient's age was a significant factor affecting survival. As with Laws et al., we found the best results in patients under 18 years of age in the subgroup of astrocytomas WHO II: these had a 5-year survival rate of 84% [16]. Also in patients with pilocytic astrocytomas age had the most prognostic significance. The total 5- and 10-year survival rate was 77%. Among those under 18 years of age (71.7% of all patients) the 5-year survival rate rose to 86%. In the subgroup with pilocytic astrocytoma our results are not necessarily comparable with those of other studies on surgical resection involving a higher number of lobar or cerebellar tumours [28]. In malignant gliomas our results are not satisfactory although individual patients experienced astonishing benefits over long time periods [9]. The generally better results obtained in our series as compared with the pertinent literature are partly due to the strict selection according to morphological, neuoradiological and clinical criteria. The data demonstrate the therapeutic value of IRS.

The indications for surgery or IRS of solitary cerebral metastasis have been almost identical in the past. The regression analysis of our data shows that the patients with brain metastases most likely to benefit from IRS are those with a single, well-circumscribed lesion and a latency period of over 1 year. Median survival longer than 12 months after IRS is in agreement with the results after surgery and WBRT reported in the literature [24, 26]. IRS+WBRT was not superior to IRS only in multivariate analysis. This finding is remarkable since most studies have found an important influence of WBRT on survival after surgery [26]. Therefore, it would seem that local control of the metastasis is more likely to be achieved using IRS than with surgical extirpation. In the present study IRS controlled the growth of brain metastases regardless of tumour histology, prior treatmet, or radioresistance, without any radionecrotic complications. This was in contrast to other studies using high-activity radioactive implants [25]. IRS alone as a minimally invasive method has strong advantages. Whether surgery or IRS or external radiosurgery is indicated for accessible metastases remains a controversial issue.

The more circumscribed, noninfiltrative gliomas and well-defined solitary brain metastases are the preferred cases for both surgery and IRS. Both methods entail selective destruction and removal of the tumour bulk. Whether surgery or IRS is indicated for surgically accessible tumours located superficially is a controversial issue. As the present series demonstrates, IRS can be used effectively to treat circumsribed low-grade gliomas and solitary brain metastases in particular, however, with less invasiveness, dissection of normal brain, and expense compared with open surgery.

Acknowledgements. The author gratefully acknowledges the support of P. Kleihues, Abteilung Neuropathologie, Universität Zürich, and of M. Kiessling, Abteilung Neuropathologie, Universität Heidelberg. Thanks go to H.K. Leetz, Institut für Radiologische Physik der Universität des Saarlandes, Homburg/Saar, Germany for providing the dosimetry calculations. The author is indebted to his collaborators P.C. Warnke, F.W. Kreth, F.J. Hans and Mrs. A. Korst for technical assistance. The studies were supported by the Deutsche Forschungsgemeinschaft (OS 58/2–1 and OS 58/2–2).

References

1. Anderson LL, Hsin MK, Ing-Yuan D (1981) Clinical dosimetry with 125-I. In:George FW (ed) Modern interstitial and intracavitary radiation cancer management. Masson, New York
2. Bernstein M, Gutin PH (1981) Interstitial irradiation of brain tumors: A review. Neurosurgery 6: 741–750
3. Cohadon F (1990) Indications for surgery in the management of gliomas. In: Symon L et al (eds) Advances and technical standards in neurosurgery, vol 17. Springer, Berlin Heidelberg New York, pp 189–234
4. Fike JR, Cann CE, Philips TL, Bernstein M, Gutin PH, Turowsky K, Weaver KA, Davis RL, Higgins RJ, Da Silva V (1985) Radiation brain damage induced by interstitial 125-I sources: a canine model evaluated by quantitative computed tomography. Neurosurgery 16:530–537
5. Frazier C (1920) The effects of radium emanations on brain tumors. Surg Gynecol Obstet 31:236–239
6. Groothuis DR, Wright DC, Ostertag CB (1987) The effect of I-125 interstitial radiotherapy on blood brain barrier function in normal canine brain. J Neurosurg 67:985–902
7. Groothuis DR, Lapin GD, Vriesendorp FJ, Mikhael MA, Patlak CS (1991) A method to quantitatively measure transcapillary transport of iodinated compounds in canine brain tumors with computed tomography. J Cereb Blood Flow Metab 11:939–948
8. Guthrie BL, Laws ER (1991) Management of Supratentorial Gliomas In: Karim ABMF, Laws ER Jr (eds) Glioma. Springer, Berlin, Heidelberg, pp 75–92
9. Gutin PH, Leibel SA (1985) Stereotactic interstitial irradiation of malignant brain tumors. Neurologic Clinics 3:883–893
10. Hirsch O (1952) Symptoms and treatment of pituitary tumors. Arch Otolaryngol 55:268–306
11. Hoskin P, Crow J, Ford H (1990) The influence of extent and local management on the outcome of radiotherapy for brain metastases. Int J Radiat Oncol Biol Phys 19:111–115
12. Janzer RC, Kleihues P, Ostertag CB (1986) Early and late effects on the normal dog brain of permanent interstitial Iridium-192 irradiation. Acta Neuropathol 70:91–102
13. Kreth FW, Warnke PC, Ostertag CB (1993) Interstitial Implant Radiosurgery of Cerebral Metastases Acta Neurochir Suppl 58:112–114
14. Krishnaswamy V (1978) Dose distribution around an 125-I seed source in tissue. Radiology 126:489–491
15. Larsson B (1992) Radiobiological fundamentals in radiosurgery. In: Steiner L et al. (eds) Radiosurgery: baseline and trends. Raven, New York
16. Laws ER, Taylor WF, Marvin BC, Okazaki H (1984) Neurosurgical management of low-grade astrocytoma of the cerebral hemispheres. J Neurosurg 61:665–673

17. Lindquist C, Hindmarsh T, Kihlström L, Mindus P, Steiner L (1992) MRI and CT Studies of Radionecrosis Development in the Normal Human Brain. In: Steiner L et al. (eds) Radiosurgery: baseline and trends. Raven, New York
18. Morantz RA (1987) Radiation therapy in the treatment of cerebral astrocytoma. Neurosurgery 20:975–982
19. Ostertag CB, Hossmann KA, v. d. Kerckhoff W (1982) Radiation effects of Iridium-192 implants in the cat brain. Nucl Med 21:99–104
20. Ostertag CB, Weigel K (1982) Three-dimensional CT Scanning of the Dog Brain. J Comput Assist Tom 6(5):1036–1037
21. Ostertag CB, Weigel K, Warnke P, Lombeck G, Kleihues P (1983) Sequential morphological changes in the dog brain after interstitial Iodine-125 irradiation. Neurosurgery 13:523–528
22. Ostertag CB, Warnke P, Kleihues P, Bigner D (1984) Iodine-125 interstitial irradiation of virally induced dog brain tumors. Neurol Res 6:176–180
23. Ostertag CB, Kreth FW (1992) Stereotactic interstitial radiotherapy in the treatment of gliomas. Acta Neurochir 119:53–61
24. Patchell RA, Tibbs PA, Walsh JW, Dempsey RJ, Maruyama Y, Kryscio RJ, Markesbery WR, McDonald JS, Young B (1990) A randomized trial of surgery in the treatment of single metastases to the brain. N Engl J Med 332:494–500
25. Prados M, Leibel S, Barnett CM, Gutin P (1989) Interstitial brachytherapy for metastatic brain tumors. Cancer 63:657–660
26. Sause WT, Crowley JJ, Morantz R, Rotman M, Mowry PA, Bouzaglou A, Borst JR, Selin H (1990) Solitary brain metastasis: results of an RTOG/SWOG protocol evaluation Surgery+RT versus RT alone Am J Clin Oncol 13:427–432
27. Shaw EG,Daumas-Duport C,Scheithauer BW, Gilbertson DT, et al. (1989) Radiation therapy in the management of low-grade supratentorial astrocytomas. J Neurosurg 70:853–861
28. Sheline GE (1985) The role of radiation therapy in the treatment of low-grade gliomas. Clinical Neurosurgery, Williams and Wilkins, Baltimore, pp 563–574
29. Sondhaus CA (1981) I-125: Physical properties, photon dosimetry and effectiveness. In: George FW (ed) Modern interstitial and intracavitary radiation cancer management. Masson, New York
30. Talairach J, Aboulker J, Ruggiero G, David M (1955) Essai d'un nouveau traitement des tumeurs cérébrales inopérables. Mise en place d'or radio-actif par stéréotaxie. Semin Hop Paris 31:548–653
31. Turowsky K, Fike JR, Cann CE, Higgins RJ, Davis RL, Gutin PH, Phillips TL, Weaver KA (1986) Normal brain iodine-125 radiation damage: effect of dose and irradiated volume in a canine model. Radiology 158:833–838
32. Warnke PC, Hans FJ, Ostertag CB (1993) Impact of stereotactic interstitial irradiation on brain capillary physiology. Acta Neurochir Suppl. 58:85–88
33. Weingart J, Olivi A, Brem H (1991) Supratentorial low-grade astrocytomas in adults. Neurosurg Q 1(3):141–159

*Interstitial Brachytherapy of Malignant Gliomas: The Memorial Sloan-Kettering Cancer Center Experience**

M. G. Malkin

Department of Neurology, Memorial Sloan-Kettering Cancer Center, 1275 York Avenue, New York, NY 10021,U.S.A.

Introduction

Malignant gliomas remain incurable primary brain tumors despite the dedicated efforts over many decades of hundreds of clinical scientists worldwide. Any new procedure that offers a rationale for better tumor control is seized upon and applied in the hope that theory can be translated into practice, and that treatment can be translated into longer survival. One of these new techniques is interstitial brachytherapy, the stereotactic implantation of radioactive seeds directly into the tumor. In Europe this technique has been most widely applied to the treatment of low-grade gliomas, as discussed by Dr. Ostertag at this symposium. In North America the emphasis during the past 10 years has been on the application of this method to the treatment of malignant gliomas. In 1990 at least 50 institutions in North America were licensed by the manufacturer of ^{125}I seeds to treat patients with brain tumors. This chapter reviews the experience with interstitial brachytherapy at Memorial Sloan-Kettering Cancer Center since 1986.

The rationale for brachytherapy in malignant gliomas is based upon four facts. Most malignant gliomas recur locally (Hochberg and Pruitt 1980; Wallner et al. 1989). They regrow within 2–3 cm of the original boundary of the primary tumor site in 80%–90% of cases. It is known that radiation therapy is the most effective tool at our disposal to control the growth of malignant gliomas (Walker et al. 1978), and it is also known that higher doses of radiation therapy are more effective than lower doses to achieve this aim (Walker et al. 1979). Finally, the energy characteristics of the isotopes used in brachytherapy are such that the radiation emitted falls off quickly from the margin of the tumor (Saw et al. 1989), thereby sparing normal surrounding brain tissue. With these principles in mind we set out to treat patients with malignant gliomas by the stereotactic implantation of radioactive ^{125}I seeds.

---

*Adapted from: Malkin MG (1992) Interstitial Irradiation of Malignant Gliomas. Rev Neurol (Paris) 148, 6–7: 448–453

Patients and Methods

For a patient to be eligible for brachytherapy several criteria must be met. First, the contrast-enhancing margin of the tumor must be readily visible on computed tomography (CT). Practically speaking, the physician planning brachytherapy must be able to draw a line around each image of the tumor on the CT scan with a film marker. We realize that the contrast-enhancing edge of the tumor as seen on CT scan is artificial and may not correspond to invisible nonenhancing malignant astrocytic processes that project beyond the bulk of the tumor. However, the contrast-enhancing margin of the tumor provides a reproducible target upon which to base a treatment plan and a basis to compare techniques between institutions. Patients who have had a lobectomy are not eligible for brachytherapy, but patients who have undergone gross total resection of a malignant glioma, and whose tumor bed of low attenuation is surrounded by brain of normal attenuation on CT scan, present a target which can be defined as the interface of the tumor cyst and surrounding brain. Second, patients with multifocal tumor, or with tumor that crosses the midline, are not eligible for brachytherapy. Third, patients whose tumor lies in the speech center, and who consistently are at least moderately aphasic, are not eligible for brachytherapy. We have come to this conclusion following our observation that patients who receive brachytherapy for malignant gliomas which lie in Broca's or Wernicke's area often survive a very long time but with very poor quality of life. In retrospect these patients and their families have told us that they would not have wished brachytherapy to be performed had they known of the long-term sequelae. Fourth, there is no absolute limitation to the volume of the malignant gliomas that we treat with brachytherapy, but we prefer, for improved dosimetry, to treat lesions with a volume of less than 70 cm^3. A volume of 70 cm^3 corresponds to a diameter of 5.1 cm if the tumor were spherical.

A patient who meets the above eligibility criteria is admitted to the hospital on the afternoon before the procedure. Skull radiographs (anteroposterior and lateral) are taken to verify the location of the previous craniotomy, and a peripheral venous catheter, heparin-locked, is inserted. Early on the morning of the procedure the patient receives lorazepam 1 mg intravenously and codeine 30 mg intramuscularly 30 min before the placement of the Brown-Roberts-Wells (BRW) frame. The frame is fastened to the patient's head under local anesthesia. CT is then performed immediately following the infusion (1 cm^3/s) of 150 cm^3 iodinated (60%) contrast. This scan, an example of which is shown in Fig. 1, allows us to digitize tumor attributes within a verifiable frame of reference. The Leksell system can be used interchangeably with the BRW or CRW systems (Sapozink et al. 1987; Szikla et al. 1984; Ten Haken et al. 1988).

As illustrated in Fig. 2, there is a linear relationship between the logarithm of total seed strength required in millicuries and tumor volume in cubic centimeters. Once tumor volume is calculated from the planning CT scan, the total seed strength required can be estimated and the radioactive seed inventory at the hospital searched for the requisite radioactive seeds. The microcomputer-driven treatment plan which we use, developed at Memorial Sloan-Kettering Cancer Center, is designed to

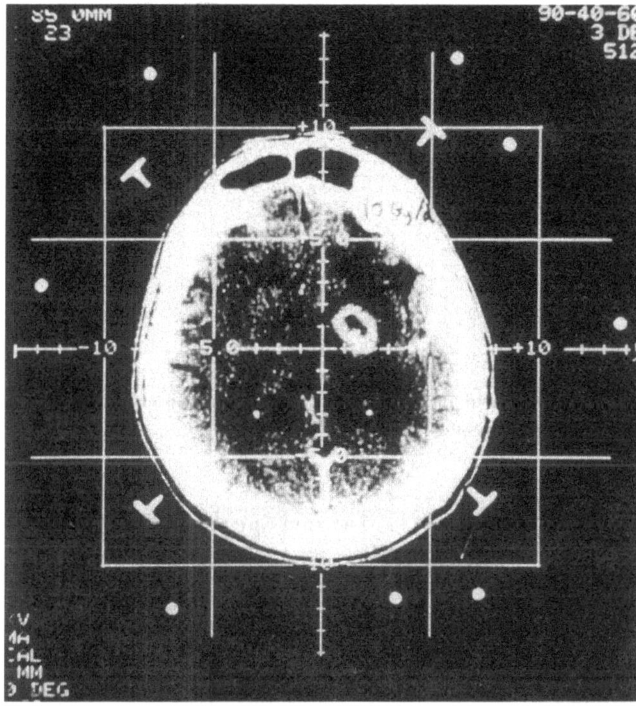

Fig. 1. CT scan of malignant glioma. Note the fiducial markings of the BRW frame, and the overlying grid, which provide a frame of reference for treatment planning. The enhancing tumor margin is well delineated from surrounding brain

provide a uniform dose rate of irradiation of 40 cGy/h to a line 0.5 cm beyond the contrast-enhancing contour of the tumor on every image where the tumor is seen on CT scan. As can be seen from Fig. 3, tumors are rarely regular spheres or ellipses but rather appear as if they were composed of a stack of coins that have been shoved side to side to create an irregularly shaped structure. A shadow of irradiation that conforms to the irregular circumference of the tumor is most efficiently cast with the aid of a computer than can perform many iterations per second. Basically, what the computer does is take a fixed number of radioactive seeds, determined by the relationship illustrated in Fig. 2, and move them within the confines of the tumor to such positions that variation of dose around the outside of the tumor is minimized. This, in turn, minimizes irradiation to normal brain far away from the tumor. We begin with a single seed per tube and then, to reduce the length of the procedure in the operating theater and the risk to the patient of multiple tube insertions, the computer combines adjacent single seeds into the same tube. A typical final array of 15 seeds in five tubes is illustrated in Fig. 4. We currently use Model 6702 ^{125}I sources manufactured by the 3-M Corporation.

When the treatment plan is finished, the patient is taken to the operating room where tube insertion is performed out under local anesthesia. We do not reopen the

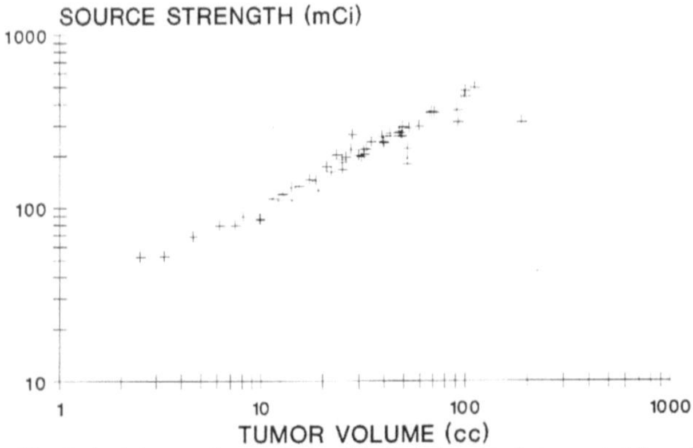

Fig. 2. Activity – volume relationship. Relationship between total seed strength required for interstitial brachytherapy and tumor volume. ^{125}I sources ($n = 59$)

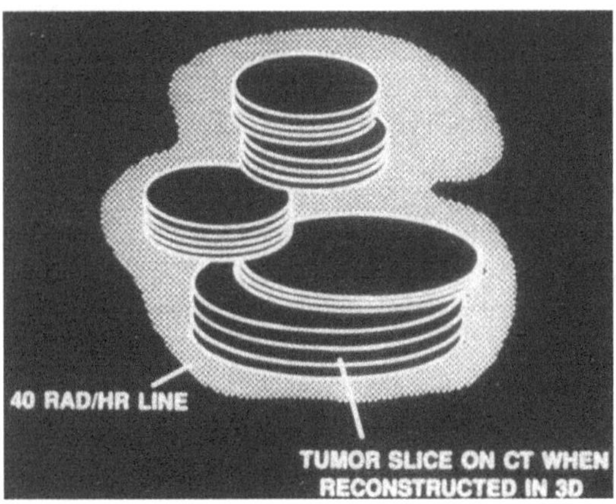

Fig. 3. Tumor volume computations versus total volume radiated at 40 rad/h. Typical reconstructed tumor shape, and prescribed brachytherapy dosimetry which conforms closely to the tumor margin, sparing "normal" brain (tumor volume, 32.7 cm^3; total volume of tissue in 40 rad/h line, 58.1 cm^3; therefore, normal tissue = 25.5. cm^3)

craniotomy but rather anesthetize the scalp with lidocaine and create paths for the tubes through twist drill burr holes. This technique offers several advantages. First, there is no need for a difficult endotracheal intubation under a low-lying BRW frame. Second, there is no need to reopen the craniotomy, thus minimizing the risk of delayed wound healing and CSF leak. Finally, a great deal of time is saved in the operating room with the use of twist drill burr holes alone. Following the insertion of tubes, dummy seeds are placed and orthogonal skull radiographs taken with a Lutz (Suetens-Gybels-Vandermuelen, SGV) box in place to verify precise tube position. Then the dummy seeds are removed and the "hot" seeds "afterloaded" in the operating room one at a time. The tubes are fastened to the scalp by silk sutures and Aron Alpha ("Krazy Glue"). The patient returns to his room on the ward and, wearing a hat lined with lead foil, is free to walk about within the hospital for such time (usually 6 days) as the tubes are in place. On the day following the implant, a CT scan with contrast is obtained.

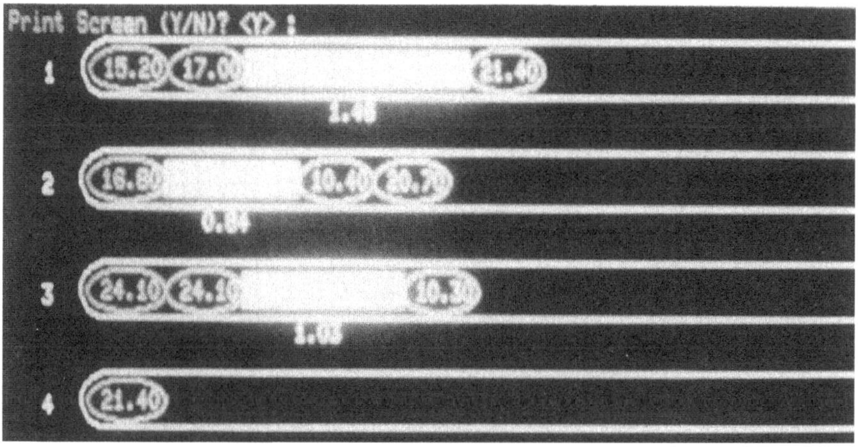

Fig. 4. Fifteen ^{125}I seeds arranged in five tubes. Individual seed strengths (in millicuries) and distance between seeds (in cubic centimeters) are shown for each tube

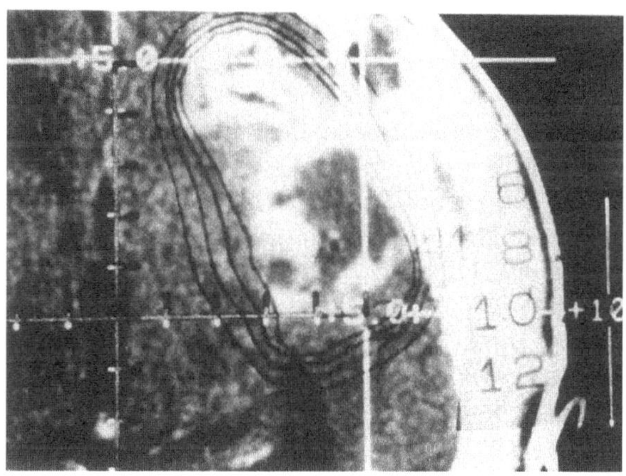

Fig. 5. Close-up of postimplant CT scan. The concentric isodose lines, proceeding from the tumor margin outward, represent 6, 8, 10, and 12 Gy/day, respectively. Note how rapidly dose rate falls off a short distance from the tumor margin

As illustrated in Fig. 5, this scan is used by the radiation physicist and radiation oncologist to verify the planned dosimetry. When the desired tumor dose has been delivered, the tubes are removed at the bedside, and silk ligatures secured to the wounds. Provided there is no CSF leak or fever, the patient is discharged from hospital 24–36 h later.

Results

From December 1986 through January 1991 we treated 56 patients with malignant gliomas using brachytherapy. Mean number of seeds has been 11, range 4–26. Mean number of tubes has been 6, range 2–18. Mean radiation dose 0.5 cm beyond the

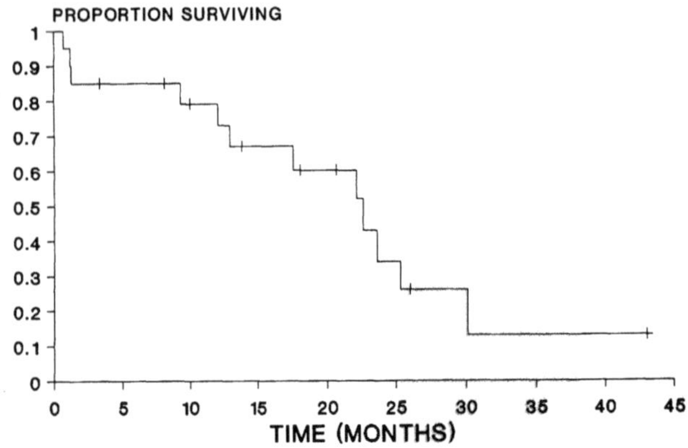

Fig. 6. Survival of patients (n = 20) with GBM treated with interstitial brachytherapy following resection, before further external beam radiation and chemotherapy. Analysis was performed using the Kaplan-Meier method

enhancing tumor edge was 5972 cGy, range 5320–7030. Mean dose rate has been 37 cGy/h, range 23–50. Mean duration of tubes in the brain has been 6.9 days, range 4.8–10.7. Mean total volume of brain irradiated has been only 67 cm^3 per patient, range 11–184.

We have treated two groups of patients, an "up-front" group (n = 20), and a group treated at recurrence (n = 36). Results are considered separately for each group.

All patients treated up-front had glioblastoma (GBM). Seventeen had had resections, and three biopsies only. Their mean age was 56, range 32–73. Their mean Karnofsky performance score (KPS) at the time of brachytherapy was 78, range 50–100. Their mean tumor volume was 37 cm^3, range 5–100. Eighteen patients went on to receive a further 6000 cGy external beam radiation therapy following the implant, and 17 of the 20 went on to chemotherapy, usually intravenous carmustine, following brachytherapy. At last follow-up, the mean KPS for the living patients was 66, range 30–100. Median survival for this group was 22 months as shown in Fig. 6.

Of the 36 patients treated at recurrence, 24 had GBMs, and 12 anaplastic astrocytomas. Thirty-four had undergone resections, all had been irradiated, and 22 had received chemotherapy prior to recurrence and implant. Mean age was 43, range 7–69. Mean KPS at implant was 73, range 50–100. Mean tumor volume was 43 cm^3, range 6–187. Following the procedure, ten patients proceeded to further chemotherapy. Mean KPS at last follow-up for the living patients was 65, range 40–100. Median survival for this group of patients was 10 months, as illustrated in Fig. 7.

It is usual following brachytherapy for intense inflammation and radiation necrosis to develop at the tumor site as a consequence of the intense dose of radiation administered. Clinically, the patient may develop focal signs relevant to the site of the tumor, or symptoms due to intracranial hypertension. CT and magnetic resonance imaging scans may show increased contrast enhancement with surrounding cerebral edema (Kumar et al. 1988). Symptoms and signs can generally be controlled with corticosteroids. However, in 24 patients (43%) in our series, 27 craniotomies were

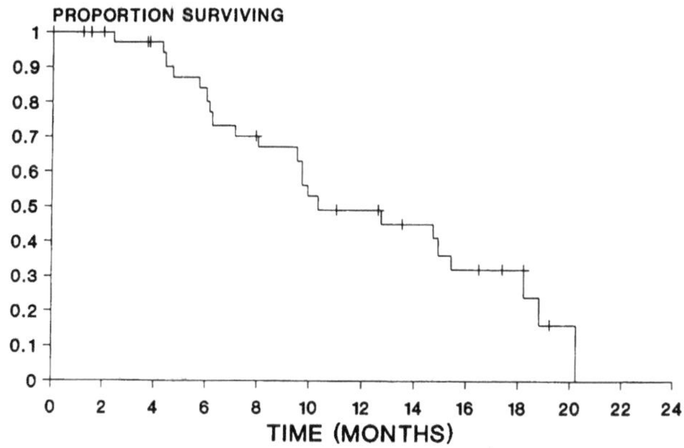

Fig. 7. Survival of patients ($n = 36$) with malignant glioma treated with interstitial brachytherapy at recurrence. Analysis was performed using the Kaplan-Meier method

performed 1–25 months after brachytherapy because the expanding contrast-enhancing mass lesion at the site of the original tumor was refractory to the effects of corticosteroids. The incidence of reoperation was no different in patients treated up-front or at recurrence. Age, KPS, tumor volume, total implant dose, and dose rate did not influence the likelihood of reoperation or survival. The mean time from brachytherapy to reoperation was 6 months in these patients. Of the 27 reoperation specimens 25 were available for pathological review at our institution. In 18 substantial radiation necrosis was observed with minimal anaplastic tumor; in 5 only radiation necrosis was noted;and in 2 only anaplastic tumor was seen. We view reoperation as integral to this procedure, not as a complication. The intent of our treatment is to produce tumor necrosis using focused radiation therapy. We hope that the effect of this can be managed by the patient's own macrophages, and helped with corticosteroids, but we recognize that in almost half of patients surgery will be needed, and ultimately beneficial, to the patient's welfare and survival (Gutin et al. 1987).

We have noted complications with this treatment. Of our 56 patients, one died within 30 days of the implant from *Pneumocystis* pneumonia and *Aspergillus* septicemia. Therefore, our 30-day mortality rate is 2%. In five patients (9%) the technique has resulted in permanent neurological deficit. In two of these patients the reason was tube misplacement, and in three patients the reason was a neurological deficit produced when an effort was made to remove tumor at the time that tubes were removed. These five complications occurred early in our experience. Refinements in our treatment planning software, and neurosurgical expertise, have prevented tube misplacement, and we have come to realize that there is no good reason to remove tumor immediately after tubes are removed. Other side effects which have not resulted in permanent patient morbidity have included tube misplacement in three, CSF leak in four, *Staphylococcus aureus* meningitis in two, aseptic meningitis in two, catheter wound infection in two, asymptomatic epidural hematoma in two, subgaleal effusion in two, and status epilepticus (in a patient with antecedent seizures) in one. To prevent perioperative infection, all patients are treated with intravenous Oxacillin from the time they enter the operating theater until 24 h after the tubes have been removed.

Discussion

We believe that there is a place for interstitial brachytherapy in the treatment of malignant gliomas both at recurrence and shortly after diagnosis. Interstitial irradiation of malignant gliomas is not a cure for this cancer and is applicable to only about 30% of all patients with malignant gliomas. Nevertheless, our experience in treating malignant gliomas at recurrence is very similar to that reported by the investigators at the University of California at San Francisco (Larson et al. 1990) and thus validates their conclusion of the usefulness of brachytherapy for malignant gliomas that recur locally. The virtual doubling of median survival in our experience (22 months versus the usual 12 months) for GBM up-front using brachytherapy is encouraging. It remains to be seen whether the addition of brachytherapy to surgery, external irradiation, and chemotherapy, administered shortly after diagnosis, improves survival and quality of survival in patients with malignant gliomas. To this end, we are participating in a national phase III prospective randomized clinical trial performed by the Brain Tumor Cooperative Group and funded by the National Cancer Institute. In this protocol (BTCG 87–01) patients with malignant gliomas verified at craniotomy are randomly assigned to receive brachytherapy (as outlined in this paper) followed by teletherapy (6000 cGy tumor dose) and carmustine (200 mg/m^2 intravenously every 8 weeks 8 doses) versus the same external irradiation and chemotherapy but without brachytherapy. In other words, BTCG Protocol 87–01 is designed to answer the question "Does brachytherapy add to the effect of external beam radiation therapy and chemotherapy for newly diagnosed malignant gliomas?" The criteria for patient exclusion from Protocol 87–01 are similar to those described above; in addition, patients with a second primary malignancy, children, patients with a KPS below 50, and those who have received prior antineoplastic therapy are excluded. This trial is still open to patient accrual. A similar study is underway at the University of Toronto (Bernstein et al. 1990). Chemotherapy is not used in the Toronto trial, and the brachytherapy is administered following external beam radiation therapy rather than before.

Those involved in the use of brachytherapy for malignant gliomas have already begun to ask questions whose answers may well come before the end of the decade. Will brachytherapy with hyperthermia be more effective than brachytherapy alone? Should brachytherapy be administered with a radiation sensitizer, or with a chemotherapeutic agent (e.g., cisplatin) thought to act as a sensitizer? Which lesions should be treated with brachytherapy as described in this paper, and which could be equally well treated with stereotactic radiosurgery ("gamma knife" or stereotactic linear accelerator)? The author remains optimistic that our experience to date with brachytherapy, and the answers to the questions just raised, will materially benefit the lives of patients with malignant gliomas in the near future.

References

Bernstein M, Laperriere N, Leung P, McKenzie S (1990) Interstitial brachytherapy for malignant brain tumors: preliminary results. Neurosurgery 26:371–380
Gutin PH et al (1987) Recurrent malignant gliomas: survival following interstitial brachytherapy with high-activity iodine-125 sources. J Neurosurg 67:864–873
Hochberg FH, Pruitt A (1980) Assumptions in the radiotherapy of glioblastoma. Neurology 30: 907–911
Kumar PP, Good RR, Jones EO, Skultety FM, Leibrock LG, McComb RD (1988) Contrast-enhancing computed tomography ring in glioblastoma multiforme after intraoperative endocurietherapy. Cancer 61:1759–1765
Larson DA, Gutin PH, Leibel SA, Phillips TL, Sneed PK, Wara WM (1990) Stereotaxic irradiation of brain tumors. Cancer 65:792–799
Sapozink MD, Moeller JM, McDonald PM, Heilbrun MP (1987) Improved precision of interstitial brain tumor irradiation using the BRW CT stereotaxic guidance system. Int J Radiat Oncol Biol Phys 13:1753–1760
Saw CB, Suntharalingham N, Ayyangar KM, Tupchong L (1989) Dosimetric considerations of stereotactic brain implants. Int J Radiat Oncol Biol Phys 17:887–891
Szikla G, Schlienger M, Blond S, Daumas-Duport C, Missir O, Miyahara S, Musolino A, Schaub C (1984) Interstitial and combined interstitial and external irradiation of supratentorial gliomas Results in 61 cases treated 1973 1981. Acta Neurochir Suppl 33:355–362
Ten Haken RK, Diaz RF, McShan DL, Fraass BA, Taren JA, Hood TW (1988) From manual to 3-D computerized treatment planning for 125I stereotactic brain implants. Int J Radiat Oncol Biol Phys 15:467–480
Walker MD et al (1978) Evaluation of BCNU and/or radiotherapy in the treatment of anaplastic gliomas. J Neurosurg 49:333–343
Walker MD, Strike TA, Sheline GE (1979) An analysis of dose-effect relationship in the radiotherapy of malignant gliomas. Int J Radiat Oncol Biol Phys 5:1725–1731
Wallner KE, Galicich JH, Krol G, Arbit E, Malkin MG (1989) Patterns of failure following treatment for glioblastoma multiforme and anaplastic astrocytoma. Int J Radiat Oncol Biol Phys 16: 1405–1409

Aggressive Oligodendroglioma: A Chemosensitive Tumor

J. G. Cairncross

Departments of Clinical Neurological Sciences and Oncology, University of Western Ontario and Victoria Hospital, and the London Regional Cancer Centre, 790 Commissioners Road East, London, Ontario, N6A 4L6, Canada

Introduction

Aggressive oligodendrogliomas, tumors that are symptomatic, enlarging, enhancing, and usually but not always anaplastic (Fig. 1), respond to chemotherapy. PCV, a regimen that includes procarbazine, lomustine (CCNU), and vincristine, is predictably effective, but other drugs have anti-oligodendroglioma activity. Cooperative group trials will be necessary to determine the most effective drug or drug combination and to explore fully the role of chemotherapy in the treatment of this uncommon glioma.

Background

Anaplastic gliomas are incurable cancers. Surgery and radiotherapy (RT) prolong life [24], and there is some evidence that adjuvant treatment with nitrosourea-based chemotherapy augments tumor control [9,25]. In the case of recurrent tumors reoperation [27] and brachytherapy [10] help some patients, but, once again, chemotherapy has proved to be of only modest benefit, with low response rates and short response durations [13]. The search for effective antiglioma chemotherapy continues with only occasional signs of progress [16, 20]. It is in this context that recent reports of "successful" chemotherapy for oligodendroglioma [4, 5, 18, 22] and mixed tumors containing oligodendroglial elements [8] are both encouraging and welcome. This chapter reviews our experience with chemotherapy for aggressive oligodendroglioma, highlights that of others, and suggests avenues for future clinical and basic research.

Recurrent Anaplastic Oligodendroglioma

Macdonald and I became interested in chemotherapy for oligodendroglioma in 1985 when a patient with recurrent right frontal anaplastic tumor and ipsilateral cervical lymph node metastasis responded to carmustine (BCNU) and a patient with a recurrent right parietal anaplastic tumor responded to PCV (Table 1). (Note: mini-

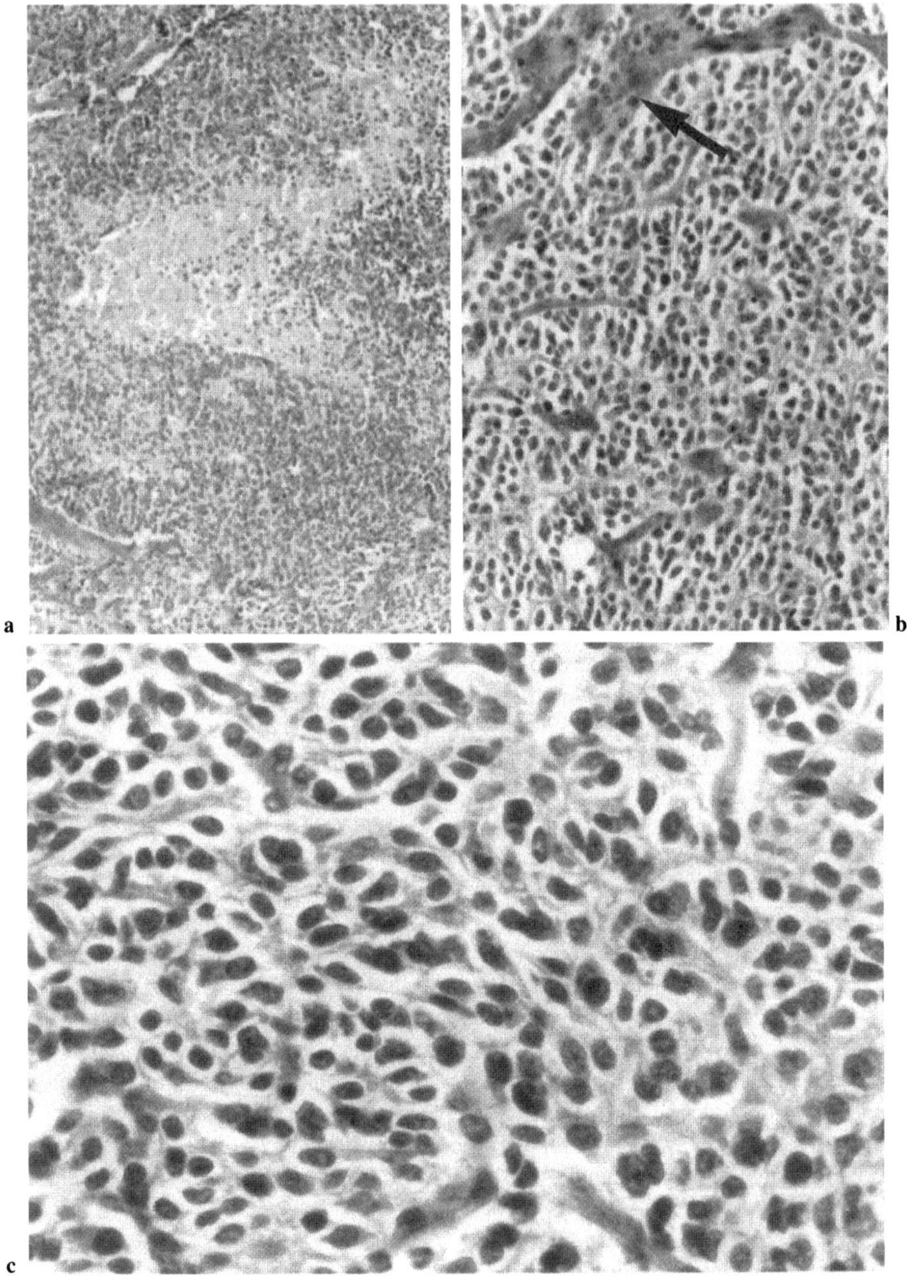

Fig. 1a-c. Photomicrographs (H&E) of an oligodendroglioma with anaplastic features. **a** Small chevron-shaped area of necrosis in a hypercellular tumor (x 100). **b** Hyperplastic tumor vessel (arrow; x 360). **c** Neoplastic cells with pleomorphic nuclei and perinuclear halos (x 500)

Table 1. PCV chemotherapy regimen

Drug(s)	Dosage and Schedule	Frequenzy
Lomustine	110 mg/m^2 po; day 1	
Vincristine[a]	1.4 mg/m^2 IV; day 8	
		q 8 weeks
Procarbazine	60 mg/m^2/day po; days 8–21	
Vincristine[a]	1.4 mg/m^2 IV; day 29	

[a] Maximum dose, 2 mg.

mum criteria for response: > 50% reduction in tumor size [17].) We were struck by the completeness and durability of these responses, began to wonder whether anaplastic oligodendrogliomas were especially chemosensitive, and decided to treat these tumors in a uniform way, separate from other malignant gliomas. Over the next few years we observed that oligodendrogliomas that had regrown after one or more resections and RT invariably responded to chemotherapy [4]. These tumors were clinically aggressive, contrast enhancing, histologically anaplastic. and relatively pure (for a detailed review of these patients see [4, 5]). Briefly, we saw responses – two complete and eight partial – in ten consecutive patients with recurrent anaplastic tumors. One patient responded to BCNU, one to diaziquone (AZQ), and the others to PCV. The partial responses were often dramatic with near total regression of large enhancing tumors [4]. The responses to PCV were usually prompt, often evident after one or two cycles of treatment. The median duration of response in these previously irradiated patients was 15 months (range 8–36 months).

"Salvage" Chemotherapy

Patients with recurrent anaplastic tumors responded to chemotherapy, especially PCV, but were not cured. All relapsed – three while receiving chemotherapy, and the others had late relapses. We retreated seven patients with "salvage" chemotherapy (for a detailed review of these patients see [5]). AZQ and cisplatin were ineffective in four patients (two each). PCV produced a partial response for 12 months in the patient who had previously responded to AZQ. This patient had also received adjuvant BCNU, teaching us that some patients with recurrent tumors would respond to PCV despite prior nitrosoureas. Inadequate bone marrow reserve precluded further chemotherapy when this man's tumor recurred for a third time. Two patients who had previously responded to PCV had brief partial responses to intravenous melphalan. Inadequate bone marrow reserve limited our ability to give full doses of melphalan and may have compromised their treatment.

Newly Diagnosed "Aggressive" Oligodendroglioma

Encouraged by successful chemotherapy for recurrent oligodendroglioma, we began to treat new aggressive tumors with chemotherapy prior to local RT and again observed responses [18]. By "aggressive" we mean anaplastic tumors or nonanaplastic ones displaying clinical and radiological evidence of aggressiveness, namely increasing symptoms, growth, and enhancement. Pre-RT chemotherapy is feasible, effective, and for those with residual tumor after surgery affords an opportunity to assess the tumor's response to drugs alone. This treatment approach may or may not be superior to radiation alone or other less aggressive early treatment strategies. Intensive initial treatment seems logical, but we are proceeding cautiously because some have stated that the behavior of oligodendrogliomas cannot always be reliably predicted by their histological appearance [21], and others have argued that potentially toxic treatment may be inappropriate for indolent gliomas [3]. We recommend chemotherapy after initial surgery for patients with aggressive oligodendrogliomas, especially when there is evidence of residual enhancing tumor, and because there is no way to assess response, consider delaying chemotherapy when the scan is "clean." We do not recommend chemotherapy for patients with nonenlarging, nonenhancing, nonanaplastic (i.e., indolent) tumors.

Procarbazine, CCNU, Vincristine

PCV, developed by Levin et al. [14], is effective treatment for aggressive oligodendrogliomas but other alkylating agents including BCNU, AZQ, melphalan, and thiotepa have anti-oligodendroglioma activity [2, 4, 22]. There is no way at this time to judge the effectiveness of PCV relative to the others. We think it may be more effective than AZQ, and Levin et al. [15] have reported that patients with moderately aggressive anaplastic gliomas (i.e., nonglioblastoma) live longer after adjuvant treatment with PCV, than BCNU. PCV, melphalan, and thiotepa may be equally effective. The CNS Cancer Consortium, a cooperative brain tumor group led by Schold, conducted a phase II study of intravenous melphalan (40 mg/m^2 intravenously, every 4 weeks) for recurrent anaplastic glioma and observed that oligodendrogliomas were more likely to respond (55%) than nonoligodendrogliomas (11%) [2]. This important finding, and a case report by Saarinen et al. [22], describing a complete response to high-dose thiotepa in a heavily pretreated patient, provide further evidence that aggressive oligodendrogliomas are chemosensitive.

Clinical Trials

The National Cancer Institute of Canada's (NCIC) Clinical Trials Group has just concluded a phase II study of "intensive PCV" for patients with measurable, newly diagnosed or recurrent, contrast-enhancing, relatively pure anaplastic oligodendroglioma. The overall response rate will approach 80% with approximately 40%

complete responses. Intensive PCV was more toxic than standard-dose PCV, but there were no instances of nadir sepsis or bleeding in this study. The CNS Cancer Consortium has accrued additional patients with oligodendroglioma to its trial and will soon report a definitive analysis of intravenous melphalan.

Mixed Gliomas

The patients we reported and those studied by NCIC had relatively pure oligodendrogliomas, that is to say, tumors containing at most a minor astrocytic element (i.e., %). Since oligoastrocytomas, like oligodendrogliomas, appear to arise from the O-2A (i.e., oligodendrocyte type 2 astrocyte) branch of the glial lineage [1, 6], Hochberg predicted that these tumors would also be sensitive to chemotherapy. Indeed, Glass et al. [8] have recently demonstrated that oligoastrocytomas also respond predictably to PCV.

Future Directions

If correct, our observations and those of others [2, 8, 22] raise several interesting questions; for example, what is the best treatment for newly diagnosed patients, how can the treatment of recurrent tumor be improved, do aggressive tumors in children also respond to chemotherapy, why are oligodendrogliomas and oligoastrocytomas chemosensitive? It is clear from our work that new treatment approaches are needed for oligodendrogliomas that recur after RT. Recurrent tumors respond to PCV and other cytotoxic drugs but inevitably regrow. Dose intensification coupled with strategies for "preserving" bone marrow may be critical to better control of recurrent disease. The stage may soon be set for trials that compare treatments for newly diagnosed patients. Since comparative studies are expensive, require large numbers of patients, and take years to complete, it is critical that investigators join forces and ask a good question.

The ability to predict accurately a tumor's behavior is critical to prudent treatment decisions at diagnosis, this is especially true when using potentially toxic therapies. We are reluctant to overtreat indolent tumors but do not want to undertreat potentially aggressive ones, especially if by doing so curability is compromised. Can conventional light microscopic analysis of these tumors be augmented? We are currently reexamining the ability of clinical, radiological, and pathological features present at diagnosis to predict the future behavior of oligodendrogliomas (i.e., will they be indolent or aggressive?). Perhaps newer techniques such as DNA ploidy and S-phase fraction analysis by flow cytometry, glucose utilization by positron emission tomography, biochemical profiles by magnetic resonance spectroscopy, uptake of radiolabeled nucleosides [11, 19], or expression of proliferation markers such as Ki-67 [12] will be helpful prognostically and, together with the tumor's histology, guide treatment decisions.

Why might aggressive oligodendrogliomas and mixed tumors containing oligodendroglial elements be sensitive to chemotherapy? The answer to this question may lead to better therapies for all malignant gliomas. Perhaps, for example, they are O^6-alkylguanine DNA alkyltransferase deficient and unable to repair the damage to DNA caused by CCNU and procarbazine [23]. Indeed, there is some data in the literature to support this speculation [7,26]. Oligodendrogliomas respond to alkylating agents, but which of the many cytotoxic drugs, or combinations, is best? This important question can be addressed in clinical trials but might be answered earlier if human oligodendroglioma cell lines, perhaps grown as xenografts in nude mice, were available to screen drugs.

Macdonald and I are increasingly convinced that aggressive oligodendroglioma is a chemosensitive tumor. The observation that aggressive oligoastrocytomas are also chemosensitive is an important new finding [8]. We believe future studies in the laboratory and clinic will elucidate the biochemical basis of their responsiveness and define an important role for chemotherapy in the treatment of these gliomas.

References

1. Bishop M, de la Monte SM (1989) Dual lineage of astrocytomas. Am J Pathol 135:517–527
2. Brown M, Cairncross JG, Vick NA, Macdonald DR, Friedman HS, Dropcho EJ, Schold SC Jr (1990) Differential response of recurrent oligodendrogliomas versus astrocytomas to intravenous melphalan. Neurology 40 [Suppl 1]:397–398 (abstr)
3. Cairncross JG, Laperriere NJ (1989) Low-grade glioma:to treat or not to treat? Arch Neurol 46:1238–1239
4. Cairncross JG, Macdonald DR (1988) Successful chemotherapy for recurrent malignant oligodendroglioma. Ann Neurol 23:460–464
5. Cairncross JG, Macdonald DR (1991) Chemotherapy for oligodendroglioma – progress report. Arch Neurol 48:226–227
6. de la Monte SM (1989) Uniform lineage of oligodendrogliomas. Am J Pathol 135:529–540
7. Frosina G, Rossi O, Arena G, Gentile SL, Bruzzone E, Abbondandolo A (1990) O^6 Alkylguanine–DNA alkyltransferase activity in human brain tumors. Cancer Lett 55:153–158
8. Glass J, Hochberg FH, Gruber ML, Louis DN, Smith D, Rattner B (1992) The treatment of oligodendrogliomas and mixed oligodendroglioma – astrocytoma with PCV chemotherapy. J Neurosurg 76:741–745
9. Green SB, Byar DP, Walker MD, Pistenmaa DA, Alexander E Jr, Batzdorf U, Brooks WH, Hunt WE, Mealey J Jr, Odom GL, Paoletti P, Ransohoff J, Robertson JT, Selker RG, Shapiro WR, Smith KR, Wilson CB, Strike TA (1983) Comparisons of carmustine, procarbazine, and high-dose methyl prednisolone as additions to surgery and radiotherapy for the treatment of malignant glioma. Cancer Treat Rep 67:121–132
10. Gutin PH, Leibel SA, Wara WM, Choucair A, Levin VA, Philips TL, Silver P, DaSilva V, Edwards MS, Davis RL, Weaver KA, Lamb S (1987) Recurrent malignant gliomas:survival following interstitial brachytherapy with high-activity iodine-125 sources. J Neurosurg 67:864–871
11. Hoshino T, Rodriguez LA, Cho KG, Lee KS, Wilson CB, Edwards MSB, Levin VA, Davis RL (1988) Prognostic implications of the proliferative potential of low-grade astrocytomas. J Neurosurg 69:839–842
12. Kleihues P, Sarioglu A, Shibata T, Yasargil GM (1989) Ki-67 expression in the multiform glioblastoma:correlation between growth fraction and patient survival. Clin Neuropath 8:206 (abstr)
13. Kornblith PL, Walker MD (1988) Chemotherapy for malignant gliomas. J Neurosurg 68:1–17
14. Levin VA, Edwards MS, Wright DC, Seager ML, Pischer-Schimberg T, Townsend JJ, Wilson CB (1980) Modified procarbazine, CCNU and vincristine (PCV-3) combination chemotherapy in the treatment of malignant brain tumors. Cancer Treat Rep 64:237–241

15. Levin VA, Silver P, Hannigan J, Wara WM, Gutin PH, Davis RL, Wilson CB (1990) Superiority of post-radiotherapy adjuvant chemotherapy with CCNU, procarbazine, and vincristine (PCV) over BCNU for anaplastic gliomas:NCOG 6G61 final report. Int J Rad Oncol Biol Phys 18:321–324
16. Longee DC, Friedman HS, Albright RE, Burger PC, Oakes WJ, Moore JO, Schold SC Jr (1990) Treatment of patients with recurrent gliomas with cyclophosphamide and vincristine. J Neurosurg 72:583–588
17. Macdonald DR, Cascino TL, Schold Sc Jr, Cairncross JG (1990) Response criteria for phase II studies of supratentorial malignant glioma. J Clin Oncol 7:1277–1280
18. Macdonald DR, Gaspar LE, Cairncross JG (1990) Successful chemotherapy for newly diagnosed aggressive oligodendroglioma. Ann Neurol 27:573–574
19. Morimura T, Kitz K, Budka H (1989) Proliferation markers for human brain tumors. Clin Neuropath 8:206 (abstr)
20. Poisson M, Chiras J, Fauchon F, Debussche C, Delattre JY (1990) Treatment of malignant recurrent glioma by intra-arterial, infra-ophthalmic infusion of HECNU 1-(2-chloroethyl)-1-nitroso-3-(2-hydroxyethyl) urea. A phase II study. J Neuro-Oncol 8:255262
21. Rubinstein LJ (1972) Tumors of the nervous system. Armed Forces Institute of Pathology, Washington, D.C. (Fascicle 6)
22. Saarinen UM, Pihko H, Makipernaa A (1990) High-dose thiotepa with autologous bone marrow rescue in recurrent malignant oligodendroglioma:a case report. J Neuro-Oncol 9:5762
23. Schold SC Jr, Brent TP, von Hofe E, Friedman HS, Mitra S, Bigner D, Swenberg JA, Kleihues P. O^6-Alkylguanine-DNA alkyltransferase and sensitivity to procarbazine in human braintumor xenografts. J Neurosurg 70:573–577
24. Walker MD, Alexander E Jr, Hunt WE, MacClarty CS, Mahaley MS, Mealey J Jr, Norrell HA, Owens G, Ransohoff J, Wilson CB, Gehan EA, Strike TA (1978) Evaluation of BCNU and/or radiotherapy in the treatment of anaplastic gliomas. A cooperative clinical trial. J Neurosurg 49:333–343
25. Walker MD, Green SB, Byar DP, Alexander E Jr, Batzdorf U, Brooks WH, Hunt WE, MacCarty CS, Mahaley MS, Mealey J Jr, Owens G, Ransohoff J, Robertson JT, Shapiro WR, Smith KR, Wilson CB, Strike TA (1980) Randomized comparisons of radiotherapy and nitrosoureas for the treatment of malignant glioma after surgery. N Engl J Med 303:1323–1329
26. Wiestler O, Kleihues P, Pegg AE (1984) O^6-Alkylguanine-DNA akyltransferase activity in human brain and brain tumors. Carcinogenesis 5:121–124
27. Young B, Oldfield EH, Markesbery WR, Haack D, Tibbs PA, McCombs P, Chin HW, Maruyama Y, Meacham WR (1981) Re-operation for glioblastoma. J Neurosurg 55:917–921

Chemotherapy of Malignant Gliomas

P. Krauseneck[1] and B. Müller[2]

[1]Neurologische Klinik, St.-Getreu-Str. 14-18, 96049 Bamberg, Germany
[2]Neurologische Universitätsklinik, Kopfklinikum Würzburg, Josef-Schneider-Str. 11, 97080 Würzburg, Germany

Introduction

Cure of primary malignant brain tumors today may be expected only in childhood in about 50% of medulloblastomas or primitive neuroectodermal tumors (PNETs), whereas in most other childhood tumors and in adults after 5 years a finally lethal relapse must be accounted for. The concept of primary multimodal treatment of brain tumors aims, however, at cure. Until now there is no controlled trial to compare overall survival after adjuvant postoperative chemotherapy with a palliative chemotherapy beginning only at the time of relapse.

More precise and more objective evaluation criteria have created better possibilities for systematic clinical trials. Large, multicenter, randomized studies could determine the value of therapeutic modalities, identify prognostic factors, and broaden the knowledge of pathobiology of the CNS tumors. Nevertheless the therapeutic efficacy remains only modest and – even with the great advantages in molecular biology and immunology enabling us to use cytokines and specially educated lymphocytes, e.g., lymphokine activated killer cells or tumor infiltrating lymphocytes, in the treatment of malignant brain tumors – a breakthrough is not to be expected within the near future.

A realistic goal, however, in a major percentage of patients is a longer lasting remission or at least a delay of further progression. Since about one-third of patients do not recieve a measurable benefit from chemotherapy, it is always necessary to weigh possible complications, toxicity, and quality of life against the possible gain in survival, particularly if an adjuvant chemotherapy is considered.

Because individual needs are highly important in this process of decision making, in our opinion an essential task of the physician consists in counseling the patient and his relatives very extensively to enable them to take part in the decision.

Intrinsic brain tumors are the most common (40%) of all brain tumors in adults, and 80% of them are malignant gliomas, i.e., mainly glioblastomas (80%), anaplastic astrocytomas (10%–15%), anaplastic oligodendrogliomas (2%–8%), and a few anaplastic mixed gliomas. Therefore a large body of data from randomized clinical studies is available for these entities, documenting spontaneously rapidly progressing course and efficacy of surgery, radiotherapy, and chemotherapy. For other rare malignant intrinsic brain tumors, however, well-controlled data on natural course and treatment are lacking [31, 33, 39]. In this chapter we therefore concentrate on the problems with malignant gliomas.

Pecularities of Chemotherapy of Malignant Brain Tumors

Space Limitation

Because of the strict volume restriction in the skull usually secondary effects of the tumor, particularly brain edema and disturbed CSF flow, are much more important for the clinical symptoms than local infiltration or destruction by the tumor itself. This leads to two consequences: (a) Before starting chemotherapy (or any another intensive treatment modality) usually treatment of brain edema and sometimes a shunt procedure to allow CSF flow are necessary. In the first approach treatment of edema is usually highly effective in alleviation of symptoms. (b) There is not much time for the chemotherapy to manifest efficacy unless the tumor is resected or halted by radiotherapy since tumor doubling in malignant gliomas, for instance, can take place in a few weeks. Therefore palliative surgery is often needed.

Lymph Drainage

No own lymph vessels exist in the brain. This in parts explains the fact that intrinsic, even highly malignant brain tumors only extremely rarely develop regional metastases. The lack of lymph vessels is also one of the main reasons that necroses in the brain can hardly be dissolved and may have to be surgically removed to avoid an increase in brain edema and space occupation.

Blood-Brain Barrier

The blood-brain barrier restricts the passage of most molecules from the vessel lumen into the brain parenchyma or CSF. Essentially only water and small inert and lipophile molecules up to a molecular weight of 200 may passively penetrate this barrier. For some substances, such as glucose, specific transport mechanisms exist. Another important part is the concentration gradient for a given substance. Therefore the physicochemical properties of a substance do not strictly correlate with its blood-brain barrier penetration in vivo [6, 23] (Table 1). The barrier is disturbed in the tumor area, but this is highly variable depending on the structure of the tumor region and also on the nature of the given tumor: Primary brain tumors are supplied by the original brain vessels, and therefore the barrier is well preserved in the infiltration area where the tumor invades normal brain tissue, whereas in the necrotic center of at least larger tumors a barrier virtually does not exist. Cytostatic drugs may

Table 1. CSF – penetration of antineoplastic agents

Substance	CSF-penetration	Remarks
Nitrosourea compounds	++	
Dianhydrogalactitol	++	
Dibromodulcitol	++	
Procarbazine	++	
Hydroxurea	++	
Aziridiniylbenzoquinone	++	
Cytosine-Arabinoside	++	only with prolonged infusion 2 h
5-Fluorouracil	++	equivocal
Methotrexate	-/+	only with high-dose administration
Etoposide	-/+	only with high-dose administration
Teniposide	-/+	equivocal
Dacarbazine	(+)	low penetration in animals
Cyclophosphamide	+/-	only maternal substances,
Ifosfamide	+/-	but not the active metabolites
Actinomycine C	–	
Doxorubicin	–	
Bleomycin	–	
Mitoxantrone	–	
Cisplatin	–	
Vincaalkaloids	–	
Interferons	–	

++, 20–30% of serum-level achieved in CSF; +, cytotoxically sufficient levels in CSF achievable; only very poor CSF-levels achievable (approx. 0%–2% of serum-level).

therefore reach the necrotic sector of a tumor rather well but only poorly the actively proliferating and infiltrating cells in the periphery. This explains why a good clinical efficacy may not be expected from a drug not penetrating the blood-brain barrier, although such a drug may be able to induce tumor regression [32, 50].

Neurotoxicity

Besides their general cytotoxicity on proliferating cells some of the cystostatic drugs have specific neurotoxic effects limiting their applicability. These side effects may become life threatening with high-dose treatment or, albeit rarely, intrathecal administration of chemotherapy. In the framework of standardized therapy modalities it may be difficult to differentiate the spectrum of neurotoxic side effects from infections, cerebral ischemia, or – most commonly – tumor progression. This may well interfere with assessing the therapeutic efficacy. Acute side effects such as fever, disorientation, and mental disorders/psychosis are in general reversible within a few days. In this context the acute hearing loss after administration of cisplatinum – although infrequent – constitutes an exception because improvement is questionable. Systemic as well as local administration of interferon-α (or, to a lesser extent, interferon-β) may cause acute and severe neurotoxicity, which seems to be only partially reversible. It appears from the literature that chronic neurotoxic effects are found predominantly in the peripheral nervous system, such as with administration of vinca alcaloids, cisplatinum, and, rarely, of the epipodophyllotoxin derivatives teniposide (VM26) and etoposide (VP16). Chronic cerebral neurotoxicity accompanies almost exclusively along brain irradiation and is seen as cortical atrophy or toxic leukencephalopathy with or without mental changes of all degrees of severity. Inflammatory leukencephalopathy was recently described with 5-fluorouracil and levamisole [28].

In our studies we observed acute mental changes with long-term oral administration of procarbazine and also with antimetabolites (adenine arabinoside, cytosine arabinoside, 5-fluorouracil, methotrexate) given intravenously, particularly in patients with heavy tumor burden [5, 7, 11, 17, 24, 30, 40, 41, 52, 62].

Local Growth and Extent of Surgery

A close connection of the tumor to the CSF pathways or the brain surface points to the risk of spreading of single tumor cells into the CSF. In these cases we perform CSF monitoring and prophylactic intrathecal cytostatic treatment in order to avoid tumor dissemination via the CSF pathways. To distinguish a postoperative tumor rest from surgically induced changes early contrast medium enhanced series (within 48 h after surgery) of computed tomography (CT) or magnetic resonance imaging (MRI) are necessary and allow a substantial diagnosis. MRI is much more sensitive in this regard [4, 18]. This provides a much better guidance of therapy.

Timing of Chemotherapy

For theoretical reasons chemotherapy should be given as early as possible after surgery. Although the feasibility and safety of pre- and intraoperative chemotherapy is proven [10,19], wound healing is generally waited for, and treatment is begun simultaneously with radiotherapy on days 10–14 after surgery. Provided prophylaxis of brain edema is carried out with corticosteroids (15–25 mg prednisone equivalent per day), no acute adverse effects of simultaneous administration of radiotherapy and cytostatic treatment are to be expected. Whether the risk of late sequelae (leukencephalopathy!) is slightly higher in this setting is not known.

Duration of Chemotherapy

There are no comparative studies regarding the necessary length of chemotherapy when no tumor is seen in the CT scan. Many large randomized studies (US-BTSG, BTCG, German-Austrian Study) prescribed treatment for 1 year; in San Francisco a period of 2 years was taken, and the EORTC BTSG treated only two cycles, i.e., 3 months. We analyzed a recent series in our clinic treated 0.5 years and compared it to the corresponding study population of our former randomized study and did not see any disadvantage for the shorter treatment period. However, these are preliminary results. With remaining tumor in the CT scan cytostatic treatment must be continued until remission or regrowth. Alternative drugs may have high efficacy in single patients with progressive tumors; therefore another chemotherapy protocol may be applied in relapse/progression.

Results of Chemotherapy of Anaplastic Gliomas and Glioblastomas

Overview of Results of Intravenous Therapy:

In the early 1970s the American Brain Tumor Study Group (BTSG) demonstrated with their second randomized multicenter trial the relative effects of surgery, radiotherapy, and carmustine (BCNU) chemotherapy [60] (Table 2); BCNU was effective but less so than radiotherapy. The main effect of BCNU was not a prolongation of median survival but multiplying the rate of long-term survivors, i.e., the percentage of patients living longer than 18 months after diagnosis. These results were essentially confirmed by further studies of the BTSG and other groups. With better radiotherapy and more consequent chemotherapy the median survival of the combination of radiotherapy plus BCNU reached 52 weeks, and the rate of 18-months survivors was increased to 20%–35% [38, 45]. 5-year survival was reported only anecdotically. In the German-Austrian study it was 8%, 15% for grade 3 tumors, and 4% for glioblastomas [34]. Thus in general chemotherapy has a clearcut effect in up

Table 2. Clinical trials with adjuvant chemotherapy for malignant gliomas (for extensive overview see [31,33,39])

Drugs	n	Age	KPS	% 4	MST(wk)	Reference
BCNU	72	57	?	90	34	[60][a]
	147	57	70	89	50	[22][a]
CCNU	59	62	?	41	43	[15][a]
	94	47	66	41	52	[57][a]
MeCCNU	91	54	60	82	43	[61][a]
PCZ	153	56	70	89	47	[22][a]
ACNU	27	59	?	33	61	[53][a]
BCNU+VCR	17	58	?	76	44	[51]
CCNU+PCZ+VCR+MT	35	51	50	60	64	[29][a]
CCNU+VM26	61	53	60	28	58	[16][a]
BCNU+PCZ	176	56	73	79	50	[49][a]
BCNU+PCZ/HU+VM26	168	56	72	78	59	[49][a]
BCNU+VM26	259	55	75	81	53	[34][a]

(n = number of patients, KPS = Karnofsky performance status, % 4 = percent of glioblastomas WHO grade 4, MST = median survival time, [a] = randomized trial); HU, hydroxyurea.

to one-third of these patients, a modest effect in another one-third and no measurable effect in the last one-third.

The question of whether symptomatic treatment with corticosteroids – frequently dramatically improving signs and symptoms – adds to the prolongation of median survival was answered by another study of the BTSG showing no effect of routinely administered high dose methylprednisolone on survival [22].

In randomized studies other single-agent chemotherapy was no more or even less effective than BCNU.

European studies from the EORTC-Brain Tumor Study Group [14, 15, 26] and the Scandinavian and Italian groups [25, 44] argue for a slightly less efficacy of CCNU, whereas American studies demonstrated comparable effectiveness of methyl-CCNU [61] or procarbazine [16, 22, 26]. Nimustine (ACNU) used in Japan and Germany achieved also comparable results [8, 58, 59].

In smaller clinical trials or phase II studies evaluating response, a number of other substances proved efficacious. PCNU – another nitrosourea, i.e., 1-(2-chloroethyl-3-(2,6-dioxo-3-piperidyl)-1-nitrosourea – was not better than BCNU [21]. Other alkylating agents such as cyclophosphamide not penetrating the blood-brain-barrier have no proven efficacy in malignant gliomas. In other intrinsic brain tumors such as medulloblastomas, however, they apparently are efficient. Blood-brain-barrier penetrating alkylating drugs such as the hexitols dianhydrogalactitol (DAG), dibromodulcitol (DBD), and diacetyl-DAG are possibly as effective as the nitrosoureas but are not extensively investigated [3, 14]. Hydroxyurea may play a role as radiosensitizer, but the data of the San Francisco group are not unequivocal [37]. Intravenous cisplatinum produced responses, but no additional effect in combination with radiotherapy was seen [26]. Aziridinylbenzoquinone (AZQ), a lipophilic, specially designed anthrachinone was only moderately effective in various trials (e.g., [23, 54]). For other anthrachinones early promising reports could not be confirmed [20, 46].

The antimetabolites have at least limited efficacy as shown for 5-fluorouracil (e.g., [1]), 6-mercaptopurin [63], high-dose – but not low-dose – methotrexate [12] and cytosine arabinoside [27]. Our experience with cytosine arabinoside is very promising, but the drug has considerable hematotoxicity and some reversible neurotoxicity. Mitotic poisons also have some therapeutic potential, which was shown for vincristine only in earlier trials with less strict evaluation criteria [2]. VM26 and VP16 have been rather well documented in recent years [16, 56]. In a randomized trial VM26 showed, even in addition to BCNU, a marginal but statistically significant advantage over BCNU alone [34]. For a variety of other substances remissions have been described [33, 39]. However, none of these has been more promising than those above and therefore no subsequent trials have been reported.

Among the biological response modifiers interferon-α and -β and in a few cases interferon-γ and interleukin-2 with or without lymphokine-activated killer cells have been tested in small series. No convincing data of more than modest activity against malignant gliomas have been reported (e.g., [9, 13, 39, 43]). Interferon-α and -β may have response rates of 15% but certainly have considerable toxicity in patients with brain tumors.

In contrast to other human malignancies which have experienced significant therapeutic advances with polychemotherapy, treatment with combinations of cytostatic drugs has not yet achieved major improvement in gliomas. Levin et al. [36] reported superiority of combined procarbazine, CCNU, and vincristine (PCV) over BCNU alone. but the study design was not free from possible flaws. In the German-Austrian trial there was a significant (but modest) prolongation of the free interval and – only for the group with Karnofsky performance status (KPS) of at least 70% – of the median survival with BCNU plus VM26 in comparison to BCNU alone [34]. Response rates were only slightly higher with different, rationally designed polychemotherapy schedules than with single-drug therapy [39]. It must also be considered that polychemotherapy may lead to even worse results, adding undue toxicity to an already rather toxic regimen with simultaneous radiotherapy and chemotherapy. Thus, surprisingly, in the German-Austrian study the certainly moderately toxic combination of BCNU and VM26 yielded slightly shorter survival in the group with low KPS (50%–60%) [34], and the significance of this interaction of patients' general condition with the intensity of chemotherapy was high. This must be born in mind, and it makes aggressive schedules such as "8 drugs in 1 day" [47] questionable.

The design of better and risk-adapted polychemotherapy protocols is one of the possibilities to achieve better results in the near future in terms of survival, quality of life, and avoidance of unjustified toxicity. In this context the search for better definition of individual prognosis and risk profile plays an important role, and one additional prognostic factor may be in vitro chemosensitivity of a given tumor. A systematic randomized study in the United Kingdom is under way (D.G.T. Thomas, personal communiction). Various other approaches to improve chemotherapy of gliomas promise better results in the future: (a) new drugs with better therapeutic ratio or with new modes of action, such as calcium-antagonists, enzyme inhibitors, and invasion inhibitors; (b) cytokines and growth factors; and (c) monoclonal antibodies.

Standard Treatment

As standard treatment today adjuvant monotherapy with BCNU in addition to resection and radiotherapy is established, as is the PCV regimen in other centers (Table 3). Because of the high and only partially predictable pulmonary toxicity of BCNU this drug should be replaced by ACNU or as second choice CCNU, since the moderate efficacy of chemotherapy does not justify the risk of a lethal complication (pulmonary fibrosis) – in about 4% of patients in the German-Austrian-Glioma Study [34] with BCNU.

The standard protocols are those using monotherapy with ACNU, BCNU, CCNU, or procarbazine:

ACNU Monotherapy. Dosage: 100 mg/m^2, intravenously (bolus injection), only day 1 every 6 weeks. Toxicity is similar to that with other nitrosourea compounds: Delayed hematotoxicity with leukocyte and thrombocyte nadir in the 5th/6th week. Varying

Table 3. Median survival times (MST) and long term survivors (LTS); (more than 18 months) with single modality treatment in malignant gliomas (from [60])

MST	%	LTS
Surgery	17 weeks	0
Surgery + BCNU	25 weeks	0
Surgery + Radiotherapy	38 weeks	5
Surgery + Radiotherapy + BCNU	40 weeks	19

cumulative bone marrow toxicity beginning usually after five or six cycles as with other nitrosoureas and only rarely limiting further cytostatic treatment. Pulmonary fibrosis has not been described with this dosing, but thrombopenia seems to be more pronounced than with BCNU.

BCNU Monotherapy. Dosage: 200 mg/m^2 on day 1, or 80 mg/m^2 per day on days 1–3, per infusion (about 20 min), starting 10–14 days after resection, simultaneously with radiotherapy. Interval: 6 (–8) weeks, if leukocytes 4000/µl and platelets $\geq$ 100 000/µl. The most critical side effect of BCNU is the development of an interstitial pneumonia/pulmonary fibrosis occurring rarely after only one single cycle and sometimes progressing until death even after discontinuation of BCNU. Even frequent routine pulmonary function tests were not sufficient to prevent this severe side effect [34]. Allergic reaction to BCNU is rare.

CCNU Monotherapy. Dosage: 130 mg/m^2, orally, only day 1 every 6 weeks. Side effects, as above. The risk of pulmonary toxicity is obviously low (not well documented].

Procarbazine Monotherapy. Dosage:150 mg/m^2, orally, days 1–14, repeated every 4 weeks (for days 1–21, repeated every 6 weeks). Side effects include occasionally severe hemato- and hepatotoxicity. Often a considerable nausea and rarely allergic skin reactions are encountered.

The following protocols have been widely evaluated, including for side effects, and can be recommended as alternatives. These should be used only in patients in good condition (KPS 70%).

BCNU + VM26. This protocol is very similar to that for BCNU monotherapy (see above). In addition to the full dose of BCNU, VM26 is given intravenously in a dose of 50 mg/m^2 on days 1 and 2 over 20 min. immediately after BCNU. An increase in the VM26 dose to 100 mg/m^2 did not show higher toxicity in our own series. The BCNU + VM26 protocol has identical risks regarding pulmonary and hematological toxicity as BCNU alone. In a few cases allergic reactions to VM26 have been seen.

PCV. This protocol has been used widely in the United States but is less well documented than the other regimens. It exists in two alternative forms: (a) CCNU 110 mg/m^2, orally, day 1; procarbazine 60 mg/m^2, orally, days 8–21; vincristine

1.4 mg/m^2, intravenously, days 8 + 29, every 6–8 weeks [35, 36]; (b) CCNU 80 mg/m^2, orally, day 1; procarbazine 100 mg/m^2, orally, days 1–10; vincristine 1.4 mg/m^2, intravenously, day 1, every 6 weeks for 18 months [55]. Side effects are those of CCNU plus procarbazine and the peripheral neurotoxicity of vincristine (slight, but cumulative polyneuropathy, rarely causing paresis and then limiting further vincristine treatment).

Intra-arterial Administration

Single impressive tumor regressions have been demonstrated by direct intra-arterial injections, mainly of the nitrosoureas BCNU, ACNU, and HeCNU – 1-(2-chloroethyl)-1-nitroso-3-(2-hydroyethyl) urea – but also of cisplatinum and some other compounds. However, a large randomized trial in the United States could not verify any advantage of intra-arterial BCNU versus the conventional intravenous BCNU protocol. In contrast, serious neurotoxic side effects required reduction of the intra-arterial dose, and survival data were worse with the intra-arterial route. Therefore the trial was stopped early [50]. Because of a possible improvement of the therapeutic index tumor-brain, intra-arterial administration of a hydrophilic agent not penetrating the blood-brain barrier such as methotrexate [48] or cisplatinum [40] is theoretically propitious. Small studies and the preliminary results of the American BTCG trial showed high radiological response rates of about 35% for intra-arterial cisplatinum [40]. Because of the high risk of neurotoxicity intra-arterial therapy should be undertaken only in controlled clinical trials.

Prognostic Factors

Looking for prognostic factors is another main goal in large systematic studies. Age, histology/grade of malignancy, and general condition of the patient (KPS) have proven to be of prognostic value in nearly all trials. In one study the remainig tumor rest after surgery was also of prognostic relevance. It is not yet clear whether chemosensitivity testing adds predictive power. With malignant gliomas a clinical correlation between proliferation in vitro (methionine incorporation rate) and response to CCNU or procarbazine but not to vincristine could be demonstrated [55].

Conclusion and Aspects for the Future

Over recent years the value of chemotherapy has been broadly evaluated in supratentorial high-grade gliomas in adults. A meta-analysis by Fine et al. (cited in [39]) comprising 2400 patients in large randomized trials over the past decade shows a prolongation of survival and a substantial higher proportion of long-term-survivors (2 years) by multimodal treatment: with radiotherapy alone 41% survive 1 year, with combination of radiotherapy and chemotherapy 53%. After 2 years 16% survive with radiotherapy alone compared to 23% after combined treatment.

An intensified polychemotherapy is indicated in patients with favorable prognostic conditions. The small number of substances suitable for neuro-oncological purposes and their relatively high toxicity limit the administration of cytostatic treatment. For the time being cure of malignant glioma is not realistic, but survival of many years is possible. Improvement of chemotherapy might be achievable by developing new, blood-brain barrier penetrating substances, optimized combination of antineoplastic drugs already evaluated, extending the dose limitation by improved supportive therapy, for example, growth factors, and by avoiding neurotoxicity whereever possible.

Besides exploring new ways in basic research and clinically well-controlled phase II studies there is a need to continue large, randomized trials. Knowledge of confirmed prognostic criteria in the future will allow a risk-adapted therapy avoiding unnecessary toxicity in patients with unfavorable prognosis and accepting, on the other hand, a higher toxicity in patients with better chances. Evaluation of timing/schedule of chemotherapy, identification of additional predictive parameters, for example, chemosensitivity testing, more detailed histological and molecular biological criteria are the next steps toward offering an optimized and differentiated treatment for the individual patient. This can only be realized with intense interdisciplinary cooperation.

References

1. Adelstein DJ, Likavec MJ, Sharan VM, White RJ, Takaoka SG, Carter SG, Hines JD (1987) Intravenous 5-fluorouracil infusion and simultaneous radiotherapy in glioblastoma multiforme. ASCO Proc 6:274
2. Afra D (1973) Vincristine therapy in malignant glioma recurrencies. Neurochirurgia 16:189–198
3. Afra D, Kocsis B, Dobay J, Eckhardt S (1983) Combined radiotherapy and chemotherapy with dibromodulcitol and CCNU in the postoperative treatment of malignant gliomas. J Neurosurg 59:106–110
4. Albert FK, Forsting M, Sartor K, Kunze S (1991) Frühes postoperatives CT und MR (-/+KM) nach Exstirpation von High grade-Gliomen – Erste Ergebnisse einer prospektiven Studie. In: Firnhaber W, Dworschak K, Lauer K, Nichtweiß M (eds) Multiple Sklerose. Neuroonkologie. Konstitutionelle Dyslexie. Springer, Berlin, Heidelberg, New York (Verhandlungen der Deutschen Gesellschaft für Neurologie, vol 6), pp 284–287
5. Anderson NR, Tandon DS (1991) Ifosfamide extrapyramidal neurotoxicity. Cancer 68:72–75
6. Ausman JI, Levin VA, Brown WE, Rall DP, Fenstermacher JD (1977) Brain-tumor chemotherapy –pharmacological principles derived from a monkey brain-tumor model. J Neurosurg 46:155–164
7. Baker WJ, Royer GLJ, Weiss RB (1991) Cytarabine and neurologic toxicity. J Clin Oncol 9:679–693
8. Bamberg M, Budach V, Stuschke M, Gerhard L (1988) Preliminary experimental results with the nitrosourea derivate ACNU in the treatment of malignant gliomas. Radiother Oncol 12:25–29
9. Boethius J, Blomgren H, Collins VP, Greitz T, Strander H (1983) The effect of systemic human interferon-alpha administration to patients with glioblastoma multiforme. Acta Neurochir (Vienna) 68:239–251
10. Butti G, Knerich R, Tanghetti B, Adinolfi D, Gaetani P, Buoncristiani P, Paoletti P (1984) Perioperative carmustine chemotherapy for malignant brain tumors. Cancer Treat Rep 68:1505–1506
11. Cerny T, Meier C (1989) Neurotoxicity with cytostatic therapy:a review. Schweiz Med Wochenschr 119:1137–1147

12. Djerassi I, Kim JS, Regev A (1985) Response of astrocytoma to high-dose methotrexate with citrovorum factor rescue. Cancer 55:2741–2747
13. Duff TA, Bordon E, Bay J, Phepmeier J, Sielaff K (1986) Phase II trial for treatment of recurrent glioblastoma multiforme. J Neurosurg 64:408–413
14. Eagan RT, Creagan ET, Bisel HF, Layton DD Jr, Groover RV, Hermann RC Jr (1981) Phase-II-Studies of dianhydrogalactidol-based combination chemotherapy for recurrent brain tumors. Oncology 38:4–6
15. EORTC Brain Tumor Group (1978) Effect of CCNU on survival rate of objective remission and duration of free interval in patients with malignant brain glioma – final evaluation. Eur J Cancer 14:851–855
16. EORTC Brain Tumor Group (1981) Evaluation of CCNU, VM-26 plus CCNU and procarbazine in supratentorial brain gliomas. J Neurosurg 55:27–31
17. Forman A (1990) Recent studies on neurotoxicity and on the epidemiology of brain and nervous system tumors. Curr Opin Oncol 2:691–698
18. Forsting M, Albert FK, Kunze S, Sartor K (1992) Residual tumor after brain tumor resection? How to cut the Gordian knot with early postoperative MRI. Cancer Res Clin Oncol 118 [Suppl]:R106 (Abstract)
19. Goebel WE, Trappe AE, Weinzierl FX (1987) Perioperative cytostatische Behandlung supratentorieller maligner Hirntumoren mit BCNU unter spezieller Berücksichtigung der Tumorlage. Neurochirurgia 30:82–87
20. Green SB, Byar DP, Strike TA, Alexander E Jr, Brooks WH, Burger PC, Hunt WE, Mealey J Jr, Odom GL, Paoletti P, Pistenmaa DA, Ransohoff J II, Robertson JT, Selker RG, Shapiro WR, Smith KR Jr (1984) Randomized comparisons of BCNU, streptozotocin, radiosensitizer and fractionation of radiotherapy in the postoperative treatment of malignant glioma (study 7702). ASCO Proc 3:230
21. Green SB, Byar DP, Strike TA, Burger PC, Mahaley MS Jr, Mealey J Jr, Pistenmaa DA, Ransohoff J, Robertson JT, Selker RG, Shapiro WR, van Gilder JC (1985) Randomized phase II comparison of PCNU and AZQ for the treatment of primary brain tumor (study 8120) (BTSG Behtesda). ASCO Proc 4:143
22. Green SB, Byar DP, Walker MD, Pistenmaa DA, Alexander E Jr, Batzdorf U, Brooks WH, Hunt WE, Mealey J Jr, Odom GL, Paoletti P, Ransohoff J II, Robertson JT, Selker RG, Shapiro WR, Smith KR Jr (1983) Comparisons of carmustine, procarbazine and high-dose methylprednisolone as additions to surgery and radiotherapy for the treatment of malignant glioma. Cancer Treat Rep 67:123–132
23. Haid M, Kandekhar JD, Merrill JM, Johnson CM, Locker GY, Blough R (1987) Phase II AZQ therapy for recurrent or progressive glioma of the central nervous system – final report. ASCO Proc 6:266
24. Harmers FP, Gispen WH, Neijt JP (1991) Neurotoxic side-effects of cisplatin. Eur J Cancer 27:372–376
25. Hatlevoll R, Lindegaard K-F, Hagen S, Kristiansen K, Nesbakken R, Torvik A, Ganz JC, Mella O, Rosengren B, Ringkjöb R, Arnasson O, Lindgren S, Lipecki M, Notter G, Littbrand B, Säterborg N-E, Benediktsson G, Johansson L, Spännare B, Brun A, Berthelsen A, Busch H, Grönbaek E, Rygard J, Haase JP, Lambrethsen E, Midholm S, Sehested P, Heikkinen M, Nyström S, Taskinen P, Mäntylä M, Elgen K, Aaskoven O, Garis de ST, Jensen RH, Matheson I (1985) Combined modality treatment of operated astrocytomas grade 3 and 4. Cancer 56:41–47
26. Hildebrand J (1987) Chemotherapy of malignant supratentorial gliomas in adults: a ten year experience of the EORTC brain tumor group. In: Voth D, Krauseneck P (eds) Chemotherapy of gliomas. De Gruyter, Berlin
27. Hobert U, Krauseneck P, Bogdahn U, Neudecker T (1985) Phase I-II study of cytosine-arabinoside in malignant brain tumors. J Neurol [Suppl[7:232
28. Hook CC, Kimmel DW, Kvols LK, Scheithauer BW, Forsyth PA, Rubin J, Moertel CG, Rodriguez M (1992) Multifocal inflammatory leukencephalopathy with 5-fluorouracil and levamisole. Ann Neurol 31:262–267
29. Jellinger K, Kothbauer P, Volc D, Vollmer R, Weiss R (1979) Combination chemotherapy (COMP protocol) and radiotherapy of anaplastic supratentorial gliomas. Acta Neurochir 51:1–13
30. Kaplan RS, Wiernik PH (1984) Neurotoxicity of antitumor agents. In: Perry MC (ed) Toxicity of chemotherapy. Grune and Stratton, London, pp 365–433
31. Kornblith PL, Walker M (1988) Chemotherapy for malignant gliomas. J Neurosurg 68:1–17

32. Krauseneck P, Dommasch D (1987) Zytostatische Therapie in der Neurologie. In: Flügel KA (ed) Neurologische und psychiatrische Therapie. Perimed, Erlangen, pp 363–378
33. Krauseneck P, Mertens H-G (1987) Results of chemotherapy of malignant brain tumors in adults. In: Jellinger K (ed) Therapy of malignant brain tumors. Springer, Vienna New York, pp 349–395
34. Krauseneck P, Mertens H-G, Messerer D, Kleihues P, Bamberg M, Dittmann W, Gerhard L, Heuser K, Müller B, Makoski HB, Ransmayr G, Richter E, Schröter C, Volc D, Wiehler S (1989) Zwischenergebnissse der deutsch-österreichischen Studie zu den malignen supratentoriellen Gliomen des Erwachsenenalters. In: Fischer P-A, Baas H, Enzensberger W (eds) Gerontoneurologie, Enzephalitiden, Neurogenetik. Springer, Berlin Heidelberg New York (Verhandlungen der Deutschen Gesellschaft für Neurologie, vol 5), pp 1090–1093
35. Levin VA, Silver P, Hannigan J, Wara WM, Gutin PH, Davis RL, Wilson CB (1989) Superiority of postradiotherapy adjuvant chemotherapy with CCNU, procarbazine and vincristine (PCV) over BCNU for anaplastic gliomas: NCOG 6G61 final report. Int J Radiat Oncol Biol Phys 18:321–324
36. Levin VA, Wara WM, Davis RL, Vestnys P, Resser KJ, Yatsko K, Nutik S, Gutin P, Wilson CB (1985) Phase III comparison of BCNU and the combination of procarbazine, CCNU and vincristine administered after radiotherapy with hydroxyurea for malignant gliomas. J Neurosurg 63:218–223
37. Levin VA, Wilson CB, Davis R, Wara WM, Pischer TL, Irwin L (1979) A phase III comparison of BCNU hydroxyurea and radiation therapy to BCNU and radiation therapy for treatment of primary malignant gliomas. J Neurosurg 51:526–532
38. Lieberman AN, Foo SH, Ransohoff J, Wise A, George A, Gordon W, Walker R (1982) Long term survival among patients with malignant brain tumors. Neurosurgery 10:450–453
39. Mahaley MS Jr (1991) Neuro-oncology index and review (adult primary brain tumors). J Neurooncol 11:85–147
40. Mahaley MSJ, Hipp SW, Dropcho EJ, Bertsch L, Cush S, Tirey T, Gillespie GY (1989) Intracarotid cisplatin chemotherapy for recurrent gliomas. J Neurosurg 70:371–378
41. Merimsky O, Reider Groswasser I, Inbar M, Chaitchik S (1990) Interferon-related mental deterioration and behavioral changes in patients with renal cell carcinoma. Eur J Cancer 26:596–600
42. Mertens H-G (1982) Postoperative Strahlen- und Chemotherapie mit BCNU und VM26 bei malignen supratentoriellen Gliomen des Erwachsenenalters. Protokoll der multizentrischen Therapiestudie der deutschen Hirntumorgruppe
43. Nagai M, Arai T (1984) Clinical effect of interferon in malignant brain tumors. Neurosurg Rev 7:55–64
44. Paoletti P, Knerich R, Butti G, Adinolfi D, Locatelli D, Robustelli della Cuna G, Cordero di Montezemolo L, Schiffer D, Soffietti R, Nicolato A, Giunta F, Buoncristiani P, Scamoni C (1983) Italian cooperative study on malignant glial tumor therapy. In: Krauseneck P, Mertens H-G (eds) Therapie maligner Neoplasien des Gehirns. Perimed, Erlangen
45. Potthoff PC (1981) Ergebnisse der Therapie maligner Hirntumoren. In: Potthoff PC, Schreml W (eds) Maligne Hirntumoren. Huber, Bern
46. Pouillart P, Mathe G, Thy T (1976) Treatment of malignant gliomas and brain metastasis in adults with a combination of adriamycin, VM26 and CCNU. Cancer 38:1909–1916
47. Rozenthal JM, Robins HI, Finlay JL, Healey B, Levin AB, Steeves RA, Kohler PC, Schutta HS, Trump DL (1989) Eight-drugs-in-one-day chemotherapy in postirradiated adult patients with malignant gliomas. Med Pediatr Oncol 17:471–476
48. Shapiro WR (1986) Therapy of adult malignant brain tumors: what have the clinical trials taught us? Semin Oncol 13:38–4
49. Shapiro WR, Green SB, Burger PC, Mahaley MS Jr, Selker RG, van Gilder JC, Robertson JT, Ransohoff J, Mealey J Jr, Strike TA et al (1989) Randomized trial of three chemotherapy regimens and two radiotherapy regimens in postoperative treatment of malignant glioma. Brain Tumor Cooperative Group Trial 8001. J Neurosurg 71:1–9
50. Shapiro WR, Green SB, Burger PC, Selker RG, van Gilder JC, Robertson JT, Mealey J Jr, Ransohoff J, Mahaley MS Jr (1987) A randomized comparison of intraarterial vs intravenous BCNU for patients with malignant glioma (study 8301): interim analysis demonstrating lack of efficacy for ia BCNU. ASCO Proc 6:268
51. Shapiro WR, Young DF (1976) Treatment of malignant glioma. Arch Neurol 33:494–500
52. Shapiro WR, Young DF (1984) Neurological complications of antineoplastic therapy. Acta Neurol Scand 70 [Suppl 100]:125–132

53. Shibata S, Mori K, Moriyama T, Tanaka K, Moroki J (1987) Randomized controlled study of the effect of adjuvant immunotherapy with Picibanil on 51 malignant gliomas. Surg Neurol 27:259-263
54. Taylor S, Eyre HJ (1987) Randomized phase II trials of acivicin and fludarabine in recurrent malignant gliomas: a SWOG study. ASCO Proc 6:71
55. Thomas DGT, Darling JL, Paul EA, Mott TJ, Godlee JN, Tobias JS, Capra LG, Collins CD, Mooney C, Bozek T, Finn GP, Aribabu SO, Bullard DE, Shannon N, Freshney RI (1985) Assay of anti-cancer drugs in tissue culture: relationship of relapse free interval (RFI) and in vitro chemosensitivity in patients with malignant cerebral glioma. Br J Cancer 51:525–532
56. Tirelli U, D'Incalci M, Canetta R, Tumolo S, Franchin G, Veronesi A, Galligioni E, Trovo MG, Rossi C, Grigoletto E (1984) Etoposide in malignant brain tumors: a phase II study. J Clin Oncol 2:432–437
57. Trojanowski T, Peszynski J, Turowski K, Markiewicz P, Goscinski I, Bielawski A, Bendarzewska B, Szymona J, Dabrowska A, Lopatkiewicz J et al (1989) Quality of survival of patients with brain gliomas treated with postoperative CCNU and radiation therapy. J Neurosurg 70:18–23
58. Ushio Y, Abe H, Suzuki J, Tanaka R, Kitamura K, Miwa T, Matsutani M, Takeuchi K, Takakura K, Nomura K et al (1985) Evaluation of ACNU alone and combined with tegafur as additions to radiotherapy of the treatment of malignant gliomas – a cooperative clinical trial. No To Shinkei 37:999–1006
59. Voth D, Hüwel N, Al-Hami S, Kühnert A (1984) Mono-treatment of malignant glioma with a derivate of nitrosourea ACNU (first results). In: Voth D, Krauseneck P (eds) Chemotherapy of gliomas. de Gruyter, Berlin, pp 361–372
60. Walker MD, Alexander E Jr, Hunt WE, MacCarty CS, Mahaley MS Jr, Mealey J Jr, Norrell HA, Ransohoff J, Wilson CB, Gehan EA, Strike TA (1978) Evaluation of BCNU and/or radiotherapy in the treatment of anaplastic gliomas. J Neurosurg 49:333–343
61. Walker MD, Green SB, Byar DP, Alexander E Jr, Batzdorf U, Brooks WH, Hunt WE, MacCarty CS, Mahaley MS Jr, Mealey J Jr, Owens G, Ransohoff J II, Robertson JT, Shapiro WR, Smith KR Jr, Wilson CB, Strike TA (1980) Randomized comparisons of radiotherapy and nitrosoureas for the treatment of malignant glioma after surgery. N Engl J Med 303:1323–1329
62. Yamashima T, Yamashita J, Shoin K (1990) Neurotoxicity of local administration of two nitrosoureas in malignant gliomas. Neurosurgery 26:794–799
63. Zimm S, Ettinger LJ, Holgenberg SJ et al (1985) Phase I and clinical pharmacological study of mercaptopurine administered as a prolonged intravenous infusion. Cancer Res 45:1869–1873

Interstitial Chemotherapy with Sustained-Release Polymer Systems for the Treatment of Malignant Gliomas

A. Olivi and H. Brem

Departments of Neurosurgery and Oncology, Johns Hopkins University School of Medicine, Baltimore, MD 21205, USA

Introduction

Malignant gliomas remain poorly responsive to conventional treatment consisting of surgical resection followed by external beam radiation therapy. Moreover, systemic chemotherapy has been generally disappointing in prolonging the survival of patients with malignant brain tumors, except for those with anaplastic oligodendrogliomas, where more encouraging results have recently been reported. The significant systemic toxicity associated with the large doses of chemotherapeutic agents required and the poor delivery of anticancer agents to areas of the brain "protected" by the blood-brain barrier are likely responsible for the limited effectiveness of chemotherapy.

In order to maximize the delivery of chemotherapeutic agents to brain tumors, while minimizing the systemic toxicity, we have developed a sustained-release system consisting of biocompatible polymers impregnated with anticancer drugs. The polymers are directly implanted into the tumor site at the time of surgery thus by-passing the blood-brain barrier and providing high local concentrations of drug. The rationale for such an approach is also based on the observation that the vast majority of malignant gliomas tend to recur within 2 cm margin of the original tumor [8]. A number of polymeric systems have been studied by our group in both preclinical and clinical settings. These systems are in various stages of development, from initial trials with animal models to a placebo-controlled, double blind, prospective phase III clinical trial. A summary of our experience with these systems is presented below.

Preclinical Studies

In selecting the most effective polymer-chemotherapy system several factors must be considered: the physical properties of the polymeric devices and their safety in their interactions with biological tissues; the bioavailability of the selected drug after its incorporation in the polymeric matrix; the activity of the drug after its release from the polymers; and ultimately the efficacy of the system against brain tumors.

A sequence of rigorous preclinical studies has been developed and implemented to determine: (a) the biocompatibility and safety of implanting polymers into brain tissue; (b) the release kinetics of the drug incorporated into the polymers and its bioavailability; and (c) the efficacy of drug-loaded polymers to inhibit the in vivo growth of experimental brain tumors.

Polymers

Among the polymeric devices studied in our laboratory, two biodegradable polyanhydrides are particularly suitable for local drug delivery to the brain; the poly [bis (*p*-carboxyphenoxy) propane-sebacic acid] copolymer (PCPP-SA): and the fatty acid dimer-sebacic acid copolymer (FAD-SA). The first polymer (PCPP-SA) is the most extensively studied and is currently used with carmustine (BCNU) in clinical trials. The second (FAD-SA) was developed more recently as a more versatile delivery system for water soluble agents, such as platinum derivatives, and is being tested clinically with gentamycin for osteomyelitis.

Polyanhydride polymers react spontaneously with water in an aqueous medium to form dicarboxylic acid [10]. The degradation products are nonmutagenic, noncytotoxic, and nonteratogenic [9]. Drugs can be incorporated into the matrix of polyanhydride polymers with minimal difficulty and at low temperatures. Different shapes and configurations of polymers such as microspheres, pellets, sheets, wafers, and rods can be created. Drugs that are loaded into the polyanhydride polymers are protected from interaction with the surrounding medium prior to their release. This is essential for drugs with short biological half-lives such as BCNU (t = 13 min), which therefore can be released in active form even weeks after the implant.

The release is the result of a surface erosion degradation process which proceeds at a constant rate, thereby providing a constant rate of drug release.

Rat Brain Biocompatibility Studies

The safety and the biocompatibility of intracerebral implants of polyanhydride polymers were first studied in rat brain [1, 12]. The inflammatory reactions elicited by PCPP-SA and FAD-SA polymers were compared with those elicited by standard neurosurgical hemostatic materials (Gelfoam and Surgicel). The devices were surgically implanted through small craniotomies into the rat cerebral hemispheres. The animals were sacrificed at various time points between postoperative days 1 and 60. All animals survived to the scheduled sacrifice day without signs of neurological or systemic toxicity. On histological examination, the inflammatory reaction surrounding the polyanhydride implants was very localized and comparable to that surrounding surgicel. We concluded that the polyanhydride polymers tested were very well tolerated by the brain tissue of the rats, with no significant localized or systemic reactions.

Kinetics of Release from the Polymers

These studies were performed both in vitro and in vivo with polyanhydride polymers loaded with antineoplastic drugs including BCNU, carboplatin, and 4-hydroperoxycyclophosphamide. Drug levels of the solutions bathing the polymer, which were changed daily, were measured in vitro. Drug concentrations in the brain and surrounding the polymer implant were measured in vivo. These studies confirmed that the release of BCNU from the polymer PCPP-SA and the release of carboplatin and 4-hydroperoxycyclophosphamide from the FAD-SA were sustained for periods ranging from 2 to 4 weeks [5, 6].

Distribution Autoradiography Studies

Having established that these polymers are capable of a sustained release of anticancer drugs, we studied the distribution of BCNU released from an intracranially implanted polymer by use of autoradiography [7]. Tritiated BCNU was incorporated into cylinders of PCPP-SA polymers. These polymer-drug devices were implanted intracranially into the rabbit brain. The rabbits were sacrificed at days 3, 7, 14, and 21. The brains were removed and sectioned, and prepared for quantitative autoradiography. Approximately 50% of the area of the brain section was exposed to radiolabeled compound 3 days after BCNU-polymer implantation, 15% at 7 days, and less than 10% at 14 and 21 days post-implantation. Polymer discs containing 600 ng of BCNU produced brain tissue concentration of 6 µg BCNU at a distance of 10 mm from the disc. It was concluded that BCNU delivered by PCPP-SA reaches high local tissue concentrations in the brain for prolonged periods of time.

Efficacy Studies

Extensive studies have been performed to establish the effectiveness of the polymer chemotherapy devices in treating different rat glioma models. The efficacy of the BCNU-loaded PCPP-SA polymers was tested against the 9L rat gliosarcoma [13]. The animals underwent intracerebral implantation with tumors and were subsequently treated with a drug-loaded polymer. A group of animals received empty polymers (controls), while another group received BCNU by systemic injection. The animals treated with the drug-loaded polymer had a significantly longer survival than did those treated with empty polymers and those treated with systemic BCNU.

Similarly, the efficacy of the carboplatin-loaded FAD-SA polymers was studied on the F 98 rat glioma model [11]. The animals treated with carboplatin polymer implants had a median survival of 52 days compared with the 16 days of the control animals treated with empty polymers. Histological examination of the brains of animals receiving the polymer-drug implants at the time of death revealed significant inhibition of tumor growth in the vicinity of the polymer. The same model was used to test the efficacy of the FAD-SA polymer loaded with 4-hydroperoxycyclophosphamide. Again, survival was significantly prolonged in the group of animals treated with this system [6] The studies unequivocally confirmed the effectiveness of drug-loaded polymers in inhibiting the in vivo growth of experimental brain tumors.

Toxicity Study in Primate Brain

Before initiation of the clinical studies, further biocompatibility/toxicity tests were performed in primate brains [3, 4]. BCNU-loaded PCPP-SA polymers were implanted in the brains of 18 *Macaca fascicularis* monkeys. Again, no evidence of toxicity from the implant was observed and upon histological examination at the time of the scheduled sacrifice, only a limited localized and transient inflammatory reaction was observed in the area of the implant. Three of the 18 monkeys received concurrent radiation therapy without any deleterious effect attributed to the polymers. On the basis of these results we concluded that the PCPP-SA polymer was safe when implanted intracranially in primate brain and was suitable for trials in humans.

Clinical Studies

The promising results obtained on the preclinical studies led to the phase I-II clinical trial to investigate the safety of the BCNU-loaded PCPP-SA polymer implanted at the tumor site in patients with recurrent malignant gliomas [2].Twenty-one patients with recurrent grade III or IV astrocytomas were enrolled in this study. The inclusion criteria were: indication for the reoperation to resect recurrent mass, presence of unilateral single focus in the brain showing at least 1.5 cm enhancing volume on computed tomography and magnetic resonance imaging, Karnofsky performance score of at least 60, full course of external beam radiation therapy, and no chemotherapy during the 6 weeks prior to the enrollment. The polymer devices were surgically implanted into the resection cavity after completion of tumor debulking. Up to eight polymers, in the shape of wafers, 1.4 cm in diameter and 1 mm in thickness, were placed in the tumor bed. Three increasing concentrations of BCNU were studied: 1.93% loading dose for a surface concentration of 25 mg/mm^2; 3.85% loading dose (surface concentration, 50 mg/mm^2); 6.37% loading dose (surface concentration, 82.5 mg/mm^2). The patients were followed at regular intervals for signs of toxicity from the drug polymer implant. No patient had a significant reduction in blood cell count which would indicate systemic exposure to BCNU. No adverse reactions to the BCNU wafer treatment itself were observed. The overall median survival was 46 weeks from the reoperation and 87 weeks from the initial operation. The results of the trial established that intracranial implantation of BCNU PCPP-SA polymer into patients was a safe procedure. These patients did not exhibit toxicity related to the polymer and indeed appeared to live significantly longer than predicted based on historical controls.

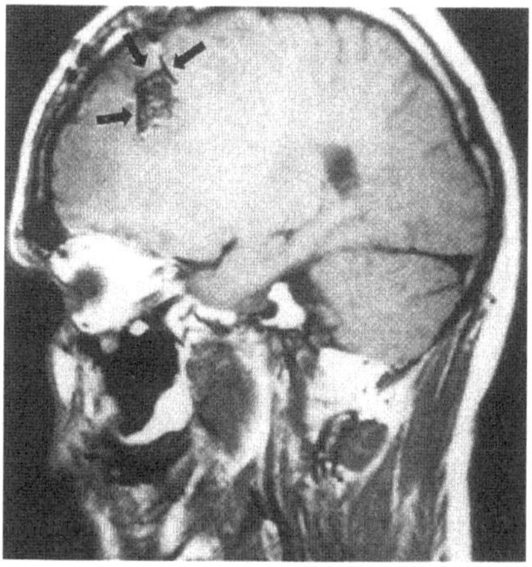
1

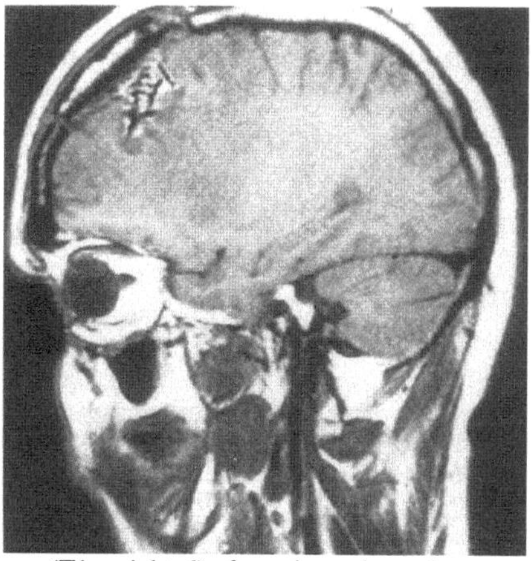
2

Fig. 1. Postoperative sagittal magnetic resonance image (T1-weighted) of a patient who underwent a left frontal craniotomy with debulking of a recurrent malignant astrocytoma and placement of polymer wafers on the tumor beds. The wafers are the hypointense structures (*solid arrows*);

Fig. 2. Postoperative magnetic resonance image of the same patient after injection of gadolinium. A small amount of enhancement is seen on the tumor bed and around the polymer wafer

Therefore, following the phase I-II trial a prospective, randomized, placebo-controlled, double-blind phase III clinical trial was conducted at 28 medical centers to test the efficacy of the BCNU-loaded polymers in patients with recurrent malignant astrocytomas. The trial included 222 patients who had failed conventional therapy. Each patient underwent a craniotomy for tumor debulking. Patients were randomized to receive either BCNU-loaded PCPP-SA polymer (3.85% loading) or empty PCPP-SA polymer. The polymer implants were placed on the surface of the cavity formed by the tumor resection. Imaging studies of these patients immediately after the polymer implant showed the presence of the polymers in the tumor bed (Figs. 1, 2).The results of the phase III clinical studies are currently being analyzed and should be completed in a few months.

Final Considerations

Our experience suggests that interstitial chemotherapy by means of implantable biodegradable polymers can be used safely for the treatment of human brain tumors. The biodegradable polymer PCPP-SA loaded with BCNU has been studied most extensively. It is not only effective against several animal models, but also was shown to be safe when used in patient phase I-II clinical trial. Even in the recently completed phase III clinical trial no significant adverse reactions have been reported. The effectiveness of this treatment of patients affected by recurrent malignant gliomas is currently being analyzed. A variety of potential future applications of drug-polymer implants are under investigation including other chemotherapeutic agents, corticosteroids, radiation sensitizers, angiogenesis inhibitors and other biological response modifiers. The capability of these systems to provide high local concentrations of the selected drug in areas normally protected by the blood-brain barrier may prove to be useful for the treatment of a variety of central nervous system diseases.

References

1. Brem H, Domb A, Lenartz D, Dureza C, Olivi A, Epstein I (1992) Brain biocompatibility of a biodegradable controlled release polymer consisting of anhydride copolymer of fatty acid dimer and sebacic acid. J Controlled Release 19:325–330
2. Brem H, Mahaley S, Vick NA, Black KL, Schold C, Burger PC, Friedman AH, Ciric IS, Eller TW, Cozzens JW, Kenealy JN (1991) Interstitial chemotherapy with drug polymer implants for the treatment of recurrent gliomas. J Neurosurg 74:441–446
3. Brem H, Tamargo RJ, Olivi A, Pinn M, Wharam M, Epstein J (1994) Controlled delivery using biodegradable polymers for chemotherapy with and without radiation therapy in the monkey brain. Neurosurg in press
4. Brem H, Tamargo RJ, Pinn M, Chasin M (1988) Biocompatibility of a BCNU-loaded biodegradable polymer: a toxicity study in primates. American Association of Neurological Surgeons, Toronto, p. 381
5. Chasin J, Domb A, Ron E, Mathiowitz E, Langer R, Leong K, Laurencin C, Brem H, Grossman S (1990) Polyanhydrides as drug delivery systems In: Chasin M, Langer R (eds) Biodegradable polymers as drug delivery systems. Marcel Dekker, New York, pp. 43–70
6. Domb A, Bogdansky S, Olivi A, Judy K, Dureza C, Pinn ML, Colvin M, Brem H (1991) Controlled release of water soluble and hydrolytically unstable anticancer drugs from polymeric implants. Polym Prepr 32 (2):219–220
7. Grossman SA, Reinhard C, Colvin OM, Chasin,M, Brundrett R, Tamargo RJ, Brem H (1992) The intracerebral distribution of BCNU delivered by surgically implanted biodegradable polymers. J Neurosurg 76:640–647
8. Hochberg F, Pruitt A (1980) Assumptions in the radiotherapy of glioblastoma. Neurology 30:907–911
9. Leong KW, Brott BC, Langer R (1985) Bioerodible polyanhydrides as drug-carrier matrices I: characterization, degradation, and release kinetics. J Biomed Mater Res 19:941–955
10. Leong KW, D'Amore P, Marletta M, Langer R (1986) Bioerodible polyanhydrides as drug-carrier matrices II: biocompatibility and chemical reactivity. J Biomed Mater Res 20:51–64
11. Olivi A, Domb A, Lenartz D, Dureza C, Goodman JH, Pinn M, Brem H (1991) Treatment of F-98 rat glioma with local controlled release of carboplatin from a biodegradable polymer. American Association of Neurological Surgeons, April 1991, New Orleans, p. 526
12. Tamargo RJ, Epstein JI, Reinhard CS, Chasin M, Brem H (1988) Brain biocompatibility of a biodegradable controlled-release polymer in rats. J Biomed Mater Res 23:253–266
13. Tamargo RJ, Myseros JS, Epstein JI, Yang MB, Chasin M, Brem H (1993) Interstitial chemotherapy of the 9L gliosarcoma: controlled release polymers for drug delivery in the brain. Cancer Res 53:329–333

*Primary Central Nervous System Lymphoma**

L. M. DeAngelis

Department of Neurology and Neuroscience, Cornell University Medical College, New York, and Department of Neurology, Memorial Sloan-Kettering Cancer Center, 1275 York Avenue, New York, NY 10021, USA

Introduction

Primary central nervous system lymphoma (PCNSL) is a non-Hodgkin's lymphoma which arises within and is confined to the central nervous system. For many years this tumor was called microglioma, reticulum cell sarcoma, or perivascular sarcoma, but the lymphocytic origin of the malignant cell which comprises this neoplasm is now well established [1–3]. While it is clear that PCNSL is a malignant lymphocytic tumor, how and why a lymphoma develops within the CNS which lacks lymph nodes and lymphatics remains an unanswered question.

Until recently, PCNSL has been a rare tumor, accounting for only 0.5%–1.2% of all intracranial neoplasms; it is associated with a variety of congenital, acquired, and iatrogenic immunodeficiency states [2, 4, 5]. The highest incidence has been reported in patients with the acquired immunodeficiency syndrome (AIDS) where it is seen in 1.9%–6% of patients [6, 7]. However, a recent epidemiological study revealed a threefold increase in the incidence of this tumor in otherwise apparently normal individuals which could not be attributed to new diagnostic techniques or the adoption of a uniform nosology [8]. The reason for this marked rise in PCNSL is unknown, but physicians are seeing these patients with increased frequency. At Memorial Sloan-Kettering Cancer Center, we have seen a 17-fold increase in PCNSL in the 5 years between 1985–1990 compared to the previous 20 years.

*Portions of the text are reprinted from *Principles and Practice of Oncology. Update Series*, DeVita VT, Hellman S, Rosenberg SA (eds), Lippincott, Philadelphia, PA. with permission from the publisher.

Clinical Features

General

PCNSL affects all ages, from the very young to the elderly. Its peak incidence occurs in the 6th and 7th decades in immunocompetent patients and younger in immunosuppressed patients [9]. Among apparently immunocompetent individuals, there is a 3:2 male to female ratio. By definition, PCNSL excludes the presence of systemic lymphoma. Extensive testing of newly diagnosed patients with PCNSL, using abdominal,pelvic, and chest computed tomography (CT) and bone marrow biopsy, has never revealed systemic lymphoma [10]. The absence of systemic tumor in virtually all patients confirms the primary nature of this brain tumor even though the cell of origin is not neuroectodermal.

Brain

Most PCNSLs present with symptoms of an intracranial mass lesion. The specific presenting symptoms and signs reflect the location of the tumor, with focal cerebral deficits occurring in about half of patients [9]; however, there are some differences in the presentation of PCNSL from other brain tumors. Because PCNSL involves the frontal lobes frequently and multiple lesions are often seen, changes in personality and level of alertness are common presenting symptoms. Headaches and symptoms of increased intracranial pressure are also seen frequently. Seizures are less common than in patients with other types of brain tumors, occurring in only 10% of patients as a presenting sign, because most PCNSLs are more likely to involve deep structures. Symptoms are usually present only for a short duration, weeks to a few months, before a diagnosis is made.

PCNSL is usually disseminated within the nervous system at diagnosis. Brain lesions are multifocal in roughly half of immunocompetent patients. Multiple lesions often cause diagnostic confusion with brain metastases, particularly since 13% of PCNSL patients have a history of a prior systemic malignancy [11]. Multiple lesions may be connected to each other by tumor which has infiltrated the brain microscopically but is not apparent on CT or magnetic resonance imaging (MRI) scan; however, the majority of patients with multiple masses appear to have multifocal disease with no continuity among the lesions. Many lesions are periventricular, and thus tumor cells can easily gain access to the CSF. The reported incidence of meningeal seeding by PCNSL varies from 0% to 25% [12–15], but if a vigorous search is conducted, a positive cytology is seen in one-third of patients and a suspicious cytology is obtained in another one-third [10]. Therefore, at least 67% of patients have definitive or probable leptomeningeal lymphoma, and this is probably still an underestimate. At autopsy 100% of patients have leptomeningeal tumor either from direct invasion into the ventricular system by periventricular tumor or by local involvement of the leptomeninges overlying a cortical lesion.

Despite the high incidence of a positive CSF cytology, few patients have clinical symptoms or signs of leptomeningeal lymphoma, such as cranial neuropathies, painful lumbosacral radiculopathies, or hydrocephalus. Therefore, the absence of these clinical features is no guarantee that PCNSL has not involved the leptomeninges. CSF needs to be examined in every patient, preferably before corticosteroids have been started. Furthermore, we assume that all patients have demonstrable or microscopic CSF involvement at diagnosis, and include treatment of the CSF in our therapeutic regimen.

Eye

The eye, a direct extension of the nervous system, is another site of multifocal disease in PCNSL. Ocular involvement does not imply the presence of systemic lymphoma. Typically, PCNSL involves the vitreous, retina, or choroid, but optic nerve infiltration can also occur [16–18]. Of all patients with PCNSL 20% have ocular disease at diagnosis, the majority detected only by careful ophthalmological examination [10,18]. Ocular lymphoma can present with blurred vision or floaters or be clinically silent. A cellular infiltrate of the vitreous can be visualized only by slit-lamp examination, and choroidal or retinal lesions often require indirect ophthalmoscopy. Cells in the vitreous offer a diagnostic opportunity, and lymphoma can be identified in vitrectomy specimens [17]. In some patients the disease begins in the eyes, with a nonspecific uveitis which may begin unilaterally. Most eventually develop bilateral disease although it may be asymmetric. The uveitis typically does not respond to conventional ophthalmological treatment, and this is often the first clue that the observed cellular infiltrate represents malignant lymphoma. As many as 80% of patients with ocular lymphoma eventually develop cerebral lymphoma although there may be a several year latency [17, 18]. Any patient with ocular lymphoma should have cranial MRI with gadolinium and lumbar puncture and, if negative, followed closely.

Leptomeninges

Primary leptomeningeal lymphoma in the absence of a parenchymal brain mass is rare, accounting for approximately 7% of PCNSLs [15, 19, 20]. Patients can present with a progressive lumbosacral root syndrome, cranial neuropathies, increased intracranial pressure, confusion, or a combination of these symptoms. Symptoms are usually present for only 2–3 months before diagnosis, but an occassional patient can have symptoms for 1–2 years before the diagnosis is made [19]. Diagnosis is established by demonstration of malignant lymphocytes in the CSF or on meningeal biopsy.

The CSF invariably shows an elevated protein concentration, and a lymphocytic pleocytosis often in excess of 100 cells/mm3; CSF glucose is low in about one-third of patients. Myelography may reveal intradural nodules and gadolinium MRI of the head or spine may show meningeal enhancement or hydrocephalus but no brain tumors.

Spinal Cord

Primary spinal cord lymphoma is even less common than primary leptomeningeal lymphoma [15, 21–23]. Lymphoma in the spinal cord parenchyma can occur in isolation or with brain lymphoma. Patients present with painless bilateral limb weakness, usually involving the legs; sensory symptoms and signs may initially follow a radicular pattern, but eventually a sensory level may be found. CSF may be normal or have a mildly elevated protein concentration with a few lymphocytes. Prognosis has been poor, with patients surviving only a few months from the onset of symptoms, but this is often due to the fact that the diagnosis was not made until autopsy, and that no appropriate therapy was administered.

Diagnostic Tests

CT/MRI

The CT/MRI of PCNSL is usually quite distinctive, and the diagnosis may be suspected on the basis of the radiographic appearance alone. On the precontrast CT the tumor is usually iso- or hyperdense. This corresponds to an isointense signal on the pregadolinium T1-weighted MRI. After contrast administration, PCNSL densely and diffusely enhances on both CT and MRI (Fig. 1) [24–26]. The lesions often have indistinct borders, and the amount of surrounding edema is quite variable. Unlike brain metastases or malignant gliomas, ring enhancement is rarely seen. The MRI sometimes reveals additional lesions not seen on CT.

While prominent contrast enhancement of tumor is typical in patients with PCNSL, 12% (10/85) of our patients have had nonenhancing lesions on CT/MRI at some time during the course of their illness [27]. Nonenhancing tumor may occur at diagnosis or at relapse, and half of patients had a simultaneous enhancing lesion on the same scan (Fig. 1). Corticosteroids were not responsible for diminution of enhancement in the majority of patients. Nonenhancing tumor may cause significant diagnostic problems, but also has important therapeutic implications, suggesting that tumor resides behind an intact blood-brain barrier (BBB; discussed below).

Lumbar Puncture

Lumbar puncture should be part of the diagnostic evaluation of every patient with PCNSL. The protein concentration is elevated in 85% of patients although rarely above 150 mg/dl [12, 14, 28, 29]. The glucose concentration is usually normal but can be low when florid leptomeningeal tumor is present. A CSF pleocytosis is seen in more than half of patients, and always consists of lymphocytes, either reactive or malignant (see below). An unequivocally positive CSF cytology eliminates the need for brain biopsy confirmation of a PCNSL. This may be particularly important in the immunosuppressed or desperately ill patient at increased risk for a surgical compli-

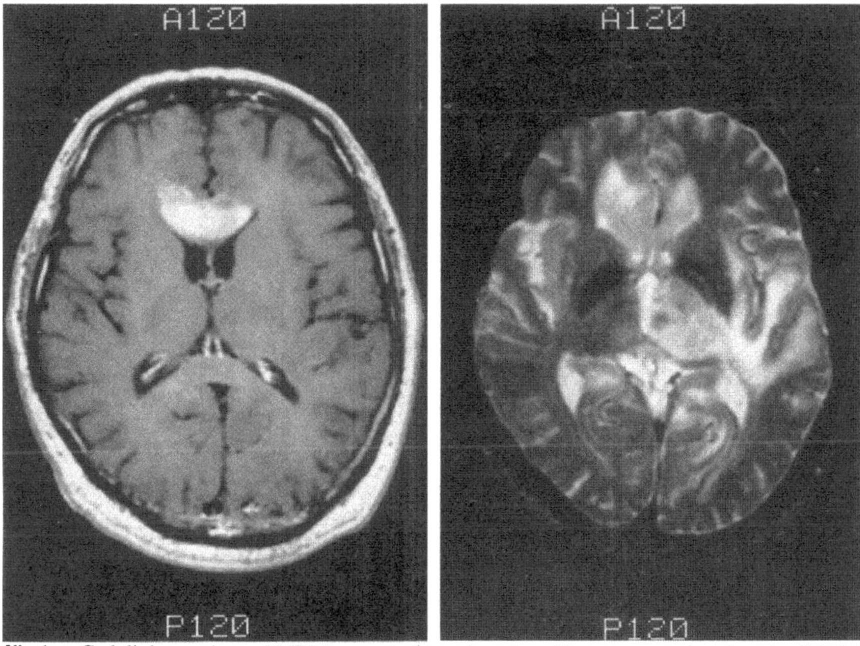

a b

Fig. 1. a. Gadolinium-enhanced MRI demonstrating a densely and homogeneously enhancing PCNSL lesion involving the corpus callosum. Note the relative lack of edema surrounding the mass. **b** T2-weighted MRI of the same patient revealing two lesions

cation. Occasionally immunohistochemical stains of CSF demonstrate a monoclonal population of cells establishing the neoplastic nature of the pleocytosis even if the cells appear cytologically benign [30]. Tumor markers, such a b_2-microglobulin, lactate dehydrogenase isoenzymes and b-glucuronidase can, when the level is elevated, provide circumstantial evidence for tumor invasion of the meninges.

Molecular Biological Techniques

As in systemic lymphomas, detection of immunoglobulin gene rearrangement may be helpful diagnostically, particularly if small tissue samples are obtained by stereotactic biopsy, and a histological diagnosis is not certain [31]. These techniques have been successfully applied to PCNSL both for diagnostic purposes and to establish clonality [32].

Pathology

PCNSL is a non-Hodgkin's lymphoma, usually of a high-grade malignant subtype [13, 15]. The majority are diffuse histiocytic lymphomas, diffuse mixed histiocytic-

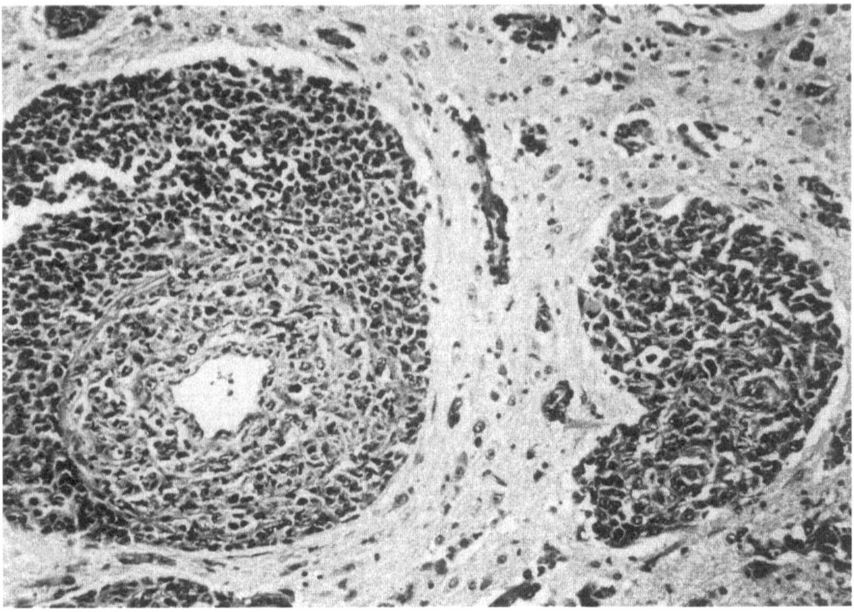

Fig. 2. A pathological specimen of PCNSL demonstrating perivascular tumor growth

lymphocytic lymphomas or diffuse poorly differentiated lymphocytic lymphomas according to the Rappaport classification. Comparable Working Formulation definitions are diffuse large cell; large cell, immunoblastic; and lymphoblastic lymphoma.

PCNSL usually has a characteristic vasocentric growth pattern with tumor infiltrating the brain parenchyma between involved blood vessels (Fig. 2). Tumor margins are poorly defined, and extend a substantial distance from an obvious mass lesion; in addition, tumor is often found in multiple regions throughout the CNS parenchyma. Neither necrosis nor hemorrhage are dominant histological features.

Several investigators have demonstrated the B-cell nature of this tumor using immunohistochemistry to demonstrate monoclonal heavy or light immunoglobulin chain production or to identify B-cell markers [3, 15, 33]. Immunoglobulin gene rearrangement has also been shown [32]. Recent reports suggest a rising incidence in the number of T-cell PCNSLs. This may be a result of newer immunohistochemical techniques, or it may be an artifact of the difficulties in interpreting immunohistochemical studies. In both the CSF and the tumor itself, these neoplasms are often accompanied by a reactive pleocytosis, in the case of the spinal fluid, or a reactive lymphocytosis surrounding the tumor [34]. The number of reactive cells can differ among patients, and they are not seen in every case. These reactive cells are always T-cells and can make interpretation of special stains difficult. For the most part, one can clearly distinguish the cytologically malignant cells, which are usually B-cells, from the reactive lymphocytes, which are T-cells. With diagnostically difficult specimens, immunohistochemical stains are often employed in an effort to clarify the situation, and for this reason, an appreciation of these two cell populations is important.

Response to treatment is not related to pathological subtype or the cell of origin; however, most series contain so few patients in any given category that it is possible that a relationship has been missed, and further prospective studies with a large number of patients may reveal differences comparable to those seen for systemic lymphomas. At this time, all PCNSLs are treated in the same manner regardless of subtype or cell of origin.

Management

The appropriate management of a patient with PCNSL requires a correct diagnosis. This may be difficult because the clinical presentation of PCNSL is not distinctive, and other primary and secondary brain tumors are much more common; however, the method outlined below can aid in the approach to a patient who harbors this tumor.

When neurological symptoms and/or signs first develop, CT or MRI should be performed. If a mass lesion(s) is discovered, the CT/MRI appearance may strongly suggest the diagnosis of PCNSL, for example, multiplicity of lesions, a deep or periventricular location, diffuse and dense contrast enhancement, poorly defined borders, and relatively little edema surrounding the mass are all characteristics of PCNSL. In addition, the clinical setting in which the tumor arises may point to the diagnosis (e.g., an immunocompromised patient). If PCNSL is a strong diagnostic consideration, corticosteroids should be withheld unless the patient is in immediate danger of herniation, a rare situation. Corticosteroids may alter or even eliminate the ability to establish the diagnosis pathologically. Histological confirmation is essential, and the diagnosis can be accomplished with stereotactic biopsy but may also be done by lumbar puncture demonstrating leptomeningeal lymphoma or slit-lamp examination documenting lymphomatous cells in the vitreous, which can be confirmed by vitreous biopsy or aspirate. Therefore, a spinal tap and ocular examination should be performed prior to a neurosurgical procedure in an effort to obtain evidence of the tumor type without subjecting the patient to surgery. If the patient required the immediate use of corticosteroids, or if PCNSL was not considered originally, and the patient was placed on corticosteroids, a repeat CT should be perfomed to evaluate for possible resolution or significant shrinkage of the lesion(s). This would indirectly substantiate whether the tumor is a lymphoma since no other intracranial tumor disappears after treatment with corticosteroids alone; however, nonneoplastic contrast-enhancing processes such as multiple sclerosis or sarcoidosis can resolve after steroid administration. For this reason, biopsy should still be attempted if the lesion(s) is reduced in size but still evident; however, nondiagnostic tissue is frequently obtained after corticosteroids. A steroid trial may be considered in a patient too ill to undergo stereotactic biopsy, or when the risk of the procedure is too great; however, every effort to obtain histological confirmation should be made. Once the diagnosis is certain, appropriate treatment can be instituted.

Using the clinical staging criteria developed for systemic lymphomas, PCNSL corresponds to stage IE, i.e., disease confined to a single extra-nodal site. Systemic stage IE disease has a 100% complete response rate and a 70% 10-year survival, or cure, rate with focal radiotherapy (RT) [35]. Surprisingly, the prognosis for PCNSL is poor. Despite the highly responsive nature of PCNSL to any initial treatment, median survival is only 12-18 months with corticosteroids and cranial RT [28, 36–39]. There is only a 3%–4% 5-year survival rate, a prognosis similar to that of glioblastoma multiforme [14, 29]. This short survival is due to recurrence of PCNSL after an initial response to cranial irradiation. Relapse occurs primarily in the brain, often in regions remote from the original site but within the prior radiation port, and also occurs in the leptomeninges and eye. Systemic lymphoma is found in only 7%–8% of autopsied patients, and the vast majority of these patients have a single focus of clinically silent disease thought to represent a systemic metastasis from recurrent nervous system tumor [14, 28].

Because of its current poor prognosis, new approaches to the treatment of PCNSL are essential. With the recently increased number of patients with PCNSL, new therapeutic strategies can be devised and tested in a relatively timely fashion. Recent developments using chemotherapy have already shown promise. In the next section, each therapeutic modality and its current and potential therapeutic role will be discussed.

Therapy

Corticosteroids

A unique feature of PCNSL in comparison to other brain tumors is its exquisite sensitivity to corticosteroids. At least 40% of patients have a significant shrinkage or disappearance of tumor masses on CT after administration of corticosteroids [10, 15, 38, 40]. Conversely, if contrast-enhancing lesions disappear after corticosteroids, the diagnosis of PCNSL is highly probable although multiple sclerosis and sarcoid are also possible. This apparent remission is due to a direct cytotoxic effect of the corticosteroids; biopsy following steroid administration often yields normal, necrotic, or nondiagnostic tissue. This is comparable to the cytolytic effect of corticosteroids on systemic lymphoma and is the reason why corticosteroids are an important component of all combination chemotherapy regimens. Clinically, disappearance of PCNSL lesions is accompanied by improvement which may last long after the corticosteroids have been discontinued. There are isolated reports of patients being cured or having prolonged survival after treatment with steroids alone [40]. However, achievement of clinical improvement after the administration of corticosteroids does not require resolution or diminution of tumor as many patients have amelioration of symptoms without any detectable change in tumor size on CT. Regardless of apparent tumor regression, steroid-induced remission is short lived in the majority of patients and should not be considered definitive treatment.

Surgery

Surgery is important to confirm the histological diagnosis, but it has no therapeutic role. Mean survival of patients with PCNSL with supportive care alone is 1.8–3.3 months [1, 4, 28]. Surgical resection adds little, prolonging the average survival to only 3.3–5 months [28, 38, 41, 42]. Unlike malignant glioma, where extensive resection is an important component of therapy, surgical extirpation is usually ineffective in PCNSL because of its multifocal and infiltrative nature. Furthermore, the deep location of many PCNSLs leaves the patient susceptible to severe postoperative deficits if a complete resection is attempted [10]. In our experience this has been particularly true in patients who have minimal neurological deficits preoperatively. Therefore, stereotactic biopsy is the method of choice for documenting the diagnosis which also allows for biopsy of deep lesions which could not be approached safely with conventional surgery.

Radiotherapy

Whole brain radiotherapy (WBRT) combined with corticosteroids has been the conventional treatment for PCNSL, yielding median survivals of 12–18 months. There have been no prospective studies to ascertain the optimal dose or fractionation of WBRT in the treatment of this disease. Extrapolation from treatment regimens of comparable systemic lymphomas suggest that 4200 cGy is probably necessary to achieve local control [43]. In systemic disease the fractionation schedule and elapsed time appear less important than the total dose, and this appears to be the case with PCNSL as well [37, 43]. While most retrospective studies suggest that survival is improved with doses greater than 4000 cGy of WBRT, not all authors agree. Sagerman et al. recommended a total dose greater than 3500 cGy, and Berry et al. noted improved survival with doses of 5000 cGy or more [36, 37]. However, Woodman et al. did not find any difference in survival when patients received 4000 cGy or less [38]. Nevertheless, the current recommendation is for patients to receive 4000-5000 cGy WBRT, often with a 1000–1500 cGy boost to the tumor bed [29, 44].

The primary treatment of ocular lymphoma is radiotherapy to the posterior two-thirds of the globe [16, 18, 45]. Because of the rarity of this condition, few patients have been treated for this complication, and therefore, few data exist as to the optimal dosage; however, 3500–4500 cGy over 4–5 weeks is the recommended total dose. Because ocular lymphoma is predominately a binocular process, both eyes should be irradiated, even when only monocular disease can be detected on slit-lamp examination. Most patients experience both symptomatic improvement and resolution of cells in the vitreous after radiotherapy; however, some have vitreal clearing without improved vision, and others may not improve at all. The incidence of ocular toxicity from radiotherapy in this disease is not known, but may increase with improved survival since many of the complications are delayed. Conjunctivitis, retinal atrophy, vitreous hemorrhage, and cataract formation have all been reported in PCNSL patients after ocular radiotherapy [45].

Craniospinal irradiation has been proposed as the initial therapy of PCNSL because of the high incidence of clinically evident meningeal tumor at recurrence and the invariable demonstration of leptomeningeal infiltration at autopsy. Few data exist to evaluate this approach, although in the few patients treated with neuraxis RT there is a suggestion of improved survival over WBRT alone [46]. However, irradiation of such a large portion of the bone marrow compromises the patient's ability to tolerate subsequent systemic chemotherapy which might be required at relapse. Administration of intrathecal chemotherapy at diagnosis effectively treats leptomeningeal lymphoma, and is associated with less systemic toxicity.

Chemotherapy

No large prospective trials have examined the role of chemotherapy in either relapsed or initial disease. Nevertheless, important information has accumulated which documents the sensitivity of PCNSL to systemic chemotherapy, and this suggests that it will play an increasingly important role in the treatment of this tumor in the future.

A primary consideration in the interpretation of existing data and design of chemotherapy trials for PCNSL is the function of the BBB within regions of bulk tumor and in remote regions which contain microscopic disease. The normal BBB excludes hydrophilic compounds, including most chemotherapeutic agents, from entering cerebral tissue. As evidenced by the prominent contrast enhancement seen on CT/MRI, PCNSL mass lesions have an impaired BBB. This suggests that drugs which are not usually considered candidates for treatment of cerebral tumors may be effective in this disease, and in fact several examples support this concept [41, 47, 48]. However, parenchymal tumor always exists behind an intact BBB, and drug penetration into the CSF is essential for the treatment of leptomeningeal lymphoma. While tumor bulk can be appreciated on contrast enhanced CT/MRI, autopsy specimens always show microscopic lymphoma in regions which appear completely normal radiographically, even on T2-weighted MRI [27]; these areas of tumor have a normal BBB, and therefore their treatment requires the use of drugs which can penetrate an intact BBB. Furthermore, drugs which can not penetrate the BBB or CSF have been reported to produce remissions of gross parenchymal brain lymphoma but often lead to subsequent and rapid leptomeningeal relapse [48].

Therefore, PCNSL should be treated with a combination of agents known to have efficacy against lymphoma, which can penetrate the intact BBB, and delivered in doses or routes which assure adequate coverage of the leptomeninges.

Recurrent PCNSL

Systemic chemotherapy was first used for patients with recurrent PCNSL. High-dose intravenous methotrexate (MTX; 3–10 g/m^2) was used as a single agent and produced complete and lasting remissions from recurrent parenchymal disease [49, 50].

Recurrences after MTX could also respond to additional, but often higher doses of MTX, and usually for a shorter period of time. Frick et al. reported a patient with parenchymal brain involvement by a systemic lymphoma which occurred in the setting of a systemic relapse; high-dose cytosine arabinoside (ara-C; 3 g/m^2) produced a short-lived but complete remission of both the cerebral and systemic disease [51].

Primary Chemotherapy

Randomized prospective therapeutic trials are difficult in PCNSL because of the small numbers of patients encountered in most centers. Nevertheless, a variety of chemotherapeutic schedules, usually in combination with WBRT, have been used as the initial treatment of PCNSL. There is very limited experience with any single regimen, but there is an overall suggestion that chemotherapy improves survival. Loeffler et al. treated ten patients, five with cranial irradiation and five with RT plus chemotherapy; each received a different protocol although four of the five received intrathecal MTX [52]. Median survival was 44 months in those treated with RT plus chemotherapy compared to 14 months in those treated with RT alone. Three of the ten patients survived 2 years or longer, and all had received chemotherapy. Kawakami et al. also reported improved survival with the addition of chemotherapy either cyclophosphamide, doxorubicin, vincristine and prednisone (CHOP) or nimustine [1-(4-amino-2-methylpyrimidine-5-yl) methyl-3-(2-chlorethyl)-3-nitrosourea hydrochloride; ACNU] to WBRT [41]. Recent studies have focused on the use of standard combination chemotherapy regimens for systemic lymphomas for the treatment of PCNSL. While some reports suggest that CHOP added to WBRT enhances survival, enthusiasm must be tempered by the rapid and frequent multifocal brain and leptomeningeal recurrences seen after CHOP [47, 48, 53, 54]. Brada et al. treated ten patients with cyclophosphamide, doxorubicin, methotrexate at 400 mg/m^2, vincristine, bleomycin, and prednisone (MACOP-B) and RT, but there was no improvement in survival over patients treated with WBRT alone [55]. PET studies of two of these patients demonstrate that areas of bulky tumor which have an abnormal BBB, regain the permeability of normal brain within 5 weeks of the start of treatment demonstrating a rapid reconstitution of the BBB with the use of chemotherapy [56]. These reports suggest that PCNSL is a chemo-sensitive neoplasm; however, failure of many regimens, particularly those adapted from systemic lymphoma, may be attributed to the fact that none of the agents or the dosages used permit drug penetration through an intact BBB. While the optimal choice, sequence, and combination of appropriate agents for efficacious treatment of PCNSL has yet to be determined, an essential component of therapy must included adequate drug delivery behind a normal BBB where microscopic disease always resides.

The potential obstacle that the BBB presents to systemic chemotherapy has led to novel methods of treatment using BBB disruption with mannitol followed by intra-arterial MTX and intravenous cyclophosphamide, procarbazine, and dexamethasone [57]. This combination is effective whether or not it is combined with cranial irradiation. In a series of 16 patients treated with this chemotherapeutic regimen as the primary therapy, using cranial RT at recurrence, the median survival was 44.5 months. The most promising feature of this regimen is its apparent success in 6 of the 16 patients who achieved a remission with chemotherapy alone, thus eliminating the potential neurological morbidity associated with cranial RT; however, 10 patients relapsed and required WBRT.

At Memorial Sloan-Kettering Cancer Center we treated 31 patients with PCNSL using systemic chemotherapy which penetrates the BBB, including vigorous treatment of the leptomeninges in all patients. We used preradiation intravenous MTX (1 g/m^2) combined with intrathecal MTX (12 mg/dose) via an Ommaya reservoir, and post-radiation high dose ara-C (3 g/m^2); corticosteroids were used to control neurological symptoms [10]. All MTX was completed prior to radiotherapy to minimize the known potential for combined neurotoxicity of radiation and MTX. We reported a disease-free median survival of 41 months, a significant difference from the median of 10 months seen in those treated with WBRT alone [58]; additional follow-up reveals a median disease-free survival of 51 months in those treated with chemotherapy plus cranial RT. These results are at least comparable to those achieved by BBB disruption because conventional agents were administered in high-doses known to penetrate the nervous system. Furthermore, our regimen is substantially easier to administer and potentially less toxic to normal brain.

As with systemic lymphoma which has spread to the leptomeninges, meningeal infiltration by PCNSL responds to intrathecal MTX [59]. MTX can be instilled into the subarachnoid space via an Ommaya reservoir or lumbar puncture. The Ommaya reservoir assures drug entry into the CSF since the lumbar route often deposits drug in the sub- or epidural space; the Ommaya reservoir also offers superior drug distribution as well as easy administration, and consequently is the preferred method [60]. Intra-Ommaya MTX produces a sustained therapeutic concentration of MTX for a minimum of 24 h [60]. Intrathecal ara-C has also been used for leptomeningeal lymphoma, but is often used after MTX failure. High intravenous doses of either MTX or ara-C can yield therapeutic concentrations of drug in the CSF, and may represent an alternative to intrathecal therapy [61, 62]. The intravenous route also offers the advantage of treating both parenchymal brain and leptomeningeal disease simultaneously.

There are few examples of ocular lymphoma being treated with chemotherapy. Barr et al. used cyclophosphamide and then vincristine in one patient with metastatic ocular lymphoma without effect [63]. Sullivan and Dallow reported a patient with a systemic histiocytic lymphoma and a ciliary body metastasis who had both a systemic and an ocular remission after treatment with procarbazine, lomustine (CCNU), and vincristine [64]. Baumann et al. reported a patient with lymphomatous uveitis who relapsed after ocular irradiation [65]. Treatment with intravenous ara-C (500 mg) and MTX (200 mg) had no effect; however, high-dose ara-C, 3 g/m^2, produced a complete response which was long-lasting. Furthermore, therapeutic ara-C levels were documented in both aqueous and vitreous humor 90 min after completion of the infusion. Strauchen et al. treated six patients with primary ocular lymphoma with high-dose ara-C and obtained a response in five [66]. While the role of chemotherapy in the treatment of ocular involvement by PCNSL remains to be clarified, these reports suggest that some agents or combination regimens may prove useful in the future.

Long-term treatment-related neurological toxicity has not previously been an issue in this disease because of short survival. However, delayed toxicity may become a problem if survival is improved with newer approaches to treatment [67]. In addition, chemotherapy, particularly with agents such as MTX and ara-C, can potentiate neurological toxicity from cranial irradiation which remains the cornerstone of treatment for this tumor. It can be anticipated that these agents will be widely used in the initial design of treatment protocols for PCNSL because of their specific advantages, namely intrathecal and high-dose intravenous administration. The enhanced toxicity seen when chemotherapy is combined with WBRT is usually related to the total dose of the drugs being administered, and it is hoped that a regimen can be designed to maximize the therapeutic effect but minimize the potential toxicities.

References

1. Burstein SD, Kernohan JW, Uihlein A (1963) Neoplasms of the reticuloendothelial system of the brain. Cancer 16:289–305
2. Rubinstein LJ (1972) Tumors of the central nervous system. Atlas of Tumor Pathology; Second Series, Fascicle 6. Washington, D.C.: Armed Forces Institute of Pathology, 215–234
3. Taylor CR, Russell R, Lukes RJ et al (1978) An immunohistological study of immunoglobulin content of primary central nervous system lymphomas. Cancer 41:2197–2205
4. Jellinger K, Radaskiewicz TH, Slowik F (1975) Primary malignant lymphomas of the central nervous system in man. Acta neuropath (Berlin), Suppl VI, 95–102
5. Zimmerman HM (1975) Malignant lymphomas of the nervous system. Acta Neuropath(Berlin) Suppl VI:69–74
6. Rosenblum ML, Levy RM, Bredesen DE et al (1988) Primary central nervous system lymphoma in patients with AIDS. Ann Neurol 23(Suppl):S13–S16
7. Welch K, Finkbeiner W, Alpers CE et al (1984) Autopsy findings in the acquired immune deficiency syndrome. JAMA 252:1152–1159
8. Eby NL, Grufferman S, Flannelly CM et al (1988) Increasing incidence of primary brain lymphoma in the US. Cancer 62:2461–2465
9. DeAngelis LM, Yahalom J, Rosenblum M, et al (1987) Primary CNS lymphoma: Managing patients with spontaneous and AIDS-related disease. Oncology 1:52–59
10. DeAngelis LM, Yahalom J, Heinemann M-H et al (1990) Primary CNS lymphoma: Combined treatment with chemotherapy and radiotherapy. Neurology 40:80–86
11. DeAngelis, LM (1991) Primary central nervous system lymphoma as a secondary malignancy. Cancer 67:1431–1435
12. Schaumburg HH, Plank CR, Adams RD (1972) The reticulum cell sarcoma-microglioma group of brain tumors. A consideration of their clinical features and therapy. Brain 95:199–212
13. Letendre L, Banks PM, Reese DF et al (1982) Primary lymphoma of the central nervous system. Cancer 49:939–943
14. Murray K, Kun L, Cox J (1986) Primary malignant lymphoma of the central nervous system. J Neurosurg 65:600–607
15. Hochberg FH, Miller DC (1988) Primary central nervous system lymphoma. J Neurosurg 68:835–853
16. Appen RE (1975) Posterior uveitis and primary cerebral reticulum cell sarcoma. Arch Ophthalmol 93:123–124
17. Char DH, Ljung B-M, Miller T et al (1988) Primary intraocular lymphoma (ocular reticulum cell sarcoma) diagnosis and management. Ophthalmology 95:625–630

18. Rockwood EJ, Zakov ZN, Bay JW (1984) Combined malignant lymphoma of the eye and CNS (reticulum-cell sarcoma). J Neurosurg 61:369–374
19. Lachance DH, O'Neill BP, Macdonald DR, et al (1991) Primary leptomeningeal lymphoma: report of 9 cases, diagnosis with immunocytochemical analysis, and review of the literature. Neurology 41:95–100
20. Scott TF, Hogan EL, Carter TD et al (1990) Primary intracranial meningeal lymphoma. Amer J Med 89:536–538
21. Bruni J, Bilbao JM, Gray T (1977) Primary intramedullary malignant lymphoma of the spinal cord. Neurology 27:896–898
22. Hautzer NW, Aiyesimoju A, Robitaille Y (1983) "Primary" spinal intramedullary lymphomas: a review. Ann Neurol 14:62–66
23. Mitsumoto H, Breuer AC, Lederman RJ (1980) Malignant lymphoma of the central nervous system: a case of primary spinal intramedually involvement. Cancer 46:1258–1262
24. Cellerier P, Chiras J, Gray F, et al (1984) Computed tomography in primary lymphoma of the brain. Neuroradiology 26:485–492
25. Schwaighofer BW, Hesselink JR, Press GA et al (1989) Primary intracranial CNS lymphoma: MR manifestations. AJNR 10:725–729
26. Thomas M, Macpherson P (1982) Computed tomography of intracranial lymphoma. Clinical Radiology 33:331–336
27. DeAngelis LM (1992) Primary central nervous system lymphoma (PCNSL) presenting as a non-enhancing lesion on MR scan. Neurology 42(Suppl 3):389
28. Henry JM, Heffner RR, Dillard SH et al (1974) Primary malignant lymphomas of the central nervous system. Cancer 34:1293–1302
29. Littman P, Wang CC (1987) Reticulum cell sarcoma of the brain. Cancer 35:1412–1420
30. Li C-Y, Witzig TE, Phyliky RL et al (1986) Diagnosis of B-cell non-Hodgkin's lymphoma of the central nervous system by immunocytochemical analysis of cerebrospinal fluid lymphocytes. Cancer 57:737–744
31. Hu E, Horning S, Flynn S et al (1986) Diagnosis of B cell lymphoma by analysis of immunoglobulin gene rearrangements in biopsy specimens obtained by fine needle aspiration. J Clin Oncol 4:278–283
32. Kumanishi T, Washiyama K, Nishiyama A et al (1989) Primary malignant lymphoma of the brain: demonstration of immunogloubulin gene rearrangements in four cases by the Southern blot hybridization technique. Acta Neuropathol 79:23–26
33. Nakhleh RE, Manivel JC, Hurd E et al (1989) Central nervous system lymphomas. Immunohistochemical and clinicopathologic study of 26 autopsy cases. Arch Pathol Lab Med 113:1050–1056
34. Ng CS, Chan JKC, Hui PK et al (1989) Large B-cell lymphomas with a high content of reactive T-cells. Hum Pathol 20:1145–1154
35. Vokes EE, Ultmann JE, Golomb HM et al (1985) Long-term survival of patients with localized diffuse histiocytic lymphoma. J Clin Oncol 3:1309–1317
36. Berry MP, Simpson WJ (1981) Radiation therapy in the management of primary malignant lymphoma of the brain. J Rad Oncol, Biol, Phys 7:55–59
37. Sagerman RH, Collier CH, King GA (1983) Radiation therapy of microgliomas. Radiology 149:567–570
38. Woodman R, Shin K, Pineo G (1985) Primary non-Hodgkin's lymphoma of the brain. A Review. Medicine 64:425–430
39. Freeman CR, Shustik C, Brisson M-L et al (1986) Primary malignant lymphoma of the central nervous system. Cancer 58:1106–1111
40. Singh A, Strobos RJ, Singh BM et al (1982) Steroid-induced remissions in CNS lymphoma. Neurology(Ny)32:1267–71
41. Kawakami Y, Tabuchi K, Ohnishi R et al (1985) Primary central nervous system lymphoma. J Neurosurg 62:522–527
42. Mendenhall NP, Thar TL, Agee OF et al (1983) Primary lymphoma of the central nervous system. Computerized tomography scan characteristics and treatment results for 12 cases. Cancer 52:1993–2000
43. Cox JD, Koehl RH, Turner WM et al (1974) Irradiation in the local control of malignant lymphoreticular tumors (non-Hodgkin's malignant lymphoma). Radiology 112:179–185
44. Leibel SA, Sheline GE (1987) Radiation therapy for neoplasms of the brain. J Neurosurg 66:1–22

45. Margolis L, Fraser R, Lichter A et al (1980) The role of radiation therapy in the management of ocular reticulum cell sarcoma. Cancer 45:688–692
46. Rampen RHJ, van Andel JG, Sizoo W et al (1980) Radiation therapy in primary non-Hodgkin's lymphomas of the CNS. Europ J Cancer 16:177–184
47. Stewart DJ, Russell N, Atack EA et al (1983) Cyclophosphamide, doxorubicin, vincristine, and dexamethasone in primary lymphoma of the brain: A case report. Cancer Treat Rep 67:287–291
48. Stewart DJ, Russell N, Dennery M et al (1984) Cyclophosphamide, adriamycin, vincristine and dexamethasone in the treatment of bulky central nervous system lymphomas. J Neuro-Onc 2:289
49. Ervin T, Canellos GP (1980) Successful treatment of recurrent primary central nervous system lymphoma with high-dose methotrexate. Cancer 45:1556–1557
50. Abelson HT, Kufe DW, Skarin AT et al (1981) Treatment of central nervous system tumors with methotrexate. Cancer Treat Rep 65(Suppl 1):137–140
51. Frick JC, Hansen RM, Anderson T et al (1986) Successful high-dose intravenous cytarabine treatment of parenchymal brain involvement from malignant lymphoma. Arch Intern Med 146:791–792
52. Loeffler JS, Ervin TJ, Mauch P et al (1985) Primary lymphomas of the central nervous system: patterns of failure and factors that influence survival. J Clin Oncol 3:490–494
53. Socie G, Piprot-Chauffat C, Schlienger M et al (1990) Primary lymphoma of the central nervous system. An unresolved therapeutic problem. Cancer 65:322–326
54. Lachance DH, Gockerman J, Halperin E, et al (1992) Cyclophosphamide, doxorubicin, vincristine, and prednisone (CHOP) for primary central nervous system lymphoma (PCNSL): Short-duration response, multi-focal intracerebral recurrence preceding radiotherapy. Neurology (Suppl 3) 42:343
55. Brada M, Dearnaley D, Horwich A et al (1990) Management of primary cerebral lymphoma with initial chemotherapy: Preliminary results and comparison with patients treated with radiotherapy alone. Int J Radiation Oncology Biol Phys 18:787–792
56. Ott RJ, Brada M, Flower MA et al (1991) Measurements of blood-brain barrier permeability in patients undergoing radiotherapy and chemotherapy for primary cerebral lymphoma. Eur J Cancer 27:1356–1362
57. Neuwelt EA, Goldman DL, Dahlborg SA et al (1991) Primary CNS lymphoma treated with osmotic blood-brain barrier disruption: Prolonged survival and preservation of cognitive function. J Clin Oncol 9:1580–1590
58. DeAngelis LM, Yahalom J, Thaler HT et al (1992) Combined modality treatment for primary CNS lymphoma. J Clin Oncol 10:635–643
59. Herbst KD, Corder MP, Justice GR (1976) Successful therapy with methotrexate of a multicentric mixed lymphoma of the central nervous system. Cancer 38:1476–1478
60. Shapiro WR, Young DF, Mehta BM (1975) Methotrexate: distribution in cerebrospinal fluid after intravenous, ventricular and lumbar injections. N Engl J Med 293:161–166
61. Pitman SW, Frei E (1977) Weekly methotrexate-calcium leukovorin rescue: effect of alkalinization on nephrotoxicity; pharmacokinetics in the CNS; and use in CNS non Hodgkin's lymphoma. Cancer Treat Rep 61:695–701
62. Slevin ML, Piall EM, Aherne GW et al (1983) Effect of dose and schedule on pharmacokinetics of high-dose cytosine arabinoside in plasma and cerebrospinal fluid. J Clin Oncol 1:546–551
63. Barr CC, Green WR, Payne JW et al (1975) Intraocular reticulum-cell sarcoma: clinico-pathologic study of four cases and review of the literature. Survey of Ophthal 19:224–239
64. Sullivan SF, Dallow RL (1977) Intraocular reticulum cell sarcoma: its dramatic response to systemic chemotherapy and its angiogenic potential. Ann Ophthalmol 9:401–406
65. Baumann MA, Ritch PS, Hande KR et al (1986) Treatment of intraocular lymphoma with high-dose Ara-C. Cancer 57:1273–1275
66. Strauchen JA, Dalton J, Friedman AH (1989) Chemotherapy in the management of intraocular lymphoma. Cancer 63:1918–1921
67. Merchut MP, Haberland C, Naheedy MH et al (1985) Long survival of primary cerebral lymphoma with progressive radiation necrosis. Neurology 35:552–556

Epidermal Growth Factor Receptor Expression in Human Malignant Glioma: In Vitro and In Vivo Effects of Application of Monoclonal Antibodies to the Epidermal Growth Factor Receptor

M. Westphal[1], W. Hamel[1], D. Zirkel[1], H. D. Herrmann[1], T. Bilzer[2], G. Reifenberger[2], R. Schober[2], W. Wechsler[2], F. K. Albert[3], J. Behnke[3], G. Fries[3], D. Keller[3], M. Messing[3], and P. Stasiecki[4]

[1]Department of Neurological Surgery, University Hospital Eppendorf, Martinistr. 52, 20251 Hamburg, Germany
[2]Medizinische Einrichtungen, Moorenstr. 5, 40225 Düsseldorf, Germany
[3]For the German Multicenter Trial, EMD 55900–600
[4]E. Merck, Frankfurter Straße 250, 64293 Darmstadt, Germany

Introduction

Antibodies against the receptor for epidemal growth factor (EGF-R) have long been expected to turn out to be anticancer agents (Mendelsohn et al. 1988). The overexpression of EGF-R is the most constant pathological cell biological feature of human malignant gliomas of the astrocytic lineage (Bigner et al. 1988; Libermann et al. 1985). Such overexpression may be due to gene amplification of the EGF-R gene on chromosome 7 (Bigner and Vogelstein 1990) but may also be present in the absence of gene amplification due to other mechanisms (Chaffanet et al. 1992). An antibody against the extracellular domain of the EGF-R has been generated several years ago, called MAb 425 (Rodeck et al. 1987) and has been developed into a therapeutic compound (EMD 55900). The effects of this antibody as well as others on cell proliferation have been studied in cell culture and in xenotransplants, with contradicting results (Aboud-Pirak et al. 1988; Bigner et al.1988; Rodeck et al. 1987; Werner et al. 1988). It was thought that the antibody might be effective by inhibiting the autocrine self-stiumulation of tumor cells which is afforded by the concomitant secretion of transforming growth factor-α (TGF-α), a homologue to EGF and overexpression of EGF-R (Di Marco et al. 1989). It has yet to be confirmed that this mechanism contributes substantially to the sustained cell proliferation seen in brain tumors. For this interaction to be at all relevant, it has been shown that certain quantitative requirements need to be met (Di Marco et al. 1989). There is only scant clinical evidence that the expression of EGF-R in gliomas due to gene amplification is associated with worse prognosis (Hurtt et al. 1992), and in cell lines it has been shown that despite the presence of the constituents of the autocrine loop for EGF/TGF-α there is little dependence of the cells on this loop for autostimulation of proliferation (Westphal et al., 1993).

Therefore, in addition to interfering with cell proliferation, two other aspects need to be considered when expecting clinical efficacy of the antibody, namely interference with cell migration and activation of immune responses. Cell migration may be regulated through the EGF-R (Erickson and Turley 1987; Lund-Johanssen et al. 1990; Westermark et al. 1982) and is of great biological significance for the treatment of glioma as these tumors as a rule show an extremely infiltrative behavior. Any therapy aimed at acting locally from within the tumor cavity would benefit greatly from a pretreatment which reduces or blocks invasion of glioma cells far into the surrounding brain. An induction of an immune response would require binding of the monoclonal antibody and subsequent lysis of antibody-loaded cells in an antibody-dependent cytotoxic cytolysis with microglia most likely being the effector cells (Sutter et al. 1991).

Antibodies against the EGF-R have so far been used therapeutically as an iodinated compound in patients with malignant glioma (Epenetos et al. 1985) as well as coupled to gelonin (Hirota et al. 1989) .The antibody MAb425/EMD 55900 has also been used as a radiotherapeutic agent (Brady et al. 1990). The native antibody has been shown to be antagonistic in vitro by causing receptor down-regulation and internalization without concomitant activation of the tyrosine kinase domain (Murthy et al. 1987). The state of preclinical studies undertaken to date and the unclarified therapeutic potential of monoclonal antibodies against the EGF-R justifies the beginning of clinical trials.

Materials and Methods

Cell Culture

Fresh tumor specimens were obtained during surgery and placed immediately in Hank's balanced salt solution without calcium and magnesium. The tissue was dissected to select vital fragments no larger than pea size. The material was then minced with scissors and mechanically dispersed by rapid trituration through a disposable plastic pipet. The resulting suspension of single cells and small aggregates was added to tissue culture flasks and multiwell plates coated with an extracellular matrix derived from bovine corneal endothelial cells. The cells were maintained in Earle's modification of Eagle's minimal essential medium (MEM) with the addition of 10% fetal calf serum, glutamin 2 mM, pyruvate 1 mM, amphotericin B 2.5 µg/ml and gentamycin 40 µg/ml (Merck, Darmstadt, Germany). The cultures were maintained in 8% CO_2 in a humidified atmosphere at 37 °C. All cell lines were initiated by the described method and were permanent at the time of the experiments. The cells were detached for passaging or counting with a 0.05% trypsine, 0.04% versene solution in phosphate buffered saline. All media and supplements except when noted otherwise, were obtained from Seromed (Biochrom, Berlin, Germany). Tissue culture materials were obtained from Costar (Cambridge, MA).

Proliferation Experiments

Epidermal growth factor isolated from mouse submaxillary glands was added every second day to serum-free cultures of glioma cells in doses ranging between (100 nM) and (60 pM) in quadruplicates for each dose. The cells were counted after 4 days after tryptic detachment in a Coulter Counter. Either monoclonal antibody EMD 55900 (150 nM) was added as a single dose, and the cells were left for 4 days, or the addition was repeated after 2 days. Suramin (Germanine, Bayer 205, Bayer, Leverkusen, Germany) was added at 200 µg/ml concentration as a single addition as in previous studies (Westphal et al. 1991).

Migration Assays

Cells from stock cultures of the cell lines were detached with trypsin and layered on top of soft agar and left to form spontaneous spheroids. These spheroids were picked, seeded onto 24-well culture dishes and left to attach for 2 h. Thereafter either serum-free medium or medium containing 10% fetal calf serum was added. EGF, EMD 55900, or suramin was added immediately in the same concentrations as in the proliferation experiments and the migration of cells away from the spheroids assessed every day.

Southern Blot Analysis

High molecular weight DNA was prepared from the cell lines and tested for degradation before digestion with the selected restriction enzymes. DNA (10 µg) was digested and then separated on a 0.6% agarose gel. The DNA was transferred onto Hybond N+ (Amersham, Arlington Heights, IL) or GeneScreenPlus (NEN, Wilmington, DE) nylon filters with 0.4 M NaOH/1.0 M NaCl (alkaline blotting). Filters were prehybridized and hybridized at 42°C in formamide, 5 x SSC, 5 x Denhardt's solution, 50 mM $NaPO_4$ (pH 6.5) 30 mM Tris HCl (pH 8.5), 0.1% sodium dodecyl sulfate, and 100 µg salmon sperm DNA. Additionally, 5% dextran sulfate was added. Washes carried out done under high stringency conditions (0.2 SSC at 65 °C).

Two different cDNA probes were used for the EGF-R, one encoding the whole receptor and one encoding a 0.8-kb *Eco*RI cDNA fragment. The probes were radiolabeled with [α^{32}P]-dCTP and [α^{32}P]-dATP (50 Ci each) by random priming using a labeling kit (Amersham, Arlington Heights, Il). Unincorporated label was removed by filtration through a Sephadex G-50 column (Pharmacia, Gaitersburg, MD). At least 10^6 cpm/ml of purified probe were added to the hybridization solution.

Phosphotyrosine Western Blotting

Onto each well of a 24-well cluster dish 150 000 cells were seeded (Costar, Cambridge, Mass. USA) and left overnight. The attached confluent cells were then starved for 4 h in Dulbecco's modified Eagle's medium with only 0.1% fetal bovine serum. The medium was then replaced with fresh medium with or without 5ng/ml recombinant EGF. After an incubation period of 15 min at 37 °C, the cells were lysed in 100 µl of an ice cold lysis buffer which contained protease inhibitors as well as phosphatase inhibitors. The lysate was cleared from debris by centrifugation after which 30 µl of supernatant was separated on a 4%–12% sodium dodecyl sulfate polyacrylamide gel electrophoresis. The gels were blotted onto PVDF membranes (Millipore, Bedford, MA) by semidry blotting. The membranes were blocked with 4% of bovine serum albumin/TBST for 1 h and subsequently incubated with an antiphosphotyrosine monoclonal antibody (UBI, Lake Placid, NY) for 2 h. After incubation with the secondary antibody (goat anti-mouse conjugated to alkaline-phosphatase; Promega, Madison, WI) the blot was developed with NBT/BCIP.

Analysis of the EGF-R

The content of EGF-R in the experimental cell lines was assayed by enzyme-linked immunosorbent assay (ELISA) using a monoclonal antibody as well as by FACS analysis.

Patient Selection and Trial Design

Only patients were admitted into the clinical trial who had undergone previous removal of a primary malignant glioma, had received a full course of irradiation and were reoperated on for recurrent tumor. Only patients who had a Karnofsky performance score of 60 or higher and appeared as if they would benefit from another surgical debulking procedure were eligible. All patients gave informed consent according to guidelines supervised by the regional ethics committees, from which permission was obtained by each of the centers participating in the trial. The recurrent tumors had to be, again, high-grade glioma and also had to show a positive EGF-R status after immunocytochemical staining with EMD 55900 with routine methods.

Of 45 patients who were evaluated immunohistochemicaly, 25 were suited to go onto the treatment protocol but only 10 were treated. The other patients either failed because of their low EGF-R expression or were ineligible because of the clinical course of the disease.

Each patient was to receive three weekly doses of 40 mg EMD 55900 during an infusion period of 1 h over a total period of 4 weeks. During that time all major laboratory parameters and the clinical performance were closely monitored.

Results

In Vitro Studies Concerning EGF-R Expression in Glioma Cell Lines

All glioma cell lines used as experimental systems had EGF-R as determined by FACS, ELISA, and northern blot gene expression analysis. In comparison with standard control cell lines WI-38 (normal expression), SK-Br-3 (elevated expression, approximately 90 000 receptors/cell), and MDA-MB-468 (high level of overexpression 10^6 receptors/cell), three of the cell lines had more than 90 000 receptors per cell (NCE-G44, NCE-G55 and NCE-G62). The EGF-R gene was analyzed by Southern blot after restriction enzyme digest of chromsomal DNA. No gross rearrangement was seen with a set of different enzymes (Fig. 1).

The cell lines were incubated in the presence and absence of EGF (5 g/ml) and lysed at the end of the incubation. After western blotting of cell lysates and incubation with an antiphosphotyrosine monoclonal antibody it was seen that the 170-kDa band had an increased intensity in the EGF treated cells of all lines (Fig. 2) thus indicating that EGF-R phosphorylation occurs in response to the addition of external EGF. In all cell lines, however, there is already some baseline activity, indicating that there is some EGF-R phosphorylation without external stimulation, probably due to the secretion of TGF-a which is also made by all the cell lines (Hamel et al., in press). Yet it cannot be excluded that this tyrosine phosphorylation represents also activation of other protein tyrosine kinases (receptors) of similar molecular weight.

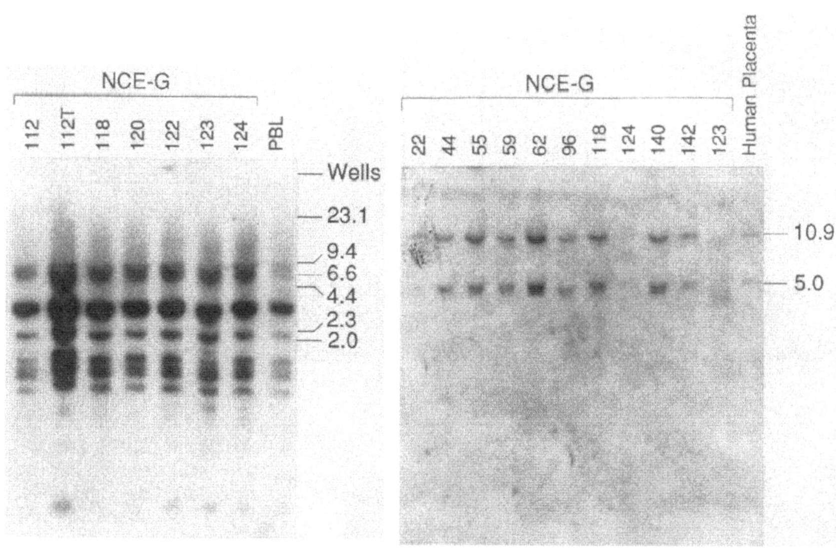

a b

Fig. 1. a Southern blot analysis of high molecular weight DNA isolated from the cell lines and double-digested with *Eco*RI and *Bam*HI. After separation on a 0.8% agarose gel, the blots were probed with a labeled c-DNA probe for the entire EGF-R. **b** Southern blot of DNA digested with *Hin*dIII and probed with a 0.8-kb *Eco*RI fragment of the EGF-R cDNA

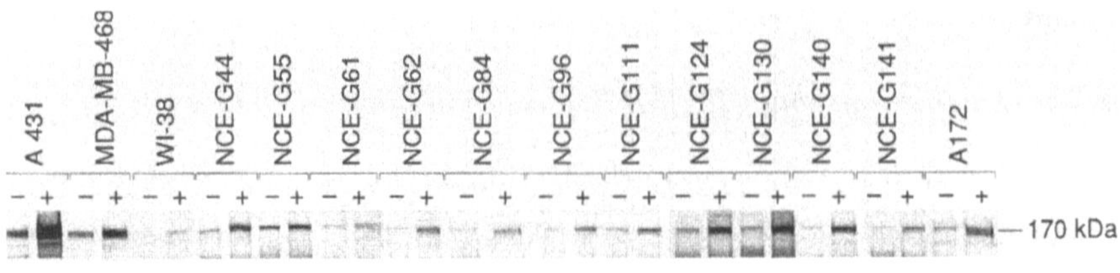

Fig. 2. Glioma cells were incubated with 5 µg/ml EGF for 15 min at 37 °C and then lysed. The cell extracts were separated on a 4%–12% polyacrylamide gel, transferred to PVDF membranes and probed with an antiphosphotyrosine antibody. The phospotyrosine contents of the 170-kDa protein after incubation with (+) and without (–) EGF is shown. Four cell lines served as controls to the panel of NCE cell lines: a 431 and MDA-MB 468 are examples for EGF-R overexpressing cell lines, and WI-38 served as a cell line with a low level of EGF-R expression

The effect of uncoupled EMD 55900 on cell proliferation was assessed by adding the antibody to serum-free or serum-containing primary cultures or cells from established cell lines (Fig. 3). In six cases in which 150 nM antibody was added either to primary cultures or second passage two cultures, an effect was seen in one case in which a 18% reduction in final cell number was seen after 4 days of incubation. Two more cases showed marginal effects with 5% and 8% decrease, however, statistically significant in quadryplicate determinations. Three cases had no effect of MAb, but suramin produced inhibition up to 50% compared to controls in all cases.

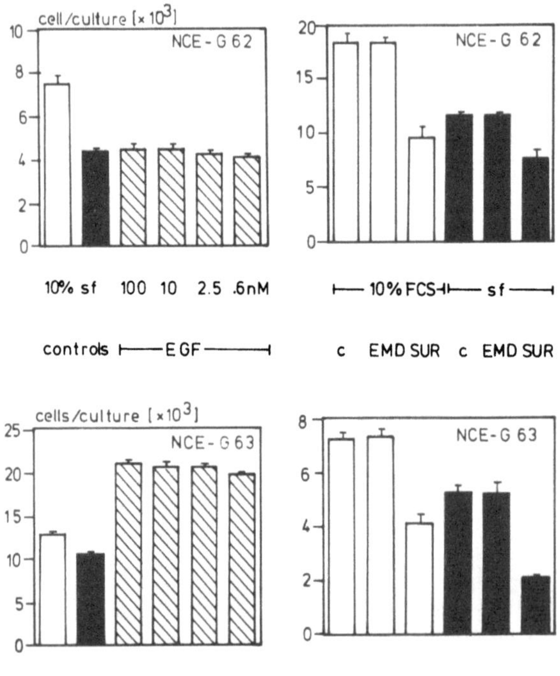

Fig. 3. Effect of EMD 55900 on cell proliferation of glioma cell lines in vitro in serum-free conditions. *Above*, NCE-G62 is derived from a glioblastoma in a child and shows the highest amount of EGF R expression determined by FACS analysis. *Below*, NCE-G63 is derived from a glioblastoma in a 52-year-old male patient. The cells were incubated with EGF as indicated for 4 days and counted on day 5 of culture. The mMAb was added in a concentration of 150 nM and left for 4 days. The same result was obtained when the addition of antibody was repeated on day 3

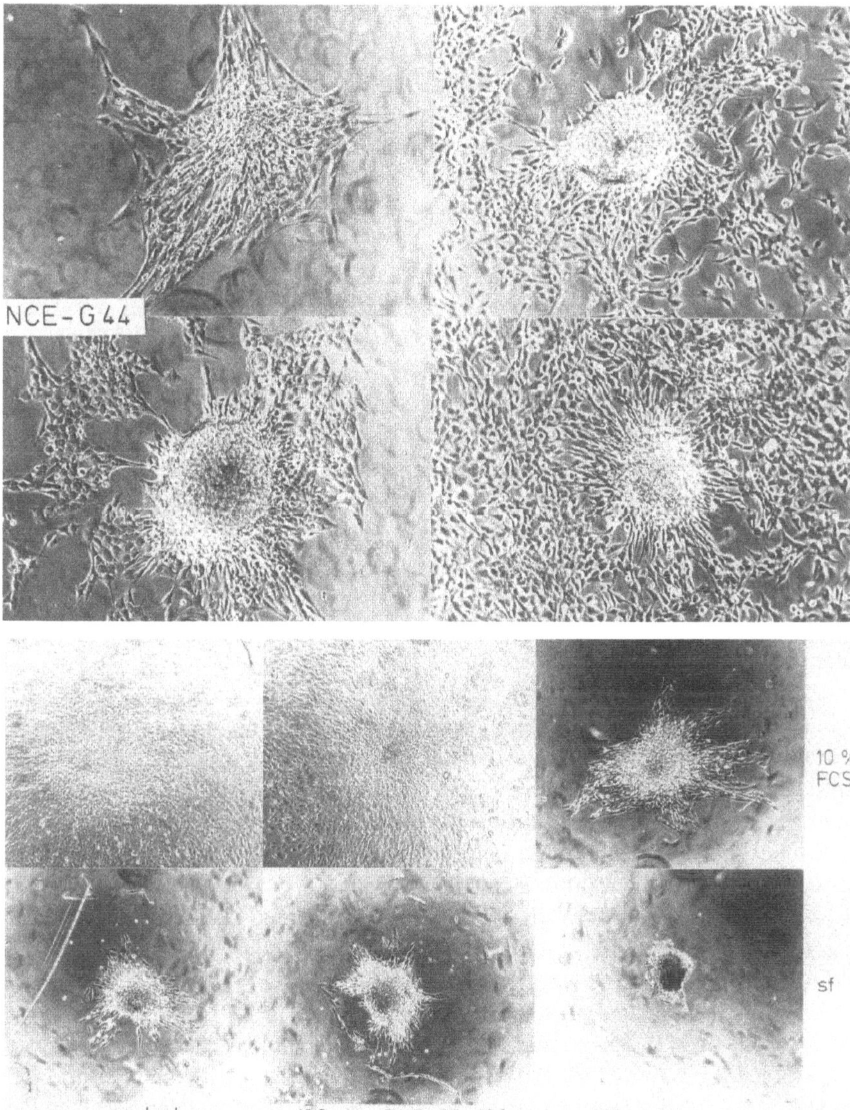

a

b

Fig. 4. a The effect of the addition of EGF to spheroids of the cell line NCE-G44 is seen in serum-free conditions to which EGF (10 nM; *top right*) fibroblast growth factor, (80 pg/ml; *bottom left*) and platelet-derived growth factor AB (5 nM; *bottom right*) were added. It can be seen that over a 4-day period, all three growth factors stimulate cell migration around the spheroid which has also grown in comparison to the serum-free control which has just flattened and shows neither migration nor dividing cells. **b** Effect of EMD 55900 on cell-migration in the spheroid culture system. Spheroids from the cell line NCE-G44 were produced as described in the text. The spheroids were maintained in medium containing 10% fetal calf serum as well as in serum-free medium. EMD 55900 was added at 150 nM and left for 3 days after which the cultures were photographed

As for the cell lines, the antibody was tested together with suramin both in serum-free and serum-containing medium. Neither a single dose or repeated addition was effective in the cultures from the cell lines. This lack of efficacy was unrelated to the number of EGF-R or the cellular responsiveness to externally added EGF, as shown in two examples. One example (the cell line NCE-G62) with a high number of EGF-R determined by FACS showed no response to EGF and was not affected by the antibody in contrast to suramin, which showed a pronounced effect at 200 µg/ml. In another example a cell with "normal" expression of EGF-R compared to the WI-38 cell line (NCE-G63) was treated the same way and showed a good response to EGF in doses as low as 1 nM. Nevertheless, the antibody by itself was again ineffective in contrast to suramin.

The same results were obtained by trying to test the efficacy against migration (Fig.4). The spheroid cell cultures were assayed again in serum containing medium and in serum-free conditions in comparison with suramin. As exemplified for one cell line, the antibody was ineffective compared to control cultures in preventing cells from migrating out. Suramin in contrast also showed an effect towards inhibiting cell migration which may be less due to interference with specific migratory mechanisms but with general reduction of vitality of the cells.

Administration of EMD 55900 In Vivo

With the idea that binding of antibody to high numbers of cell surface receptors will induce antibody-dependent cytotoxic cytolysis, the antibody was taken into human trials. The aim of this phase I study was to determine tolerability, plasma kinetics, and development of antibodies against the MAb.

With regard to plasma levels and pharmacodynamics, it was seen that a 1-h infusion of 40 mg EMD 55900 resulted in plasma levels between 6.6 and 16.6 ng/ml. These levels were also reached also after 4 weeks of administration, already indicating that human anti-mouse antibody (HAMA) levels should be very low. The plasma half-life after a 40 mg dose was found to be 16–24 h.

No severe drug-related adverse events were observed in any of the patients. There were complaints of mild, generalized itch in two patients. There was no allergic or anaphylactic reaction. During the observation interval the patients did not develop HAMA. It was advisable to extend the treatment in at least two patients in whom the antibody was believed to be efficacious based on CT evaluation.

In several patients liver enzymes (glutamic oxalo-acetic transaminase, glutamic pyruvic transaminase) were elevated (toxicity grade I). Depletion of complement was not seen. A mild increase in urinary protein, detectable as trace only, was only transient and disappeared 6 weeks after the last dose.

Although this study was conducted as a phase I trial, several clinical observations may be mentioned. One of the patients showed a very aggressive tumor with only weeks between the recurrency of the lesions which were spatially separated but most likely connected through white matter edema pathways. This patient received the antibody after the second operation being without radiological evidence of tumor at

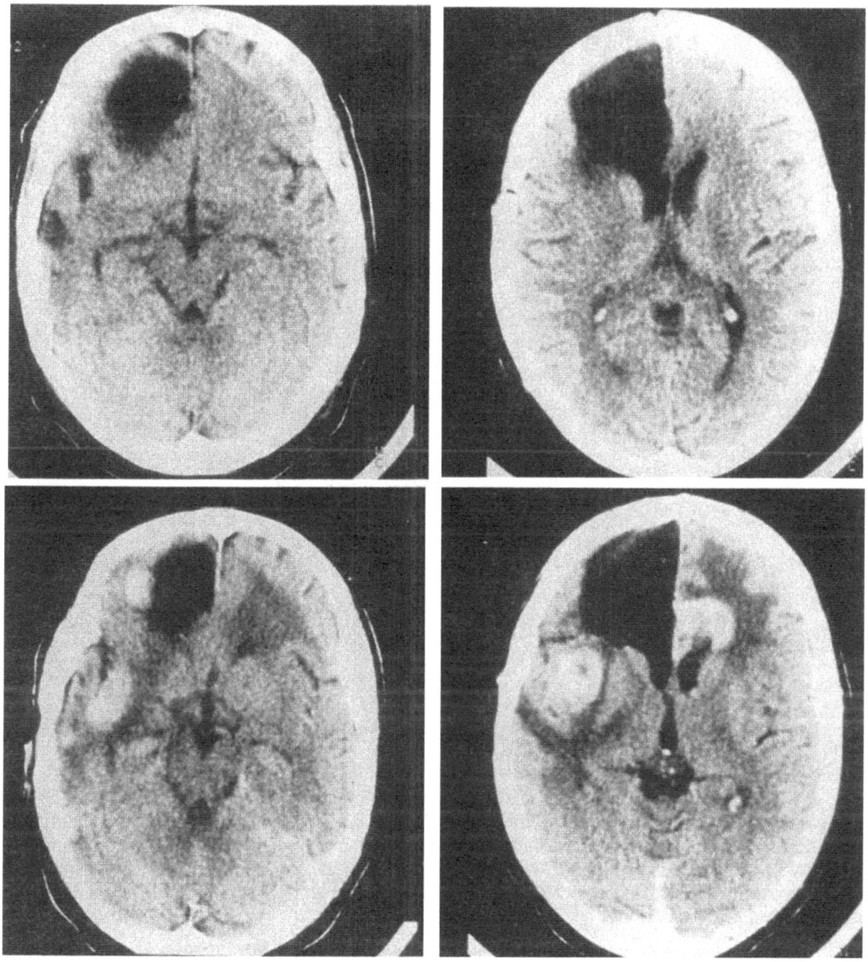

Fig. 5. CT scans of one patient at the end of EMD 55900 administration having completed the full course of the treatment (*left*) and a control CT scan 6 weeks later while the patient was still in excellent clinical condition and showed nothing but a mild memory deficit

that time. No further tumor growth was detectable at the end of the treatment. Nevertheless there were three recurrent lesions within 6 weeks after termination of the treatment (Fig. 5).

Another patient showed a hemorrhage into the cavity of the removed tumor while being treated and 3 weeks after the treatment had a MRI showing gadolinium uptake in patchy areas around the cavity (Fig. 6). This patient was reexplored and the tissue was found macroscopically to be very different from the previous operations and was thought to be mainly granulation and inflammatory reaction. Histologically, however, when the two specimens were compared, there was no difference in the appearance of the tumor except for an increase of scar tissue formation, but this was

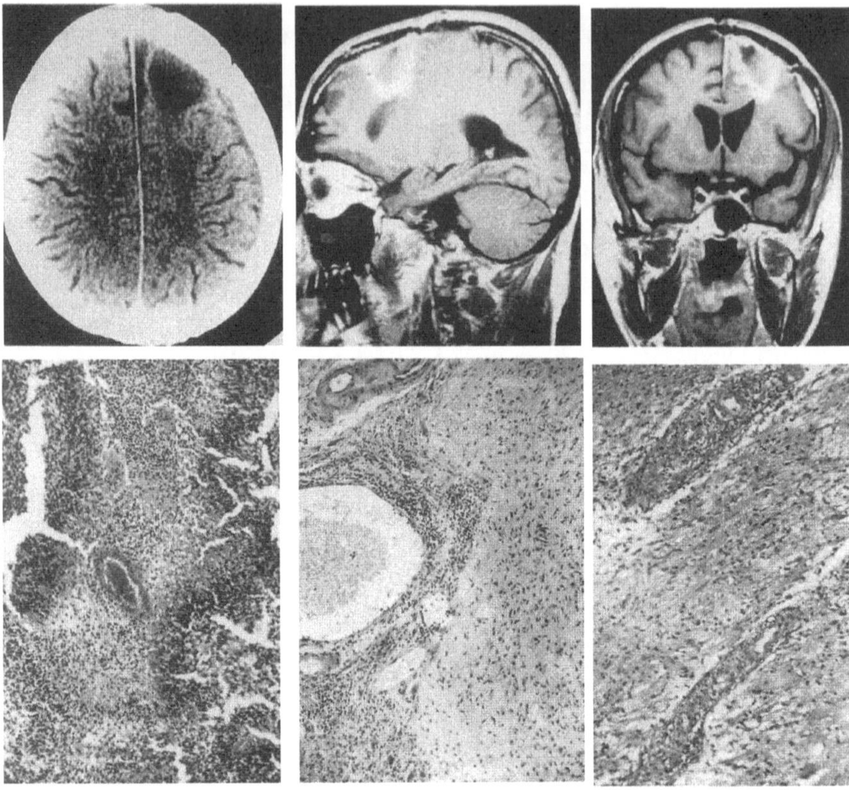

Fig. 6. MRI scans of another patient who showed gadolinium uptake around the cavity which was completely inconspicuous at the end of treatment (CT scan, *far left*). *Below*, a histological section from the recurrent glioblastoma before (*far left*, 25) is compared to two sections from the lesion removed 4 weeks after the treatment with EMD-55900 (*right*, 120). It can be seen that there is still small-cell glioblastoma after the treatment, but in addition there is a large amount of connective tissue indicating a pronounced scar formation

within the spectrum of tissue reactions seen in recurrencies and after irradiation (Fig. 6). What was even more important was the finding of persistent strong immunoreactivity with EMD 55900 in the specimen removed after the patient had received a full course of treatment. It was also in the cultures from the first recurrence of this patient that an effect of EMD 55900 was seen in vitro.

Discussion

EGF is a glial mitogen as shown in cultured purified astrocytes (Simpson et al. 1982). When cells reacquire a proliferative status as in neoplastic transformation this system appears to be reactivated with the difference that TGF-α is the ligand binding to the EGF-R which is frequently overexpressed in neoplastic cells of the astrocytic lineage (Ekstrand et al. 1991).

In this study, in contrast to other investigations, it was shown that in a panel of glioma cell lines and in primary cultures, the antibody EMD 55900 does not interfere with cell proliferation despite the presence of high numbers and functioning receptors as indicated by the increase of the phosphorylation signal in response to EGF. Suramin in contrast reduces cell proliferation in a therapeutic concentration of 200 μg/ml. Suramin in the meantime has found broad clinical application (Eisenberger and Fontana 1992) in various diseases. It has also been tested in vitro whether its effect was related to the expression of EGF-R, but it was shown to be effective regardless of the presence or absence of receptor (Olivier et al. 1990). When EGF-R was present, however, the effect of suramin appeared to be greater with increasing receptor numbers. The inefficacy of the antibody in this study in comparison with suramin is most likely unrelated to the EGF-R. Suramin has been shown to interfere with many different growth factor systems, and gliomas are known to have a multiplicity of growth factor pathways activated (Westphal et al., 1993). Since the cell lines produce also platelet-derived growth factors (Hamel et al., 1992) and many other glioma cell lines were shown to produce fibroblast growth factors and insulin-like growth factors the interference with just one system is unlikely to sufficiently inhibit cell proliferation. Another consideration concerning the ineffectiveness of antibody to inhibit cell proliferation is the activation of mature receptor molecules already inside the cell as shown for platelet-drived growth factors (Keating and Williams 1988). Although in all likelihood mature molecules are expressed only on the cell surface, this notion cannot be utterly discarded. In any case, the results are very similar to those of another study with a different antibody, antibody 528 (Werner et al. 1988), which also showed only little if any intrinsic antiproliferative activity in the dose range in which EMD 55900 was used in our in vitro experiments.

It was disappointing that no interference was observed with migration as EGF has been shown to be an important factor in glial cell locomotion (Westermark et al. 1982) and glioma invasion (Lund-Johanssen et al. 1990). Such invasion of surrounding brain is a crucial feature of gliomas and determines the surgical incurability of most lesions. It was not investigated whether EGF-induced migration was blocked but the unhindered migration in the presence of serum suggests that migration is mediated by several factors and thus any EGF-R blockade might be easily overcome.

It is likely that the antibody itself is unable to block cell proliferation. Even in early cultures the effect was only minimal and with the appropriate selection pressure it is likely that the cells will adapt in vivo to behave as the cells lines which were unaffected by EMD 55900. Thus it must be anticipated that an in vivo application of the unmodified antibody will show an effect via an antibody-mediated tumor cytotoxicity of microglia which already has been shown to be inducible in vitro (Sutter et al. 1991).

From the in vivo study it is so far only possible to conclude that the antibody is well tolerated and may have an effect when tumor is present. It must be assumed that any adjuvant treatment after total removal of the tumor as administered in most of the patients in this study will fail to produce any interaction between the tumor cells and the antibody because the blood-brain barrier has already closed. Under these conditions molecules of the size of EMD 55900 (MAb 425) will permeate only to an amount of 0.01% of their plasma concentration, as has been found with the MAb 81C6 directed against tenacsin, a glioma-associated extracellular matrix protein (Zalutski et al. 1990). Another setback to therapy with an uncoupled antibody against the EGF-R may be the heterogeneity of staining within one tumor which occurs in a large percentage of tumors (Stromer et al. 1990).

Whatever an effective mechanism of interfering with the tumor will be found to be, it is recommended to administer the antibody while tumor is still present and is shown to have substantial amount of EGF-R either by direct demonstration in a biopsy or by inference from the immunocytochemical analysis of the original tumor. Loss of EGF-R expression is a very rare event, and thus such inference appears justified. In the presence of edema molecules of the size of albumin as well as immunoglobulins are readily found in the edema fluid (Hossmann et al. 1990). Effectiveness in those studies in which radiolabeled antibody was given without determination of the level EGF-R expression (Brady et al. 1990) may just be due to the radiation delivered to the tumor by MAb molecules labeled with 125-I having leaked through the open blood-brain barrier.

There is a precedent for inhibitory and neutral effects of a monoclonal antibody to a cell surface receptor related to the EGF-R. The product of *HER2*/c-*erbB2* proto-oncogene is a cell surface receptor tyrosine kinase (Coussens et al. 1985). An antibody against the extracellular domain produced a cytostatic effect in vitro in a cell line dependent on the *HER2* expression (SK- Br-3) while another cell line with similar levels of expression (NIH 3T3) showed no change in proliferation rate (Hudziak et al. 1989).

In conclusion, it appears unlikely that MAbs against the EGF-R suffice to inhibit autocrine stimulation of cell proliferation in gliomas in vivo as already with optimal exposure in vitro, there is no effect. In vivo administration will have to tackle the problem of antibody permeability across the blood-brain barrier. From the first experiences it seems that the antibody should be used in situations when solid tumor is present and blood-brain barrier permeability is increased in the perifocal edema. Because an antibody-mediated immune-reaction is expected to be the effective principle, care must be taken to avoid steroid mediated immunosuppression (McVicar et al.1992) and maybe even provide additional immune stimulation.

Acknowledgements. This work was supported by the Deutsche Krebshilfe – Mildred Scheel Stiftung, Bonn (W 41/90/he-2), and the Heinrich Bauer Stiftung. We thank Hildegard Nausch for technical assistance. Dr. S. Reinhold (Department of Neuropathology, University Hospital Hamburg provided the histological evaluation of the patient operated for recurrence after the anti-Mab and deserves special thanks. The contribution of Sker Freist by preparing the photographical illustrations is highly appreciated. The operating-room staff are acknowledged for their cooperation. This report contains materials which represent parts of the doctorial thesis of W. Hamel which will be presented to the Fachbereich Medizin at the University of Hamburg.

References

Aboud-Pirak E, Hurwitz E, Pirak ME, Bellot F, Schlessinger J, Sela M (1988) Efficacy of antibodies to epidermal growth factor receptor against KB carcinoma in vitro and in nude mice. J Natl Cancer Inst 80: 1605–1611

Bigner SH, Burger PC, Wong AJ, Werner MH, Hamilton SR, Muhlbaier LH, Vogelstein B, Bigner DD (1988) Gene Amplification in malignant human gliomas: clinical and histopathological aspects. J Neuropath Exp Neurol 47:191–205

Bigner SH, Vogelstein B (1990) Cytogenetics and molecular genetics of malignant gliomas and medulloblastoma. Brain Pathol 1: 12–18.

Brady LW, Markoe AM, Woo DV, Rackover MA, Koprowski H, Steplewski Z, Peyster RG (1990) Iodine-125 labeled anti-epidermal growth factor receptor-425 in the treatment of malignant astrocytomas. J Neurol Sci 34:243–249

Chaffanet M, Chauvin C, Laine M, Berger F, Chedin M, Rost N, Nissou MF, Benabid AL (1992) EGF-receptor amplification and expression in human brain tumors. Eur J Cancer 28:11–17

Coussens L, Yang-Feng TL, Liao YC, Chen E, Gray A, McGrath J, Seeburg PH, Libermann TW, Schlessinger J, Francke U, Levinson A, Ullrich A (1985) Tyrosine kinase receptor with extensive homology to EGF receptor shares chromosomal location with neu oncogene. Science 230: 1132–1139

Di Marco E, Pierce JH, Fleming TP, Kraus MH, Molloy CJ, Aaronson SA, Di Fiore PP (1989) autocrine interaction between TGFa and the EGF-receptor: quantitative requirements for induction of the malignant phenotype. Oncogene 4:831–838

Eisenberger MA, Fontana JA (1992) Suramin, an active nonhormonal cytotoxic drug fir treatment of prostate cancer: compelling reasons for testing in patients with hormone-refractory breast cancer. J Natl Cancer inst 84:3–5

Ekstrand AJ, James CD, Canenee WK, Seliger B, Pettersson RF, Collins VP (1991) Genes for epidermal growth factor, transforming growth factor alpha and epidermal growth factor and their expression in human gliomas in vivo. Cancer Res 51:2164–2172

Epenetos AA, Courtenay-Luck N, Pickering D, Hooker G, Durbin H, Lavender JP, McKenzie CG (1985) Antibody guided irradiation of brain glioma by arterial infusion of radioactive monoclonal antibody against epidermal growth factor receptor and blood group A antigen. Br Med J 290: 1463–1466

Erickson CA, Turley EA (1987) The effects of epidermal growth factor on neural crest cells in tissue culture. Exp Cell Res 169:267–279

Hamel W, Westphal M, Shepard HM (1992) Proto-oncogene expression inhuman glioma derived cell lines. Int J Oncol, 1:673–682

Hirota N, Ueda M, Ozawa S, Abe O, Shimizu N (1989) Suppression of an epidermal growth factor receptor hyperproducing tumor by an immunotoxin conjugate of gelonin and a monoclonal antiepidermal growth factor receptor antibody. Cancer Res 49:7106–7109

Hossmann KA, Seo K, Szymas J, Wechsler W (1990) Quantitative analysis of experimental peritumoral edema in cats. Adv Neurol 52:449–458

Hudziak RM, Lewis GD, Winget M, Fendly BM, Shepard HM, Ullrich A (1989) p185her monoclonal antibody has antiproliferative effects in vitro and sensitizes human breast tumor cells to tumor necrosis factor. Mol Cell Biol 9:1165–1172

Hurtt MR, Moossy J, Donovan PM, Locker J (1992) Amplification of epidermal growth factor receptor gene in gliomas: histopathology and prognosis. J Neuropath Exp Neurol 51: 84–90

Keating MT, Williams LT (1988) Autocrine stimulation of intracellular PDGF receptors in v-sis.transformed cells. Science 239:914–916

Libermann TA, Nusbaum HR, Razon N, Kris R, Lax I, Soreq H, Whittle N, Waterfiled MD, Ullrich A, Schlessinger J (1985) Amplification, enhanced expression and possible rearrangement of EGF receptor gene in primary human brain tumors of glial origin. Nature 313:144–147

Lund-Johansen M, Bjerkvig R, Humphrey PA, Bigner SH, Bigner DD, Laerum O-D (1990) Effect of epidermal growth factor on glioma cell growth, migration and invasion in vitro. Cancer Research 50:6039–6044

McVicar DW, Davis DF, Merchant RE (1992) In vitro analysis of the proliferative potential od T cells from patients with brain tumor: glioma-associated immunosuppression unrelated to intrinsic cellular defect. J Neurosurg 76:251–260

Mendelsohn J, Masui H, Sunada H, MacLeod C (1988) Monoclonal antibodies against the receptor for epidermal growth factor as potential anticancer agents. UCLA Symp Mol Biol 56:307–312
Murthy U, Basu A, Rodeck U, Herlyn M, Ross AH, Das M (1987) Binding of an antagonistic monoclonal antibody to intact and fragmented EGF-receptor polypeptide. Arch Biochem Biophys 252:549–560
Olivier S, Formento P, Fischel JL, Etienne MC, Milano G (1990) Epidermal growth factor receptor expression and suramin cytotoxicity in vitro. Eur J Cancer 26:876–871
Rodeck U, Herlyn M, Herly D, Molthoff C, Atkinson B, Varello M, Steplewski Z, Koprowski H (1987) Tumor growth modulation by a monoclonal antibody to the epidermal growth factor receptor: Immunologically mediated and effector cell-independent effects. Cancer Res 47: 3692–3696
Schlegel U, Moots PL, Rosenblum MK, Thaler HT, Furneaux HM (1990) Expression of transforming growth factor alpha in human gliomas. Oncogene 5:1839–1849
Simpson Dl, Morrison R, de Vellis J, Herschman HR (1982) Epidermal growth factor binding and mitogenic activity on purified populations of cells from the cental nervous system. J Neurosci Res 8:453–462
Strommer K, Hamou MF, Diggelmann H, de Tribolet N (1990) Cellular and tumoral heterogeneity of EGF-R gene amplification in human malignant gliomas. Acta Neurochir 107:82–87
Sutter A. Hekmat A, Luckenbach GA (1991) Antibody-mediated tumor cytotoxicity of microglia. Pathobiol 59:254–258
Torp SH, Helseth E, Dalen A, Unsgaard G (1991) Epidermal growth factor expression in human gliomas. Cancer Immunol Immunother 33:61–64
Werner MH, Humphrey PA, Bigner DD, Bigner SH (1988) Growth effects of epidermal growth factor (EGF) and a monoclonal antibody against the EGF receptor on four glioma cell lines. Acta Neuropathol 77:196–201
Westermark B, Magnusson A, Heldin CH (1982) Effect of epidermal growth factor on membrane motility and cell locomotion in cultures of human clonal glioma cells. J Neurosci Res 8: 491–507
Westphal M, Herrmann HD (1989) Growth factor biology and oncogene activation in human gliomas and their implications for specific therapeutic concepts. Neurosurgery 25:681–694
Westphal M, Ackermann E, Hoppe J, Herrmann HD (1991) Receptors for platelet derived growth factor in human glioma cell lines and influence of suramin on cell proliferation. J Neuro-Oncol 11:207–213
Westphal M, Nitschke M, Nausch H, Herrmann HD (1993) Cell lines derived from human gliomas activate multiple autocrine pathways simultaneously. Int J Oncol 2:569–575
Zalutzky, MR, Moseley RP, Benjamin JC, Colapinto EV, Fuller GN, Coakham HP, Bigner DD (1990) Monoclonal antibody and a F (ab') 2 fragment delivery to tumor in patients with glioma : comparison of intracarotid and intravenous administration. Cancer Res 50:4105–4110

Target Cell Induced T Cell Activation with Bispecific Antibodies: A New Concept for Tumor Immunotherapy

H. Wolf[1], U. Freimann[2], and G. Jung[1]

[1]Labor für Rationale Immuntherapie, Medizinische Klinik III, Universität München, Klinikum Großhadern, Marchioninistr. 15, 81377 Munich, Germany
[2]Institut für Klinische Hämatologie, GSF-Forschungszentrum für Umwelt und Gesundheit, Marchioninistr. 25, 81377 Munich, Germany

Introduction

It can hardly be disputed that current treatment of malignant tumors with radiotherapy or cytotoxic drugs fails to produce cure or long-term remission in a large majority of patients, tumors of the nervous system being no exception to this rule.

Many of those seeking alternative treatment modalities have been attracted by the specificity and effectivity of the immune system. However, until today no immunotherapeutic approach has reached the state of an established treatment for malignant disease. Nevertheless it is our view that the notion of using the body's own defense mechanisms for tumor cell destruction has not lost its conceptual elegance, and that immunological research, in particular in the past 15 years, may have provided the tools and insights necessary to realize this vision.

Here we describe the development of a concept which allows the activation of resting human T cells on the surface of tumor cells. Central to this concept are bispecific constructs of two different monoclonal antibodies with specificity for both tumor cells and T cells. The tumor-specific antibody contributes target specificity, and the anti-T cell antibodies provide effectivity; these are chosen to induce the activation of the T cells and – within the bispecific constructs – to direct the activated cells toward their target.

Bispecific hybrid antibodies in this concept may be viewed as literally "hybridizing" efforts to define tumor-specific antigens and basic research aiming at understanding the function and regulation of the T cell system. While these fields have developed independently in recent years, monoclonal antibodies are of paramount importance in both:

Monoclonal Antibodies in Tumor Immunology

The most conspicious consequence of the introduction of hybridoma technology in the field of tumor immunology was the generation of a large number of monoclonal antibodies directed against tumor-associated cell surface structures. The obvious pragmatic intention of most of these efforts was to obtain reagents suited for specific in vivo targeting of tumor cells. Meanwhile monoclonal antibodies have entered the arena of both diagnosis and therapy for a number of hemapoietic and solid tumors [1], including those of the nervous system [2].

In the following we shall briefly discuss major problems for the in vivo targeting of tumor cells with monoclonal antibodies and how they might be overcome. All of these problems have been encountered in experimental clinical trials and have so far hampered therapeutic success.

Tumor Specificity

The quite extensive experience with the specificity of "tumor-specific" monoclonal antibodies accumulated up to now supports the view that antigens with an absolute specificity for the malignant state per se do not exist. After careful immunohistological testing, candidate antibodies usually turn out to exert a variable degree of cross-reactivity with nonmalignant tissue [3–5]. Nevertheless a number of antibodies have been generated with sufficiently low cross-reactivity to allow the specific targeting of tumors in humans [6]. Although not absolute, the specificity of these reagents certainly compares favorably with that of conventional cytotoxic drugs.

Tumor Heterogeneity

In most cases the expression of a given tumor-associated antigen is heterogeneous, varying for the same kind of tumor not only from patient to patient but also among different lesions of the same patient. Some investigators have suggested the use of a cocktail of different monoclonal antibodies to decrease the portion of antigen-negative cells in a given tumor. To overcome the problem of antigen heterogenicity, a therapeutic strategy with monoclonal antibodies should, ideally, provide an effector mechanism which allows the killing not only of antigen-positive cells but also of adjacent cells once the antibody has bound to its target.

Antibody Immunogenicity

Most tumor-specific antibodies are of mouse origin and elicit an immune response if applied to humans, i.e., human antibodies directed against mouse antibodies [7]. The production of anti-mouse immunoglobulin antibodies in patients can be greatly reduced if chimeric murine/human antibodies or humanized versions of mouse antibodies are used in which only the antibody binding sites of the mouse antibody are conserved, and the constant regions are exchanged by corresponding human sequences using recombinant DNA technology [8, 9] (Fig. 1a).

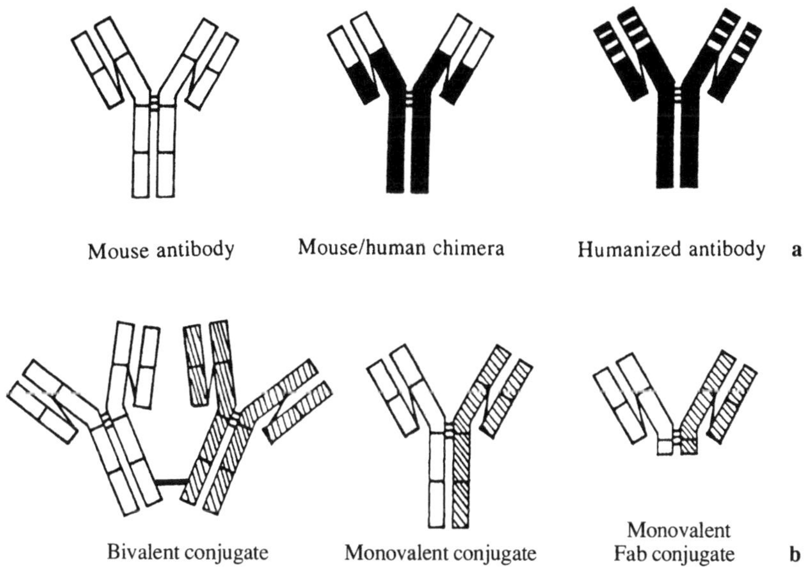

Fig. 1a,b. Natural and recreated antibodies. **a** Monospecific constructs. Depicted are the parental mouse antibody, a mouse/human chimera with murine variable regions and human constant regions, and a humanized antibody with murine complementarity-determining regions grafted into human sequences by recombinant DNA technology. **b** Three forms of bispecific antibody constructs

Pharmacokinetics of Antibodies

Numerous studies have demonstrated that after in vivo administration of radioactively labeled monoclonal antibodies usually less than 1% of the total body dose becomes specifically bound to a solid tumor. Moreover, the molecules with access to the tumor usually do not penetrate more than a few millimeters due to their large size [5, 10]. The use of antibody fragments without Fc portions may improve this situation, albeit only gradually. Conceptually, the deleterious effects of unbound or nonspecifically binding antibodies call for an antibody-mediated effector mechanism which becomes effective only after specific binding of the antibody.

Biological Effectivity of Monoclonal Antibodies

In most cases antibodies per se do not kill tumor cells, either in vitro or in vivo [11–13]. This finding underlines again the need for an effector mechanism coupled to the targeting antibody. Summarizing what has been outlined above, an antibody-mediated effector mechanism is required to meet the following three criteria: it must (a) be highly potent, (b) be effective not before but after specific binding of the targeting antibody, and (c) mediate local destruction not only of labeled but also of unlabeled cells.

Effector mechanisms used by the immune system itself (e.g., complement activation) usually meet all these criteria. However, most of the man-made strategies developed in the past 10 years for "arming" monoclonal antibodies, for example, with conventional cytotoxic drugs, highly effective toxic proteins, or radioisotopes fail to do so [1, 14].

Fortunately, recent developments in a different area of immunology have made it possible with tumor-specific antibodies to engage the T cell system, which to the best of our knowledge is central to the initiation and regulation of an immune response:

Monoclonal Antibodies in T Cell Immunology

Whereas the role of most tumor-specific antibodies is a merely "defining" one, in T cell immunology many antibodies not only define "their" surface receptor but can also profoundly manipulate its biological function by imitating or blocking the respective physiological ligand. This is best exemplified by the single most important structure on the T cell surface: the T cell receptor for antigen (TCR). Although the existence of this receptor had long been postulated, it was not before the availability of monoclonal antibody technology that it could be identified and characterized [15]. The receptor forms a multimolecular complex on the cell surface consisting of the antigen recognition part and a constant multimolecular portion termed CD3, which probably constitutes the signaling unit of the receptor.

Antibodies against the TCR/CD3 complex have profound effects on T cell function, indicating that this complex is the molecular basis not only for the specificity of the T cell system but also for the regulation of its effector function: Most anti-TCR/CD3 antibodies induce potent T cell activation provided that (a) they are "presented" to the T cell in an immobilized or multimeric form and (b) a "second signal" triggering an accessory receptor on the T cell is also present. Monoclonal antibodies can identify – and trigger – those accessory molecules, one of the most potent being a homodimeric molecule termed CD28 [16, 17]. Thus, particular monoclonal antibodies can induce effective activation of T cells in a striking analogy to what is known about "physiological" T cell activation, where the TCR/CD3 complex is triggered by peptide bound to MHC and presented by an antigen-presenting cell (APC; Fig. 2a). The APC also provides costimulation signals for the T cell. It is noteworthy that the recently identified ligand for the CD28 receptor, a molecule termed B7, is rather specifically found on cells known to function as APCs [18, 19]. Thus, the CD28/B7 receptor/ligand pair appears to constitute one (of possibly more) accessory pathways for T cell activation.

In summary, it is possible to completely mimic physiological T cell stimulation with monoclonal antibodies, thereby confirming the two-signal model for lymphocyte activation formulated for B cells over 20 years ago [20] and recently extended for T cells [21, 22]. Being initially merely a "phenomenological" model, the phenomenon has now received its molecular and functional basis.

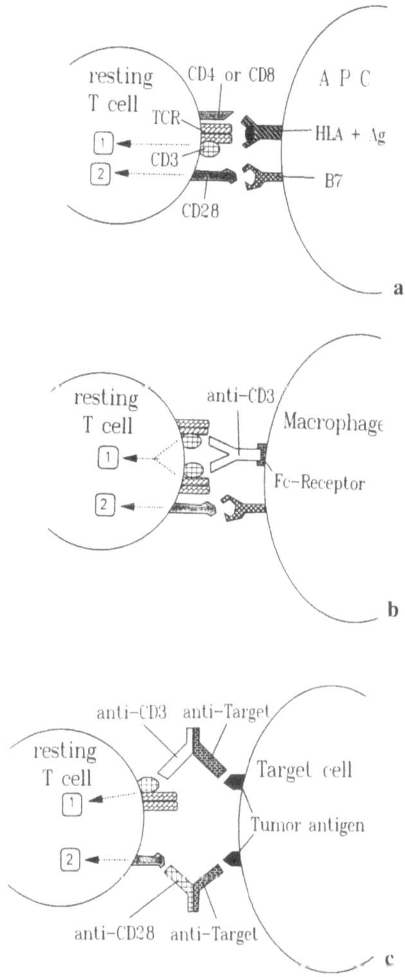

Fig. 2a–c. T cell activation according to the two-signal model. **a** Physiological recognition of antigen bound to HLA class I or class II by the antigen-specific TCR and CD8 or CD4, respectively; additional receptors on the T cell surface such as CD28, CD2 or LFA-1 bind to the respective counterreceptors on the APC (B7, LFA-3, ICAM-1) and enhance adhesion and/or signaling. **b** Antigen/HLA recognition can be mimicked by triggering the TCR/CD3 with cell-bound anti-CD3 leading to T cell activation, as long as accessory signals are provided. **c** Both antigen/HLA and accessory ligand can be mimicked by two bispecific antibody fragments, both binding to a target cell with one arm and, on the T cell side, to CD3 and CD28, respectively. Thus both bispecific constructs mediate "target cell-induced T cell activation"

Bispecific Antibodies Can Focus T Cell Function

In 1985 it was demonstrated in different laboratories that bispecific conjugates constructed of antibodies directed against tumor-specific antigens and to the TCR/CD3 complex on T cells induce lysis of the tumor cells by cloned or preactivated cytolytic T cells [23–25]. Bispecific conjugates triggering structures different from the TCR/CD3 complex were ineffective. We showed in 1986 that freshly isolated peripheral blood mononuclear cells (PBMC) stimulated with the anti-CD3 antibody OKT3 for several days effectively kill tumor cells coated with anti-tumor X anti-CD3 conjugates [26]. Unstimulated cells were ineffective. These findings established that cytolytic potential is not present in resting T cells even in those with the "lytic phenotype" (CD8-positive cells), and that lytic activity must be generated

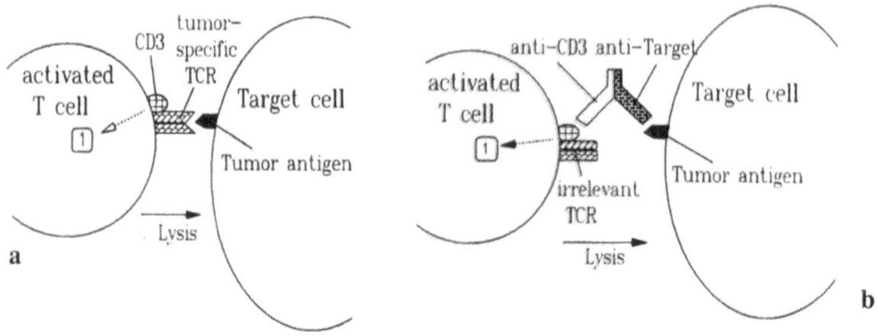

Fig. 3a,b. The effector phase of an activated cytolytic T cell. **a** A T cell with a TCR specific for a tumor-associated antigen is triggered by the tumor cell. **b** A T cell with an irrelevant specificity binds to the tumor cell via a bispecific antibody bridge, triggering tumor cell lysis. Accessory signals are not required

during the T cell activation process. Thus, in the experiments described above the role of the anti-CD3 antibody was twofold: to induce the activation of resting T cells and – as part of the bispecific conjugate – subsequently to focus the lytic potential of the activated T cells toward the tumor target cells. Although functionally linked and mediated through the TCR/CD3 receptor, the two processes differ. The effective activation of a resting cell to a lytic effector cell takes 2–3 days [27] and, according to the two-signal model, requires a costimulation signal in addition to the triggering of the TCR/CD3 complex. In the case of anti-CD3 stimulated PBMC this signal is provided by monocytes binding and "presenting" the anti-CD3 antibody via receptors for the Fc portion of the molecule [28, 29] and providing costimulation signals (Fig. 2b).

In contrast to the activation phase, the effector phase, i.e., the triggering of the lytic machinery of an activated cell, is fast and requires only the signal via TCR/CD3 (Fig. 3). In our model of anti-CD3 induced PBMC cytotoxicity we also found that the cytotoxic activity generated does not only reside in T cells but also in a probably heterogeneous population of cells negative for the T cell markers CD3, CD4, and CD8. Most likely this population is activated by lymphokines produced by the activated T cells. Its cytotoxicity is "CD3 independent", that is, it cannot be focused by anti-CD3 containing bispecific conjugates. In addition, these cells are unspecifically lytic, i.e., for unstimulated autologous lymphocytes [27, 30].

From what has been said above it is clear that any therapeutic strategy using bispecific conjugates of the kind described must provide a method for the activation of resting T cells. Several authors have suggested the use of interleukin-2 for the ex vivo activation of effector cells and the subsequent use of anti-tumor X anti-CD3 constructs to focus these cells [23, 24, 31, 32]. In our hands, PBMC activated with interleukin-2 – to a greater extent than anti-CD3 activated cells – mainly exerted "CD3-independent" cytotoxicity, which is not targetable by anti-CD3 containing conjugates. We therefore focused our efforts on a strategy which allowed the in vivo activation of T cells in a target cell dependent manner. In initial experiments we tested whether tumor target cells coated with anti-CD3 containing constructs can – as monocytes – effectively activate T cells by "presenting" anti-CD3 antibody. As

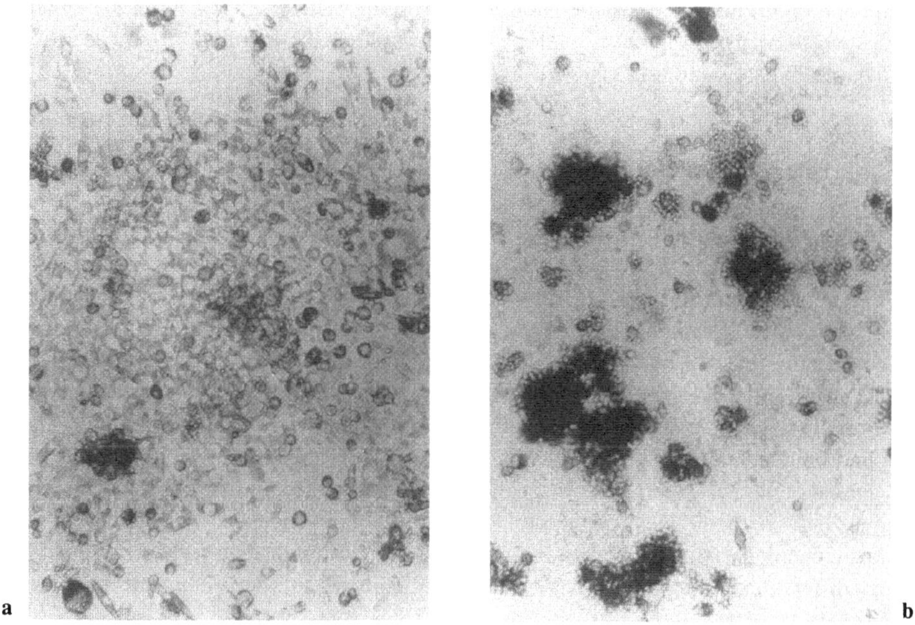

Fig. 4. Viable melanoma cells cocultered with PBMC and the bispecific F(ab')$_2$ conjugate anti-target X anti-CD3 (**a**) or a combination of anti-target X anti-CD3 and anti-target X anti-CD28 (**b**). For details see [33]

expected and as predicted by the two-signal model, this is not the case because the required costimulation signal is missing. However, if such a signal is provided using a second bispecific construct with anti-tumor X anti-CD28 specificity, effective T cell activation can occur. Thus, "attaching" an anti-CD3 and an anti-CD28 signal to the surface of a tumor cell using bispecific antibodies functionally converts this cell to an APC. This activates T cells, which then kill the conjugate-coated tumor cells (Fig. 2c). Since the activating function of the anti-CD3 containing conjugate is dependent upon its immobilization on the target cell surface, T cell activation is target cell dependent. It can be measured using various parameters such as the induction of cytolytic potential, cytokine release, or expression of interleukin-2 receptors on activated cells. Most impressively, however, it shows in mixed cultures of tumor cells and freshly isolated T cells (Fig. 4). In cultures incubated with control antibodies or anti-CD3 conjugates only, melanoma target cells continued to proliferate vigorously. The addition of the second conjugate triggering CD28 initiated T cell activation, leading to the complete destruction of the tumor cells. The combination of both conjugates does not activate T cells in the absence of the melanoma target cells [33]. Thus the above concept meets all three criteria discussed in the previous section as being required for a successful antibody-mediated effector mechanism. We expect that it allows the in situ activation of resting T cells upon in vivo administration of bispecific antibodies, provided that a sufficient number of T cells has access to the tumor. Although many of the molecular details of T cell activation remain to be elucidated, we are confident that a successful engagement of the T cell system at a given tumor in analogy to "physiological" stimulation may lead to measurable antitumor effects.

Bispecific Antibodies In Vivo

Bispecific Antibody Technology

The improvement of bispecific antibody technology is a prerequisite for successful in vivo administration. The bispecific reagents used in initial experiments were conjugates obtained by chemical cross-linking of two intact antibodies, as depicted in Fig. 1b (bivalent conjugate) [34–36]. These contructs with a molecular weight of more than 300 kDa do not appear suited for systemic in vivo administration. Using quadroma technology, i.e., the fusion of two parental hybridomas, it is possible to generate "second-generation" bispecific hybrid antibodies, univalent for each antigen (Fig. 1b, monovalent conjugate) [37]. However, a serious technical problem of this technology is the purification of the desired hybrid molecule from a mixture of ten different combinations of heavy and light chains produced by the quadroma cells [38, 39].

The concept of a target cell-induced T cell activation requires, in addition to a reduced molecular weight, the use of Fc-free reagents because Fc receptor-bearing cells such as monocytes would lead to Fc-mediated rather than target cell induced T cell activation. In recent years a technology has been introduced [40] and improved [33] which allows the production of bispecific Fab hybrid fragments (Fig. 1b, monovalent Fab conjugate) by selective reduction of the disulfide bridges in the hinge region of $F(ab')_2$ fragments. We have demonstrated that these univalent Fab hybrid reagents can mediate target cell-induced T cell activation, although – when compared to bivalent conjugates of $F(ab')_2$ fragments – with a somewhat decreased effectivity [33].

In the future recombinant DNA technology might provide the third generation of bispecific antibodies consisting of small-single chain molecules with two binding specificities in which only the hypervariable regions remain of mouse origin.

Animal Models

Several studies have demonstrated the antitumor effects of bispecific antibodies in vivo [39, 41, 42]. In two of these studies anti target X anti-CD3 constructs alone were used for the treatment of B cell tumors in mice [39, 41]; in two others ex vivo activated effector cells were also administered [42, 43]. So far, the use of an anti-CD28 antibody in mice, which circumvents the ex vivo activation of effector cells, has not been possible because it was not until recently that the mouse CD28 receptor was defined by a monoclonal antibody [44]. It was also very recently that the importance of the CD28/B7 costimulation pathway for T cell mediated tumor rejection was underlined by the finding that tumor cells transfected with the B7 gene are rejected by immunocompetent mice while the untransfected variants gave rise to tumors, eventually killing a large majority of injected animals [45].

Clinical Trials

In 1990 Nitta et al. reported the local treatment of glioma patients with anti-target X anti-CD3 Fab hybrid fragments and ex vivo activated lymphocytes [46]. Of ten patients treated initially with bispecific antibodies and effector cells eight survived more than 3 years while only two of ten treated with activated cells alone did so. Recently in the Netherlands and Italy a coordinated study was started in which anti-target X anti-CD3 hybrid antibodies are applied into the peritoneal cavity of patients with metastasized ovarial carcinoma [32, 47].

Our own efforts focus on the local administration of two bispecific constructs, an anti-target X anti-CD3 and an anti-target X anti-CD28 reagent, to patients with metastatic malignant melanoma. While most investigators in the field still prefer the use of ex vivo activated cells, we believe that the envisaged in situ engagement of the T cell system at the surface of tumor cells, as outlined above, brings us as close as currently possible to realizing the vision mentioned at the beginning of this article.

References

1. Waldman TA (1991) Monoclonal antibodies in diagnosis and therapy. Science 252:1657–1662
2. Cheung NK (1991) Immunotherapy. Neuroblastoma as a model. Pediatr Clin North Am 38:425–441
3. Pai LH, Bookman MA, Ozols RF, Young RC, Smith JW 2nd, Longo DL, Gould B, Frankel A, McClay EF, Howell S et al (1991) Clinical evaluation of intraperitoneal Pseudomonas exotoxin immunoconjugate OVB3-PE in patients with ovarian cancer. J Clin Oncol 9:2095–2103
4. Hwang KM, Fodstad, Ö, Oldham RK, Morgan AC Jr (1985) Radiolocalization of xenografted human malignant melanoma by a monoclonal antibody (9.2.27) to a melanoma-associated antigen in nude mice. Cancer Res 45:4150–4155
5. Dillman RO, Beauregard JC, Sobol RE, Royston I, Bartholomew RM, Hagan PS, Halpern SE (1984) Lack of radioimmunodetection and complications associated with monoclonal anticarcinoembryonic antigen antibody cross-reactivity with an antigen on circulating cells. Cancer Res 44:2213–2218
6. Dillman RO (1984) Monoclonal antibodies in the treatment of cancers. Crit Rev Oncol Hematol 1:357–385
7. Chatenoud L (1986) The immune response against therapeutic monoclonal antibodies. Immunol Today 7:367–368
8. Winter G, Milstein C (1991) Man-made antibodies. Nature 349:293–299
9. Plückthun A (1992) Mono- and bivalent antibody fragments produced in Escherichia coli: engineering, folding and antigen binding. Immunol Rev 130:151–188
10. Begent RHJ, Green AJ, Keep PA, Searle F, Jewkes RF, Barratt GM (1982) Liposomally entrapped second antibody improves tumor imaging with radiolabeled (first) antitumor antibody. Lancet ii:739–742
11. Press OW, Appelbaum F, Ledbetter JA, Martin PJ, Zarling Z, Kidd P, Donnall Thomas E (1987) Monoclonal antibody 1F5 (anti-CD20) serotherapy of human B cell lymphomas. Blood 69:584–591
12. Rankin EM, Hekman A, Somers R, ten Bokkel Huinink W (1985) Treatment of two patients with B cell lymphoma with monoclonal anti-idiotype antibodies. Blood 65:1373–1381

13. Schroff RW, Woodhouse CS, Foon KA, Oldham RK, Farrell MM, Klein RA, Morgan AC Jr (1985) Intratumor localization of monoclonal antibody in patients with melanoma treated with antibody to a 250,000-dalton melanoma-associated antigen. J Natl Cancer Inst 74:299–306
14. Wawrzynczak EJ, Derbyshire EJ (1992) Immunotoxins: the power and the glory. Immunol Today 13:381–383
15. Marrack P, Kappler J (1987) The T cell receptor. Science 238:1073–1079
16. Ledbetter JA, Imboden JB, Schieven GL, Grosmaire LS, Rabinovitch PS, Lindsten T, Thompson CB, June CH (1990) CD28 ligation in T-cell activation: evidence for two signal transduction pathways. Blood 75:1531–1539
17. June CH, Ledbetter JA, Linsley PS, Thompson CB (1990) Role of the CD28 receptor in T-cell activation. Immunol Today 11:211–216
18. Linsley PS, Clark EA, Ledbetter JA (1990) The T cell antigen, CD28, mediates adhesion with B cells by interacting with the activation antigen, B7/BB1. Proc Natl Acad Sci USA 87:5031–5035
19. Freeman GJ, Freedman AS, Segil JM, Lee G, Whitman JF, Nadler LM (1989) B7, a new member of the Ig superfamily with unique expression on activated and neoplastic B cells. J Immunol 143:2714–2722
20. Bretscher P, Cohn M (1970) A theory of self-nonself discrimination. Science 169:1042–1049
21. Schwartz RH (1989) Acquisition of immunological self-tolerance. Cell 57:1073–1081
22. Janeway CA Jr (1989) Immunogenicity signals 1,2,3... and 0. Immunol Today 10:283–286
23. Staerz UD, Kanagawa O, Bevan MJ (1985) Hybrid antibodies can target sites for attack by T cells. Nature 314:628–631
24. Pérez P, Hoffmann,RW, Shaw S, Bluestone JA, Segal DM (1985) Specific targeting of cytotoxic T cells by anti-T3 linked to anti-target cell antibody. Nature 316:354–356
25. Liu MA, Kranz DM, Kurnick JT, Boyle LA, Levy R, Eisen HN (1985) Heteroantibody duplexes target cells for lysis by cytotoxic T lymphocytes. Proc Natl Acad Sci USA 82:8648–8652
26. Jung G, Honsik CJ, Reisfeld RA, Müller-Eberhard HJ (1986) Activation of human peripheral blood mononuclear cells by anti-T3: killing of tumor target cells coated with anti-target-anti-T3 conjugates. Proc Natl Acad Sci USA 83:4479–4483
27. Jung G, Martin DE, Müller-Eberhard HJ (1987) Induction of cytotoxicity in human peripheral blood mononuclear cells by monoclonal antibody OKT3. J Immunol 139:639–644
28. Looney RJ, Abraham GN (1984) The Fc portion of intact IgG blocks stimulation of human PBMC by anti-T3. J Immunol 133:154–156
29. Landegren U, Andersson J, Wigzell H (1984) Mechanisms of T lymphocyte activation by OKT3 antibodies. A general model for T cell induction. Eur J Immunol 14:325–328
30. Quian JH, Titus JA, Andrew SM, Mezzanzanica D, Garrido MA, Wunderlich JR, Segal DM (1991) Human peripheral blood lymphocytes targeted with bispecific antibodies release cytokines that are essential for inhibiting tumor growth. J Immunol 146:3250–3256
31. Nitta T, Nakata M, Yagita H, Okumura K (1991) Interleukin-2 activated T cells (T-LAK) express CD16 antigen and are triggered to target cell lysis by bispecific antibody. Immunol Lett 28:31–37
32. Lamers CH, van de Griend RJ, Braakman E, Ronteltap CP, Benard J, Stoter G, Gratama JW, Bolhuis RL (1992) Optimization of culture conditions for activation and large-scale expansion of human T lymphocytes for bispecific antibody-directed cellular immunotherapy. Int J Cancer 51:973–979
33. Jung G, Freimann U, von Marschall Z, Reisfeld RA, Wilmanns W (1991) Target cell-induced T cell activation with bi- and trispecific antibody fragments. Eur J Immunol 21:2431–2435
34. Nisonoff A, Rivers MM (1961) Recombination of a mixture of univalent antibody fragments of different specificity. Arch Biochem Biophys 93:460–466
35. Hämmerling U, Aoki T, deHarven E, Boyce EA, Okol CJ (1968) Use of hybrid antibody with anti-gamma G and anti-ferritin specificities in locating cell surface antigens by electron microscopy. J Exp Med 128:1461–1469
36. Raso V, Griffin T (1981) Hybrid antibody with dual specificity for the delivery of ricin to immunoglobulin-bearing target cells. Cancer Res 41:2073–2078
37. Milstein C, Cuello AC (1983) Hybrid hybridomas and their use in immunohistochemistry. Nature 305:537–540
38. Milstein C, Cuello AC (1984) Hybrid hybridoma and the production of bi-specific monoclonal antibodies. Immunol Today 5:299–304
39. Demanet C, Brissinck J, van Mechelen M, Leo O, Thielemans K (1991) Treatment of murine B cell lymphoma with bispecific monoclonal antibodies (anti-idiotype x anti-CD3). J Immunol 147:1091–1097

40. Brennan M, Davison PF, Paulus H (1985) Preparation of bispecific antibodies by chemical recombination of monoclonal immunoglobulin G_1 fragments. Science 229:81–83
41. Weiner G, Hillstrom JR (1991) Bispecific anti-idiotype/anti-CD3 antibody therapy of murine B cell lymphoma. J Immunol 147:4035–4044
42. Garrido MA, Valdayo MJ, Winkler DF, Titus JA, Hecht TT, Perez P, Segal DM, Wunderlich JR (1990) Targeting human T lymphocytes with bispecific antibodies to react against human ovarian carcinoma cells growing in nu/nu mice. Cancer Res 50:4227–4232
43. Reid I, Lundy J, Monson J, Nelson H, Ramsay P, Ilstrup D, Donahue JH (1992) Heteroconjugated antibodies enhance lymphocyte-mediated tumor cell lysis in vitro and in vivo. Br J Surg 79:628–632
44. Gross J, St. John T, Allison JP (1990) The murine homologue of the T lymphocyte antigen CD28. Molecular cloning and cell surface expression. J Immunol 144:3201–3210
45. Townsend SE, Allison JP (1992) Tumor rejection after direct costimulation of $CD8^+$ T cells by B7-transfected melanoma cells. Science 259:368–370
46. Nitta T, Sato K, Yagita H, Okumura K, Ishii S (1990) Preliminary trial of specific targeting therapy against malignant glioma. Lancet 335:368–376
47. Mezzanzanica D, Canevari S, Colnaghi MI (1991) Retargeting of human lymphocytes against human ovarian carcinoma cells by bispecific antibodies: from laboratory to clinic. Int J Clin Lab Res 21:159–164

Subject Index

Springer-Verlag and the Environment

We at Springer-Verlag firmly believe that an international science publisher has a special obligation to the environment, and our corporate policies consistently reflect this conviction.

We also expect our business partners – paper mills, printers, packaging manufacturers, etc. – to commit themselves to using environmentally friendly materials and production processes.

The paper in this book is made from low- or no-chlorine pulp and is acid free, in conformance with international standards for paper permanency.

MIX
Papier aus verantwortungsvollen Quellen
Paper from responsible sources
FSC® C105338

If you have any concerns about our products,
you can contact us on
ProductSafety@springernature.com

In case Publisher is established outside the EU,
the EU authorized representative is:
Springer Nature Customer Service Center GmbH
Europaplatz 3, 69115 Heidelberg, Germany

Printed by Libri Plureos GmbH
in Hamburg, Germany